# THE SUNLIGHT SOLUTION

## Reclaiming Vitamin D, Reversing the Chronic Disease Epidemic, and Making America Healthy Again

**WILLIAM F. SUPPLE, JR., PhD**

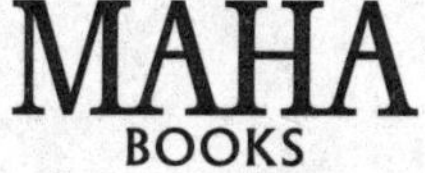

To my wife Toni, for her loving support and guidance. Thanks for being a sounding board and voice of reason as I would report to her the latest in vitamin D and sunlight research for almost the past thirty-five years.

Copyright © 2026 by William F. Supple Jr.

A portion of the proceeds goes to MAHA Action 501(c)4.

All rights reserved. No part of this book may be reproduced in any manner without the express written consent of the publisher, except in the case of brief excerpts in critical reviews or articles. All inquiries should be addressed to Skyhorse Publishing, 307 Fifth Avenue, 4th Floor, New York, NY 10016.

MAHA Books may be purchased in bulk at special discounts for sales promotion, corporate gifts, fund-raising, or educational purposes. Special editions can also be created to specifications. For details, contact the Special Sales Department, Skyhorse Publishing, 307 Fifth Avenue, 4th Floor, New York, NY 10016 or info@skyhorsepublishing.com.

MAHA Books is an imprint of Skyhorse Publishing, Inc.®, a Delaware corporation.

Visit our website at www.skyhorsepublishing.com.

Please follow our publisher Tony Lyons on Instagram @tonylyonsisuncertain.

10 9 8 7 6 5 4 3 2 1

Library of Congress Control Number: 2026937555

Cover design by David Ter-Avanesyan
Cover image credit: Getty Images

Print ISBN: 978-1-63144-090-8
Ebook ISBN: 978-1-63144-091-5

Printed in the United States of America

# CONTENTS

# DISCLAIMER

All facts presented in this book are based on publicly available published research papers, documents, and studies, the majority of which have been linked in the references. Nevertheless, in some places the author has also expressed personal opinions, where it seems to him that the facts can be assembled to form a larger, albeit partly speculative picture. The author has made every effort to clearly separate facts and such interpretations in terms of language.

The publisher and author have checked the information in this work to the best of their knowledge and belief for correctness, accuracy, and completeness sufficient for reasonable interpretation. However, neither the publisher nor the author explicitly takes any responsibility for the content of the work or for any errors.

This also applies to quantities of micronutrients, drugs, vitamins, and other supplements, as there may be differences in dosage and administration that can result from lifestyle, gender, age, body size, and possible preexisting conditions. Therefore, any use of any of the substances mentioned in this book should only be carried out after consultation with a trusted physician or other medical professional, and in any case on one's own responsibility—the publisher and author accept no liability.

The author does not endorse the contents of any of the cited websites. Reference is made to their status at the time of initial publication. All citations have been carefully checked for accuracy at the time of this writing. It is not uncommon for the content of an online source to change or even disappear completely. Unfortunately, the integrity of scientific material that is on the internet can no longer be blindly trusted.

# PREFACE

Did you know that we are in Dark Ages of medicine right now? That is a bold statement, but being bold doesn't make it any less true. For the past fifty years, citizens of the Western world have been unwitting subjects in a massive experiment to determine the effects of removing sunlight and its vitamin D from our lives. This deranged experiment is paying dividends in the form of epidemic levels of infertility, infant mortality, autism, obesity, diabetes, autoimmune disease, cancer, frailty, and neurodegenerative diseases like Alzheimer's, all resulting in decreasing life expectancy. This cradle-to-grave assault on our well-being is orchestrated by the misguided advice to avoid sunlight and its healthy life-giving vitamin D in an irrational fear of a rare skin cancer, melanoma. Melanoma is orders of magnitude rarer (22 per 100,000) than the diseases related to chronic vitamin D deficiency (e.g., breast cancer 90 per 100,000; 80 percent of Americans suffer a chronic disease). In a twisted bit of scientific irony we have since learned that use of sunscreens has no protective effect on melanoma and melanoma itself is twice as deadly among people deficient in sunlight and vitamin D, which is covered in detail in chapter 12.

Our bodies were designed around the ubiquitous role assigned to vitamin D. The presence of vitamin D receptors in and on every cell required a foolproof method of acquisition of vitamin D. That foolproof method is simply exposure to sunlight. We don't have to search, locate, catch, grow, harvest, prepare, eat, drink, or inhale vitamin D; all we have to do is go out in the sun and our skin usually makes all we need. Unfortunately, we have been advised and convinced by "experts" to shun the sun and deny our own biological hardwiring. We are now reaping the costs of that misguided advice with epidemic levels of autoimmune disease, metabolic disorders, cardiovascular disease, infertility, neurodegenerative diseases, autism, frailty, and premature death.

## HOW I BECAME INTERESTED IN VITAMIN D

Some of the best discoveries in science happen by accident. And the most far-reaching of those discoveries are simple to understand and have safe, practical applications. Furthermore, when those discoveries directly affect your life and those around you, they are especially attention-getting.

The story of my interest in vitamin D goes back to the winter of 1982 when I was in graduate school studying neuroscience at Dartmouth. Around January or February of that year, a few patches of dry skin developed on my elbows and knees. The patches grew larger and more unsightly, so I had them checked out at Dick's House, the student infirmary. The physicians there were resident medical students. The doctor examined my elbows and stated, "You have psoriasis." I was told psoriasis was an autoimmune disease that had no cure, only treatments to manage symptoms.

So began a constant battle with a persistent affliction. Nothing the dermatologists gave me ever worked. Tar creams, steroids, ointments, lotions, and proprietary dermatological concoctions. Living in Vermont, every fall, like clockwork, my skin would start to flake and got progressively worse each year with new areas on my body affected so much so that at one point up to 30 percent of my skin was affected.

I did notice over the years that the psoriasis would become less severe following trips to Florida. I thought that perhaps the salt water had a therapeutic effect. I heard about people going to the Dead Sea for saltwater treatment. So, I tried my own saltwater therapy. Nope. If anything, it made the condition worse.

Finally, in 2006, I realized that it had to be the sun that helped my skin on the trips to Florida. It was the changing of the seasons in the fall and the resultant decline of the sun that was affecting the skin. It was the move north to New Hampshire and living in Vermont and the resultant lack of sunlight that initiated and maintained the psoriasis. It was too obvious. What was it about the sun? The sun makes vitamin D in the skin. Again—too obvious. In the fall of 2006 I started taking vitamin D and within nine to ten weeks, my psoriasis was eradicated.

Over the course of that winter I experimented with various amounts of vitamin D3 supplements and found a daily amount that my skin needed to remain healthy. Since I could see the results on my skin, I could adjust how much vitamin D to take to keep the skin clear. My skin was almost like a vitamin D meter to gauge how much to take. The recommended dietary allowance (RDA) of vitamin D back then was 400 international units (IU) per day. I was taking thousands of IUs per day. The RDA of 400 IU is the bare minimum to keep your bones from crumbling. Obviously, psoriasis therapy needs much more vitamin D than the 400 IU RDA. Many with expertise in the pharmacology of vitamin D believe that this RDA amount is orders of magnitude too low. No negative consequences were observed during my yearly health examination, so I continued taking the daily high-dose vitamin D.

My wife, Toni, developed ulcerative colitis (UC) sometime around 1996. She was diagnosed with UC after a colonoscopy. She was treated with medicines with inconsistent results. Oftentimes, she claimed the medicine made the bleeding worse. This went on for around ten years, with relapses coming and going. Like me with my psoriasis, she was told her UC was an autoimmune disease with no cure.

It was just a regular Sunday morning when Toni and I were reading our respective material in the living room. I tried to read as many articles covering vitamin D as I could, and that particular day read a seemingly obscure article about vitamin D and the immune system. The article mentioned Crohn's disease and ulcerative colitis as autoimmune disease states that may be affected by vitamin D. I was alarmed to learn that UC is a major risk factor for colon cancer. I looked up from my paper and said, "Why don't you try increasing your vitamin D for your colitis?" I made the case to her that there seems to be a lot of circumstantial evidence to suggest vitamin D could help, and it certainly would not hurt. She got up, went into the kitchen and took her first high-dose vitamin D that Sunday morning. In about two weeks she announced that her symptoms had cleared!

Toni continued to take vitamin D daily for the next two years with no UC flare-ups. A few years later she had a routine colonoscopy. Her GI doctor, who had initially diagnosed the UC, reported that her tissue was now normal. She asked him what "normal" meant. He said, "normal as in free of disease, with no polyps or pathology." She then asked if she was cured. He explained that even though her tissue appeared as a person with no disease would appear, she was most likely just in remission. He then encouraged her to keep doing what she was doing.

Toni and I enjoyed the benefits of vitamin D in defeating our own personal scourges. In the fall of 2012, an ad in a local paper advertised that a local college was hosting a Crohn's and ulcerative colitis informational session. It was sponsored by a drug company, and the lead speaker was, ironically, Toni's gastroenterologist. Toni was compelled to attend as this was the opportunity to tell her story regarding vitamin D to others who might also benefit.

Toni did stand up and make her remarkable success public. Her doctor qualified her testimonial with "what works for one person may not for another . . . ," but was intrigued nevertheless.

What happened next was amazing and inspiring. A dozen or so people approached Toni after the presentation, including a mother whose twenty-year-old daughter was battling Crohn's disease. Rachel's story was one of a young woman enslaved to the symptoms of this disease. Rachel's mother made the horrific details of the disease very real when she described the slow progression of pathology, the frustration with current infusion treatments and their side effects, and the looming specter of intestinal resection surgery in her daughter's very near future. Rachel's mother was ready to try something new.

Rachel was receiving infliximab infusions and was experiencing terrible side effects and minimal relief from the symptoms it was supposed to treat. Immediately, Rachel's mother had her daughter's vitamin D levels measured. Her levels were way below minimal, essentially zero. Rachel's mother wanted to try vitamin D without any potential confounds of other treatments. She waited six weeks until the next scheduled infliximab infusion and said, "No more, we're trying something different." Rachel received several megadoses of vitamin D to get her levels up, and then started daily high-dose vitamin D.

Several weeks later, I received an enthusiastic email from Rachel's mother stating that her daughter's symptoms had subsided and that she appeared to be recovering. Several days later, Rachel and her mom dropped by to see us. Rachel recovered to the point where she felt like she had her life back. She reported that, rather than wearing adult diapers, she could now be confident enough to go on a bus trip with friends to see a show in New York City. Rachel went on to graduate from college and get a great job and is now married with two wonderful children.

So, we didn't discover vitamin D, we discovered what vitamin D can do for us.

This book has been forty years in the making. It started with my own personal experience solving a health problem, and then a scientific interest in all things vitamin D. The aha moment for me in understanding the power of vitamin D was when it was learned that virtually all cells have a receptor for vitamin D. The significance of that finding for me was that it explained why vitamin D was involved in just about every bodily system and why chronic deficiency expressed itself in so many seemingly different maladies. Anatomy determines physiology, which then determines behavior. As you'll learn in this book, afflictions from infertility to psoriasis to cancer have a common thread linking them all: immune system dysfunction due to chronic vitamin D deficiency.

In addition to this book, this interest in vitamin D led to the publishing of a Substack on all things vitamin D called Starpower.Substack.com. One of the strengths of the Substack platform is the direct interaction that readers have with the author and each other through the comments feature. A number of the topics covered in this book originated from questions and suggestions by readers of that Substack. You can go there to see some of the latest vitamin D research as time progresses and ask your questions as well.

As I stated earlier, medicine, and health care in general, has been in a dark age lasting more than five decades. We've gotten sicker and sicker despite spending more and more. The power of the sun and its vitamin D have been portrayed as poisons by modern medicine. Usually, when diseases appear, our natural tendency is to try to identify what's new that could be causing the issue. In the case of the current population-wide health decline we are experiencing, it's not what is added, what's new, it's what's missing: sensible sun exposure and vitamin D. Our avoidance of the sun and its vitamin D that we are hardwired to use in the form of vitamin D receptors on most cells is the foundation of our susceptibility to the diseases of the modern age: autoimmune disease, cancer, diabetes, metabolic disease, neurodegenerative disease, fertility dysfunction, and dysfunctional aging, among many others.

The misguided advice to shun the sun has created population-wide, epidemic vitamin D deficiencies which have directly caused the crisis of chronic disease the developed world now faces. Health and Human Service Secretary Robert F. Kennedy Jr. stated on September 4, 2025, that "the CDC now estimates that 76.4 percent of Americans now have a chronic disease, in the early 1960s it was 11 percent."[1] In 2025, these chronic diseases collectively cost the nation $4 trillion each year. Something is systemically very, very wrong with the biology of Americans, and that something is pandemic-level vitamin D starvation. It is the one, common, population-wide factor that underpins most modern disease.

Epochs in time or eras are named in hindsight and not while they are happening. During the first Dark Age, the epoch between the fifth and tenth centuries AD, contemporaries did not acknowledge or label that time the "Dark Ages." It was only in retrospect, with the benefit of hindsight, that Italian scholar Petrarch coined the term some three hundred years later in the 1330s to describe the period of time following the fall of the Western Roman Empire, that the period of cultural stagnation and disease could be seen. It is my intention with this book to bring an abrupt end to the contemporary Dark Age of Medicine we are currently suffering through as a result of removing the sun and its vitamin D from our lives, and the resultant existential health crises that have been a tragic result. This book is about revealing the ravages wrought by that starvation on our well-being more than fifty years into this sick, twisted experiment, and showing effective solutions using easy, inexpensive, and in many cases free vitamin D to eradicate those problems and Make America Healthy Again.

—William F. Supple Jr., PhD
Shelburne, Vermont

## CHAPTER 1

# THE SUN: HUMANITY'S OLDEST ALLY AND OUR MODERN BLIND SPOT

For countless millennia, humanity thrived under the sun's life-giving rays. Our ancestors instinctively understood its power, building civilizations oriented toward its light and incorporating it into their daily lives and spiritual beliefs.[1, 2] Yet, in a profound and dangerous departure from our biological heritage, modern society has been taught to fear the sun, viewing it primarily as a threat responsible for skin cancer and premature aging.[3] This distorted view has encouraged us to systematically avoid the sun, inadvertently starving our bodies of a critical, naturally produced steroid hormone: vitamin D. This is not merely a vitamin; it is a master key, fundamentally orchestrating cellular function throughout your entire body. We are not just missing out on a nutrient; we are fundamentally disrupting our biology.

### VITAMIN D: MORE THAN A VITAMIN, IT IS A POTENT HORMONE

To truly grasp the sun's importance, we must first understand vitamin D. Despite its name, it is not a vitamin at all, but a powerful secosteroid hormone that your body is designed to produce when your skin is exposed to the sun's ultraviolet B (UVB) light. This natural process begins when UVB rays (specifically light rays between 290 and 330 nM) strike the skin, converting a cholesterol-like molecule, 7-dehydrocholesterol, into pre–vitamin D3. This swiftly transforms into vitamin D3, which then travels to the liver to become 25-hydroxyvitamin D (calcidiol), the form typically measured in blood tests. But the journey isn't complete until it reaches the kidneys (and numerous other cells), where it's converted into its active, hormonal form: 1,25-dihydroxyvitamin D, or calcitriol. This active form [1,25(OH)D3], is the master key that unlocks your body's inherent potential.[4]

## THE MASTER KEY AND THE BLUEPRINT OF LIFE

The pervasive influence of vitamin D stems from its presence in the very genetic blueprint of our cells. Nearly every one of your 37 trillion cells contains a special docking station called the vitamin D receptor (VDR).[5, 6] Think of the VDR as a lock, and the active vitamin D hormone [1,25(OH) D3], as its precisely fitted key. When this key engages its lock, it transmits a potent signal directly to the cell's nucleus, the command center housing your DNA. Once inside the nucleus, the vitamin D-VDR complex locates specific regions on your DNA known as vitamin D responsive elements (VDREs). By binding to these VDREs, the complex acts as a master switch, turning genes on or off. This process, known as gene expression, dictates which proteins your cells manufacture. These proteins are the building blocks of your body and comprise what you are. These tireless workers perform functions in your body that range from combating infections to building robust bones and maintaining a sharp mind. Therefore, by regulating gene expression, vitamin D directly governs the fundamental operations of your cells, cementing its role as a true jack-of-all-trades for human health.

Beyond individual gene regulation, sunlight, through its production of vitamin D, functions as a powerful epigenetic regulator. Epigenetics describes how environmental factors, like the presence or absence of sunlight and its ensuing vitamin D, influence how your genes are expressed. While your inherent DNA sequence remains unchanged, how it is read and utilized by your cells is a dynamic process that can be influenced by many factors, including the environment. Sunlight and vitamin D don't rewrite your genetic code; they act as a conductor, guiding your cellular orchestra, dictating which genes play and at what volume. A body deprived of sunlight and vitamin D is akin to an orchestra without its conductor—the inevitable outcome is cellular discord, leading eventually to widespread disease and premature death.

There is no bypass or shortcut for the absence of sunlight and the vitamin D it produces. Our cellular machinery is intrinsically dependent on vitamin D. Decades of disregard for this fundamental biological reality has rendered Western societies increasingly susceptible to illness, frailty, and a disturbing decline in collective life expectancy and fertility. Our abandonment of the sun and its life-sustaining vitamin D is putting a large segments of the human race on a concerning trajectory toward decline and extinction.

## A PREVIEW OF THE FAR-REACHING POWER OF VITAMIN D

The presence of VDRs and VDREs throughout virtually every cell and every system in the body explains why a single hormone can exert such a broad and profound impact on health.[7] This ubiquitous presence underscores vitamin D's central role in maintaining optimal physiological function across all organ systems. We will discuss the roles of sunlight and vitamin D in each of the following systems and more, but here is a preview.

**Fertility and Reproduction:** The very capacity to create new life is intricately linked to vitamin D. VDRs are abundant in the ovaries, uterus, placenta, testes, and even on sperm cells.[8] Vitamin D orchestrates genes involved in sex hormone production (estrogen and testosterone), fosters a healthy uterine lining for successful pregnancy, and influences sperm motility.

**Immune System and Autoimmune Disease:** A robust and well-regulated immune system is your primary defense against pathogens and your safeguard against self-attack (autoimmunity). VDRs are densely distributed across all key immune cells, including T cells, B cells, macrophages, and dendritic cells.[9] Vitamin D serves as an expert immune modulator, enhancing your ability to fight infections while simultaneously calming the overactive immune responses that drive autoimmune diseases such as multiple sclerosis, psoriasis, ulcerative colitis, rheumatoid arthritis, lupus, and others.

**Cancer:** Cancer, characterized by uncontrolled cell proliferation, finds a formidable opponent in vitamin D. VDRs are present in cells of the colon, breast, prostate, skin, and numerous other tissues.[10] When activated by vitamin D, these receptors initiate genes that promote cell differentiation (guiding cells to mature and cease uncontrolled division), inhibit proliferation (curbing cell growth), and induce apoptosis (programmed self-destruction of dangerous cells).

**Cardiovascular Disease:** A healthy heart and supple blood vessels are of paramount importance for longevity. The entire cardiovascular system is rich in VDRs, which are found in the endothelial cells lining blood vessels, the smooth muscle cells within vessel walls, and the cardiomyocytes (heart muscle cells).[11] Here, vitamin D plays a vital role in regulating blood pressure, reducing systemic inflammation, and preventing the dangerous stiffening of arteries.

**Neurological Disease and Brain Health:** Your brain is far from immune to vitamin D's influence. VDRs are distributed throughout the central nervous system in both neurons and glial cells (the brain's essential support cells).[12] This explains vitamin D's profound role in protecting against neurological diseases such as multiple sclerosis, where it helps temper the immune system's attack on the nervous system, and Alzheimer's disease, where it assists in the clearance of neuroinflammatory plaques.[13] Vitamin D also contributes significantly to recovery from traumatic brain injury (TBI) and concussion by mitigating inflammation and fostering neural repair.[14]

**Muscle Function:** From peak athletic performance to the simple act of rising from a chair in old age, muscle strength is inextricably linked to vitamin D. VDRs are located directly within muscle cells.[15] Vitamin D directly stimulates the synthesis of new muscle proteins, leading to improved muscle strength, enhanced balance, and superior physical performance, thereby significantly reducing the risk of falls, particularly in older adults.[16]

**Aging and Inflammaging:** The natural process of aging is frequently accompanied by a state of chronic, low-grade inflammation, known as "inflammaging." As discussed, vitamin D is a masterful regulator of inflammation. By maintaining immune system equilibrium and optimizing cellular health across all organ systems, adequate vitamin D levels serve as a cornerstone of healthy aging, helping to defer the onset of age-related chronic diseases.[17] To deprive the body of sunlight and its vital vitamin D is to invite the health scourges that now plague humanity.

## OUR SKIN: AN EVOLUTIONARY BAROMETER

The very diversity of human skin color serves as a powerful, living testament to the nonnegotiable biological demand for vitamin D. Human skin pigmentation is a brilliant, "on-the-fly" evolutionary adaptation to varying levels of environmental ultraviolet radiation.[18] As human populations migrated away from the equatorial sun, their skin lightened over generations. This wasn't arbitrary; darker pigmentation, while excellent at protecting against UV radiation damage and preserving vital B vitamins like folate, significantly hinders vitamin D synthesis. Lighter skin is a direct evolutionary adaptation designed to maximize vitamin D production in environments with less intense sunlight.[19] Even within an individual, the ability to tan is your body's intelligent mechanism for striking a balance—providing a temporary protective shield only after sufficient vitamin D has been synthesized.

The wide spectrum of human skin color is one of the most visible and compelling proofs of our species' fundamental and nonnegotiable biological requirement for sunlight-driven vitamin D. Given that the intricate machinery to utilize vitamin D—the VDR—is present in virtually every cell in the body, it should come as no surprise that depriving the body of sunlight and its essential products, as we have systematically and unwittingly done for the last fifty years or so, has had profound and devastating health consequences.

## A HISTORY FORGED IN LIGHT: THE GREAT FORGETTING

Our ancestors evolved under the sun's unwavering gaze, their skin naturally producing vitamin D when exposed to specific frequencies of ultraviolet light. Our bodies, with their innate wisdom, seamlessly integrated this readily available natural resource into countless aspects of growth, development, and daily function. As humankind embarked on its great migrations away from the direct and consistent equatorial sun, our skin adapted. This remarkable mutation involved a reduction in melanin content, a strategic evolutionary trade-off designed to maximize essential vitamin D production in environments with less intense sunlight.[20] Over the past half-century, however, a concerted effort has led to the development and widespread adoption of technologies and public health campaigns specifically designed to virtually eliminate all cutaneously generated vitamin D synthesis.[21, 22]

## THE SUN: ANCIENT DEITY AND PRIMORDIAL HEALER

To attempt to put into context the extent of the modern perversity of sun phobia we need to take a step back to see what the ancients knew about the sun and its powers that we have apparently forgotten. Throughout recorded history, and undoubtedly long before, the sun has been a central figure in human consciousness, revered not merely as a celestial object but as a potent deity and a source of life and healing. Ancient civilizations across the globe, from the Egyptians with their sun god Ra, a personification of the midday sun and a supreme creator deity,[23] to the Incas, who worshipped Inti, the sun god from whom the Sapa Inca emperors were believed to be descended,[24] recognized the sun's indispensable role. In ancient Greece, Helios was the Titan god of the sun, often depicted driving a golden chariot across the sky,[25] while Apollo, an Olympian god, became increasingly associated with the sun and, significantly, with healing and medicine.[26] The Roman Sol Invictus, or "Unconquered Sun," became a prominent deity in the later Roman Empire, with his festival on December 25th marking the "rebirth" of the sun.[27] This deification was not mere superstition; it was an intuitive understanding of the sun's life-sustaining power.

Beyond its role in agriculture and warmth, ancient cultures recognized the sun's direct influence on health. The Greek physician Hippocrates, often hailed as the "Father of Medicine" (circa 460–370 BCE), advocated for sunbaths, or "heliosis," for various ailments, recognizing the value of sunlight in promoting health and recovery for conditions ranging from wasting diseases to promoting wound healing. Roman physicians, including Celsus and Galen, also prescribed sunbathing for conditions such as epilepsy, paralysis, and jaundice.[28] Pliny the Elder (77–79 CE) wrote extensively about the therapeutic benefits of sunlight, terming it "the greatest remedy."[29] These ancient healers observed the sun's power to invigorate, to dispel sickness, and to restore vitality. Their observations, though lacking the biochemical understanding we possess today, were astute. They saw that life flourished under the sun and withered in its absence, a fundamental truth that modern society has perilously chosen to ignore.

## HELIOTHERAPY: THE RISE AND FALL OF SUN-POWERED MEDICINE

The empirical observations of these ancient healers provided the foundation for heliotherapy—the therapeutic use of sunlight. While practiced for millennia, heliotherapy experienced a significant revival and systematization in the late nineteenth and early twentieth centuries, driven by physicians who witnessed its profound effects on diseases that defied other treatments of the era. The modern era of heliotherapy is often attributed to figures like Arnold Rikli, a Swiss physician who established a "sun cure" clinic in Austria in the mid-1850s.[30] However, it was Dr. Auguste Rollier, another Swiss physician, who truly popularized and scientifically documented heliotherapy in the early twentieth century. Starting in 1903 in Leysin, Switzerland, Rollier established high-altitude sanatoria where he primarily treated patients suffering from extrapulmonary tuberculosis (TB), such as TB of the bones, joints, and skin (lupus vulgaris).[31, 32, 33]

The justification for heliotherapy was largely empirical: Physicians observed remarkable improvements in patients exposed to sunlight, especially in alpine environments with clean air and intense UV radiation. Rollier meticulously documented his methods, emphasizing gradual, whole-body sun exposure while carefully avoiding sunburn. He noted that sunlight appeared to stimulate the body's natural defenses, improve circulation, increase muscle tone, and promote the healing of diseased tissues. Though the exact mechanism (vitamin D synthesis) was not fully understood until later, the clinical outcomes were undeniable. The justification rested on the observed power of the sun to restore health where other methods failed.

The primary application of heliotherapy in the early twentieth century was for tuberculosis and rickets. Dr. Rollier reported astonishing success rates, claiming cure rates as high as 70 to 80 percent for debilitating and often fatal surgical tuberculosis (affecting bones, joints, and lymph nodes). Photographic evidence from his clinics vividly demonstrates patients with severe tuberculous wounds and deformed joints gradually healing under the sun's rays, showcasing profound recoveries involving bone regeneration and tissue repair. Dr. Henry Gauvain in England also achieved significant success using heliotherapy for surgical tuberculosis.[34]

Independently, the connection between sunlight and rickets, a bone-deforming disease in children, was being established. In 1919, Kurt Huldschinsky, a German physician, demonstrated that exposing children with rickets to ultraviolet light from a mercury-vapor quartz lamp could cure the disease.[35] This was followed by the conclusive work of Harriet Chick and her colleagues in Vienna after World War I, who showed that sunlight (or cod-liver oil, later identified as rich in vitamin D) could prevent and cure rickets.[36] This discovery provided an important biochemical link to the sun's healing power, ultimately leading to the identification of vitamin D.

Heliotherapy was also employed for treating infected wounds, particularly during World War I, where sunlight was used as a disinfectant and to promote healing in soldiers.[37] It also found application in various skin conditions, including psoriasis and eczema.

## DECLINE OF HELIOTHERAPY

Despite its documented successes, heliotherapy began to wane in popularity within the medical community by the mid-twentieth century due to several converging factors:

**The Rise of Antibiotics:** The 1943 discovery of streptomycin, the first effective antibiotic against mycobacterium tuberculosis, revolutionized TB treatment.[38] Pharmacological interventions offered a seemingly more direct, targeted, and easily administered solution compared to the lengthy and resource-intensive process of heliotherapy.

**Focus on Specificity:** Medicine was increasingly embracing a reductionist model, seeking specific cures for specific diseases. Heliotherapy, as a broad-spectrum, holistic treatment, did not align neatly with this emerging paradigm.

**Logistical Challenges:** Operating heliotherapy clinics required specific geographical locations (sunny, high-altitude environments), specialized facilities, and prolonged patient stays, making it less scalable and more expensive in some contexts than drug-based therapies.

**Vitamin D Fortification:** The discovery of vitamin D and its role in rickets led to widespread food fortification programs (e.g., milk fortified with vitamin D), which largely eradicated rickets in many developed countries.[39] Vitamin D fortification addressed one of the most clear-cut examples of sunlight's benefit, perhaps inadvertently diminishing the perceived need for broader sun exposure.

The undeniable and lifesaving success of antibiotics caused the pendulum to swing too far, leading to the neglect of a powerful, natural therapeutic modality that addressed the body's overall physiology in a way that targeted drugs could not. The focus of medicine shifted entirely to fighting the pathogen and its symptoms, overshadowing the importance of strengthening the host—a role the sun had played for millennia.

## THE MODERN VIEW OF THE SUN: FROM HEALER TO HAZARD

The latter half of the twentieth century witnessed a dramatic and unprecedented shift in the perception of the sun. Once revered as a life-giver and healer, it was systematically recast as a dangerous carcinogen, something to be feared and meticulously avoided. This modern characterization of the sun as primarily dangerous is profoundly counter to the biological history of all living things on this planet. All life, in its myriad forms, depends directly or indirectly on the sun.[40] Photosynthesis, driven by sunlight, forms the base of most food chains. For humans, beyond the critical synthesis of vitamin D, sunlight plays a role in regulating circadian rhythms, mood, immunity, and potentially other physiological processes yet to be fully elucidated.[41, 42] To portray the sun, so fundamental to our evolution and existence, as an outright enemy is a logical and biological absurdity.

In addition to the shift toward a model of medicine based on the treatment of symptoms, the genesis of this man-made attitude of fear toward the sun is multifaceted, beginning with the dermatology profession. Starting in the mid-twentieth century, dermatology as a specialty increasingly focused on the link between sun exposure, skin aging, and skin cancer, particularly melanoma.[43] While basal cell and squamous cell carcinomas are clearly linked to cumulative sun exposure and are generally treatable and curable, melanoma, though rarer, carries a higher mortality risk. Public health campaigns, often spearheaded by dermatological associations, began to emphasize sun avoidance and the use of sunscreens as primary prevention strategies against all forms of skin cancer.[44] The message became simplified to "sun = bad," neglecting the benefits of sun exposure and the different types of skin cancer.

The broader medical community, influenced by the dermatological perspective and the prevailing risk-averse culture in public health, largely adopted this same anti-sun stance. Advice to avoid sun exposure became standard, often without consideration for an individual's vitamin D status or the broader health benefits of sensible sun exposure. The focus on minimizing one risk (skin cancer) overshadowed the potential for increasing myriad other risks associated with vitamin D deficiency.

Finally, the burgeoning fear of the sun created sun phobia and a lucrative market for sunscreen products. The sunscreen and cosmetics industry, through extensive marketing, reinforced the message that sun exposure is inherently dangerous and that daily, liberal application of sunscreen is essential for health.[45] Advertising often played on fear, depicting the sun as an aggressor from which one needs constant chemical protection. The industry promoted the idea that sunscreens allowed for "safe" sun exposure, yet the primary effect of broad-spectrum sunscreens is the highly efficient blocking of UVB radiation, the very wavelength necessary for vitamin D synthesis.[46]

This systematic vilification of the sun, driven by a narrow focus on potential skin damage, has had catastrophic and largely unacknowledged adverse consequences on public health. The primary outcome has been population-level vitamin D insufficiency. By convincing populations to shun the sun and diligently apply vitamin D-synthesis-blocking sunscreens, we have effectively engineered widespread vitamin D deficiency and insufficiency across the developed world. Estimates suggest that up to a billion people worldwide may have deficient or insufficient vitamin D levels, and most of those people live in the developed world.[47] Remember that almost all of our 37 trillion cells have receptors for vitamin D and that vitamin D has to come from somewhere. This is not a trivial matter, as vitamin D is not merely a "vitamin" but a potent secosteroid hormone essential for the proper function of virtually every system in the body. Its profound roles in immune system regulation, cardiovascular health, muscle strength and function, brain health, and healthy aging are now well-established.[48, 49, 50, 51, 52]

## THE GREAT OVERREACTION: MELANOMA, VITAMIN D, AND THE MODERN DISEASE EPIDEMIC

The modern-day fear of the sun, which has driven populations indoors and led to obsessive sunscreen use, can be characterized as a profound, pathological overreaction to the minimal risk of melanoma, coupled with a dangerous ignorance of the sun's vital benefits. Melanoma accounts for a small percentage of skin cancers but is responsible for the majority of skin cancer deaths.[53] However, the relationship between sun exposure and melanoma is far more complex than the simplistic "sun causes melanoma" narrative often portrayed. Intriguingly, melanoma often tends to occur in body areas that receive less chronic sun exposure, such as the trunk in men or the lower legs in women, and can even arise in sites that are never exposed to the sun, such as internal organs, gluteal tissue, and the soles of the feet.[54, 55, 56] Furthermore, studies suggest that individuals with chronic, regular sun exposure (like outdoor workers) have a lower risk of melanoma compared to those with intermittent, intense sun exposure (e.g., office workers who take infrequent, sun-intense vacations).[57]

More importantly, a growing body of evidence indicates that vitamin D status itself plays a critical role in melanoma prognosis. Higher vitamin D levels are associated with better prognosis (thinner melanomas) and improved survival rates, suggesting that, ironically, vitamin D itself may have protective effects against the progression and lethality of this cancer.[58, 59, 60] Therefore, the relentless campaign for sun avoidance and maximal sunscreen use, while potentially reducing the incidence of more common but less deadly nonmelanoma skin cancers, has had the devastating unintended consequence of slashing population-wide vitamin D levels and increasing the lethality of the melanomas than sun-avoidance advice was intended to prevent.

Widespread vitamin D deficiency, engineered by misguided advice creating our fear of the sun, is now emerging as a major contributing factor to the epidemics of chronic diseases that plague the modern world:[61]

- **Autoimmune Diseases:** Vitamin D is a critical modulator of the immune system. Its deficiency is strongly linked to an increased risk of autoimmune diseases such as multiple sclerosis, rheumatoid arthritis, psoriasis, inflammatory bowel disease, and type 1 diabetes.[62, 63]

- **Cardiovascular Diseases:** Low vitamin D levels are associated with an increased risk of hypertension, heart attacks, strokes, and overall cardiovascular mortality.[64]
- **Cancers:** Beyond melanoma prognosis, vitamin D deficiency has been linked to an increased risk of developing several common cancers, including colorectal, breast, and prostate cancer, and to poorer outcomes in cancer patients generally.[65, 66]
- **Metabolic Disorders:** Vitamin D insufficiency is implicated in insulin resistance, obesity, metabolic syndrome, and an increased risk of type 2 diabetes.[67]
- **Frailty and Neurocognitive Decline:** Adequate vitamin D is essential for muscle strength, bone health (preventing osteoporosis and fractures), and brain function. Deficiency is linked to increased frailty in the elderly, cognitive impairment, and potentially neurodegenerative diseases like Alzheimer's and Parkinson's.[68, 69]

Our ancestors understood the sun's power. They lived in harmony with its rhythms, benefiting from its life-sustaining energy. The modern, fear-driven narrative that has severed this ancient connection is not based on a holistic understanding of health but on a myopic focus on a single, yet rare, risk. It is time to reevaluate our relationship with the sun, guided by our evolutionary heritage and the overwhelming scientific evidence of vitamin D's critical importance, and to correct this dangerous and health-destroying overreaction.

# CHAPTER 2

# THE SUN'S GIFT UNVEILED: THE DISCOVERY OF VITAMIN D

Our human story begins under the sun. For millennia, our ancestors evolved near the equator, where their skin constantly produced a vital substance when touched by sunlight: vitamin D. Our bodies were so expertly designed to use this free and abundant resource that it became essential for our growth, development, and overall health. For those humans who migrated away from the equator into regions with less-powerful sun, their biology adapted. Over generations, skin became lighter, reducing the pigment melanin to maximize the production of essential vitamin D from weaker sunlight. However, in the last fifty years, a systematic campaign against the sun has convinced us to fear it and block its rays entirely. We have become incredibly effective at stopping our bodies from making any vitamin D at all. As a direct result, the very diseases that define modern illness—cancers, heart disease, and autoimmune disorders—are now at catastrophic levels, with no end in sight. This chapter will trace the journey of vitamin D from its discovery as a cure for a crippling bone disease to its recognition as a powerful hormone, a path lit by brilliant observation, happy accidents, and revolutionary science.

## THE SHADOW OF RICKETS: A DISEASE OF DARKNESS

The story of vitamin D starts not with a discovery, but with the widespread suffering caused by its absence. From the 1600s through the early 1900s, a devastating disease called rickets plagued the industrialized cities of Northern Europe and North America.[1, 2] Rickets causes children's bones to become soft and weak, leading to permanent deformities like bowed legs and bumps along the ribs. The industrial revolution, for all its progress, cast a literal shadow over these cities. Thick coal smoke filled the air, blocking sunlight, while families spent their days working indoors in factories and living in dark, narrow alleyways. Doctors of the time, such as Daniel Whistler and Francis Glisson, provided detailed descriptions of rickets, often calling it "the English disease," but they could not pinpoint its cause.[3] Still, there were clues. Doctors noticed that rickets was rare in children who lived in the countryside and played in the sun. They also observed that a folk remedy—cod-liver oil—seemed to help. For centuries, coastal communities in northern countries had used this oil to treat bone ailments and general poor health.[4] This traditional wisdom, though not yet understood by science, pointed the way toward a cure.

## FINDING THE "ANTI-RICKETS FACTOR": THE FIRST BREAKTHROUGHS

The early twentieth century was a golden age for nutritional science, as researchers began to identify vital amines or "vitamins"—tiny but essential nutrients. In England, Sir Edward Mellanby conducted a landmark experiment between 1918 and 1921. He raised puppies indoors, away from sunlight, and fed them a diet that he knew caused rickets. He then proved that he could prevent or cure the disease simply by adding cod-liver oil to their food.[5] Mellanby thought he had found proof that vitamin A, which was already known to be in cod-liver oil, was the cure. He was wrong.

Across the Atlantic, American biochemist Elmer McCollum at Johns Hopkins University decided to test Mellanby's theory. In 1922, McCollum took cod-liver oil and destroyed its vitamin A by bubbling hot air through it. He then fed this treated oil to rats with rickets. Remarkably, the rats were still cured. This elegant experiment proved that a second, unknown substance in the oil was responsible. McCollum named this newly discovered nutrient "vitamin D."[6]

At the exact same time, separate evidence was proving the power of sunlight. In 1919, a German doctor named Kurt Huldshinsky showed he could cure rickets in children by exposing them to ultraviolet (UV) light from a special lamp.[7] Two years later, doctors Alfred Hess and Lester Unger in New York City confirmed that simple, natural sunlight exposure could also prevent and cure the disease in children.[8]

This created a scientific puzzle: How could both a substance in an oil and invisible rays from the sun provide the same cure? The answer came from another brilliant set of experiments. In 1924, both Harry Steenbock at the University of Wisconsin and Alfred Hess at Columbia University independently discovered that they could create vitamin D by shining UV light on food.[9, 10] Steenbock famously irradiated rat food, which then protected the rats who ate it from getting rickets. This discovery was a game changer, leading directly to the practice of fortifying foods like milk with vitamin D, a public health measure that has since saved millions of children from rickets.

## ISOLATING AND UNDERSTANDING THE "SUNSHINE VITAMIN"

The next step was to identify the exact starting ingredients in our skin and food that sunlight transformed into vitamin D. German chemist Adolf Windaus led this charge. In 1927, he identified a substance in fungi and plants called ergosterol, which, when hit with UV light, turned into a form of vitamin D now known as vitamin D2 (ergocalciferol).[11, 12] For this and his related work on sterols, Windaus was awarded the Nobel Prize in Chemistry in 1928. A few years later, in the 1930s, Windaus's team identified the specific ingredient in animal skin: a cholesterol-like molecule called 7-dehydrocholesterol (7-DHC). When exposed to UV light, 7-DHC transforms into a superior form of the vitamin called cholecalciferol, or vitamin D3.[13] This is the "sunshine vitamin" our bodies are designed to make. We now know that vitamin D3, the kind made in our skin and found in animal-based foods, is more powerful and effective for humans than the D2 version from plants.[14]

## THE BIOLOGICAL POWERHOUSE: HOW OUR BODIES USE VITAMIN D

Our skin is a magnificent vitamin D factory. When UVB rays from the sun (specifically in the 290–315 nanometer wavelength) strike the skin, they provide the energy for 7-DHC to transform into a "pre-vitamin D3." Over the next several hours, your body heat naturally converts this into vitamin D3.[15]

But vitamin D3, whether made in the skin or eaten in food, is not yet active. It must be activated within the body in a two-step process to become the powerful hormone that it is.

**First Stop: The Liver.** Vitamin D from the skin travels through the bloodstream to the liver. Here, an enzyme adds a molecule to it, turning it into 25-hydroxyvitamin D, or 25(OH)D. This is the storage form of vitamin D, and it is what is measured with a blood test to determine if you are deficient.[16]

**Second Stop: The Kidneys (and Other Cells).** From the liver, 25(OH)D travels to the kidneys. Here, another enzyme adds a final piece, converting it into 1,25-dihydroxyvitamin D [1,25(OH)D], also known as calcitriol. This is the fully active, hormonal form of vitamin D.[17]

Active vitamin D works by binding to a special docking station found in nearly every cell in your body, called the vitamin D receptor (VDR). Think of the VDR as a lock and active vitamin D as the key. When the key turns the lock, it sends a signal to the cell's command center—the DNA—to turn thousands of genes on or off.[18] The fact that these VDR "locks" are found everywhere on most of the 37 trillion cells in the body, from the brain to immune cells to the heart, proves that vitamin D's job extends far beyond just building strong bones. Vitamin D is a master regulator of the entire body.

## THE IMPACT OF DISCOVERY: VICTORY AND MODERN TRAGEDY

The discovery of vitamin D led to one of the greatest public health victories of the twentieth century. By fortifying milk and other foods, including beer, nations nearly eradicated rickets.[19] However, this story has taken a tragic turn in recent decades. While we conquered rickets, a single disease of bone, we have ignored vitamin D's broader role, an arguably more important role in preventing chronic illness. This situation has occurred because the amount of vitamin D to prevent rickets is minimal compared to the amount of vitamin D that your body needs on a daily basis to function optimally and prevent disease.

Overwhelming research now links vitamin D deficiency to a higher risk for the very diseases devastating the developed world: Cancers, including those of the colon, breast, and prostate.[20] Cardiovascular diseases, such as high blood pressure and heart failure.[21] Autoimmune diseases, like multiple sclerosis, type 1 diabetes, and rheumatoid arthritis.[22] Infectious diseases, by weakening our defenses against viruses like influenza and other respiratory infections.[23] The irony is staggering. Vitamin D deficiency is now a global pandemic, precisely because we have been taught to avoid our primary source of it. Our war on the sun has left our bodies defenseless.

## MANUFACTURING VITAMIN D: FROM LAB BENCHES TO GLOBAL PRODUCTION

Commercial production of vitamin D began almost immediately after its discovery. The first form to be mass-produced was vitamin D2. Following Steenbock's discovery, factories began extracting ergosterol from yeast, purifying it, and irradiating it with UV light to create vitamin D2. This process was patented and licensed to food companies, funding decades of further research.[24]

Making vitamin D3 was initially more difficult. After Windaus identified 7-DHC in animal skin, scientists found an abundant source: lanolin, the oil in sheep's wool.[25] Today, the industrial process for making vitamin D3 remains largely the same. Cholesterol is extracted from lanolin, chemically converted into 7-DHC, and then irradiated with UV light to produce vitamin D3. This pure vitamin D3 is then stabilized and added to supplements and fortified foods.

## D2 VS. D3

It is a common misconception that vitamin D is a singular entity; in reality, there are two primary forms: vitamin D2 (ergocalciferol) and vitamin D3 (cholecalciferol). While both can contribute to vitamin D levels in the body, they are not created equal in their biological efficacy. A significant body of research consistently demonstrates that vitamin D3 is superior to vitamin D2 in its ability to raise and maintain circulating levels of 25-hydroxyvitamin D (25(OH)D), the active form of vitamin D that is measured in the blood to assess vitamin D status.[26]

This enhanced bioavailability of vitamin D3 is attributed to several factors, including its more efficient conversion in the liver and its longer half-life in the bloodstream compared to vitamin D2.[27] For example, a study of randomized controlled trials found that vitamin D3 supplementation resulted in a significantly greater increase in 25(OH)D concentrations than vitamin D2 of the same dose.[28] Regarding the magnitude of the difference, D3 is approximately 87 percent more potent in raising and maintaining serum 25(OH)D concentrations and produces two- to threefold greater storage of vitamin D than does D2.[29] This robust evidence underscores the critical importance of prioritizing vitamin D3 when considering supplementation or dietary intake for optimal vitamin D status and overall health. Plus, D3 costs pennies per dose compared to the expensive, prescription-based D2.

## FROM RICKETS TO CRICKETS

The discovery of vitamin D and our ability to manufacture it is a modern scientific marvel. Yet, this knowledge and ability exist alongside a global deficiency pandemic. Since the excitement of the discovery of vitamin D more than one hundred years ago, we have systematically ignored the life-giving benefits of the sun and its vitamin D. The vilification of our star has had profound and destructive consequences for human health, a reality we are only now beginning to confront.

# CHAPTER 3

# LESSONS FROM THE LIZARD: SUNLIGHT, BEHAVIOR, AND THE INNATE DRIVE FOR VITAMIN D

The intricate dance between an organism and its environment is a cornerstone of evolutionary biology. For millennia, life on Earth has adapted to harness the sun's energy, not just for warmth or vision, but for profound physiological processes. While humans, in their modern, technologically advanced societies, have increasingly distanced themselves from this fundamental solar connection, other creatures offer a compelling and instructive window into the innate, deeply ingrained mechanisms that govern the acquisition of vital, sun-derived compounds.

This chapter will assert that lizards, those ancient and remarkably adapted reptiles, serve as an exceptional model for understanding how behavior and physiology interact with sophisticated precision to regulate vitamin D synthesis. Their sun-basking rituals, often dismissed as mere thermoregulation, are, in fact, a powerful proxy, a behavioral manifestation of an intrinsic drive to achieve and maintain optimal vitamin D levels—a drive so important that it often outweighs significant predation risks. By examining the lizard's "vitamin D intelligence," we gain a stark and unsettling perspective on humanity's overthinking evidenced by our own shortsighted and biologically detrimental avoidance of the sun.

## ECTOTHERMY AND THE SUN'S DUAL IMPERATIVE: HEAT AND VITAMIN D

Lizards, like most reptiles, are ectothermic, meaning they rely on external heat sources to regulate their body temperature.[1] This fundamental physiological constraint dictates much of their behavior, particularly their conspicuous sun-basking activities. However, it is a profound oversimplification to view this basking solely through the lens of thermoregulation. The sun offers more than just warmth; it provides the critical UVB radiation necessary for the cutaneous synthesis of vitamin D, a secosteroid hormone absolutely essential for calcium metabolism, bone health, immune function, and, as we are increasingly understanding, a vast array of other physiological processes critical for their survival and reproductive success.[2] For lizards, therefore, sun exposure serves a dual, inseparable imperative: acquiring thermal energy and manufacturing vitamin D. Their very existence is a testament to an evolutionary bargain struck with the sun.

## SUN-SEEKING AS VITAMIN D-SEEKING: UNMASKING THE PROXY BEHAVIOR

The observable sun-basking behavior of lizards is not merely a passive response to ambient temperature but an active, physiologically driven quest to optimize vitamin D status. The lizard, in its seemingly simple act of basking, is engaging in a sophisticated form of self-regulation, a behavioral endocrinology where external actions are finely tuned to internal biochemical needs.

Lizards appear to possess an internal "vitamin D thermostat" or sensor that influences their motivation to seek out UVB radiation. When their internal vitamin D stores are low, their drive to bask in UVB-rich sunlight increases. Conversely, when their vitamin D levels are replete, their basking duration or intensity may decrease, even if thermal conditions might otherwise encourage it. This suggests a homeostatic mechanism where behavior is modulated to maintain vitamin D within an optimal physiological range.[3]

Lizards are not indiscriminate sunbathers. They demonstrate an ability to discern and preferentially expose themselves to microhabitats that offer not just warmth but also appropriate levels of UVB radiation. They can, in essence, "choose" the right kind of sunlight for their physiological needs. This selective behavior strongly implies that thermoregulation alone cannot fully explain their basking patterns.

The overt act of basking, therefore, becomes a visible proxy for an underlying, internal drive for vitamin D. The lizard isn't just seeking warmth; it is actively "dosing" itself with the necessary solar radiation to fuel a critical biochemical pathway.

## LIZARDS REVEAL THEIR VITAMIN D INTELLIGENCE

The idea that lizards actively regulate their vitamin D status through behavioral means is not mere speculation; it is strongly supported by compelling experimental research. Pioneering studies have directly tested the link between internal vitamin D status and basking behavior. In a classic experimental design, researchers have administered vitamin D injections to lizards, effectively raising their internal vitamin D levels independently of sun exposure. The results are striking and consistent: Lizards pretreated with vitamin D subsequently spend significantly less time basking in UVB-rich light compared to control lizards injected with a placebo.[4, 5] This demonstrates a clear negative feedback loop: When vitamin D levels are artificially elevated, the behavioral drive to synthesize more vitamin D via sun exposure is demonstrably reduced. Somehow, the lizard "knows" it has enough vitamin D.

**Manipulating the Solar Spectrum: UVB vs. Heat**. Further ingenious experiments have involved manipulating the spectral quality of the light sources available to lizards, decoupling heat from UVB radiation. For instance, lizards might be offered a choice between a heat lamp providing warmth but no UVB, and a UVB lamp providing the necessary radiation but less heat. Studies have shown that lizards will actively shuttle between these sources, or spend significant time under the UVB source even if it means sacrificing some thermal comfort, particularly if their vitamin D status is low.[6]

Furthermore, if deprived of UVB for extended periods, even if thermally comfortable, many lizard species will intensify their basking efforts when UVB is reintroduced, indicating a compensatory behavioral response to correct a perceived vitamin D deficit. Some studies have even shown that when provided with light sources emitting different wavelengths, lizards preferentially bask under those that include the UVB spectrum necessary for vitamin D synthesis, even if other visible or heat-producing wavelengths are equally or more available.[7] This ability to discriminate and seek out specific light spectra underscores a very sophisticated behavioral adaptation for vitamin D acquisition.

**Dietary Vitamin D and Basking**. The interplay between dietary vitamin D and basking behavior has also been investigated. Lizards fed diets deficient in vitamin D tend to increase their basking duration and intensity under UVB sources, attempting to compensate for the dietary shortfall through increased cutaneous synthesis. Conversely, those on vitamin D–replete diets may exhibit reduced basking.[8] This further supports the idea that basking is, in part, a direct behavioral response to the organism's internal vitamin D needs.

These experiments, and others like them, provide robust evidence that lizards are not passive recipients of sunlight but active managers of their vitamin D economy. Their sun-basking is an intelligent, physiologically regulated behavior.

## THE EXISTENTIAL PREDICAMENT: PREDATION RISK AS AN INDEX OF VITAMIN D'S IMPORTANCE

The drive to acquire sufficient vitamin D through sun exposure is so powerful in lizards that it often compels them to take significant, even life-threatening, risks. Basking, by its very nature, is an act of exposure. A lizard perched on a rock or log, soaking up the sun, is also highly visible to predators such as birds of prey, snakes, and mammals.

**The Trade-Off: Vital Nutrient vs. Predation.** The decision to bask involves a constant, albeit unconscious, cost-benefit analysis. The physiological imperative to synthesize vitamin D (and to thermoregulate) must be weighed against the increased risk of being caught and eaten. The very fact that lizards consistently engage in this conspicuous and risky behavior, often for extended periods, serves as a profound index of the critical importance of vitamin D to their survival and reproductive fitness.[9] If vitamin D were merely a minor nutrient, evolution would likely have favored less risky strategies for its acquisition.

**Behavioral Adaptations to Mitigate Risk**. While basking is essential, lizards have also evolved behavioral adaptations to minimize predation risk during these vulnerable periods. These include choosing basking sites with nearby escape routes, heightened vigilance, crypsis (camouflage), and adjusting basking duration based on perceived threat levels.[10] However, the fundamental need to expose themselves to sunlight remains.

**Seasonal and Temporal Risk Variation**. The predation risk associated with basking can vary seasonally and temporally. For example, during breeding seasons when energy demands (and potentially vitamin D requirements for egg production) are high, lizards might engage in more prolonged or riskier basking. Similarly, after periods of cloudy weather or brumation (reptilian hibernation) when vitamin D stores may be depleted, the drive to bask might override a higher degree of caution.

The willingness of lizards to routinely expose themselves to potentially lethal predation to acquire sunlight for vitamin D synthesis is a stark testament to the nonnegotiable importance of this hormone. It is not a luxury; it is a biological imperative for which they are willing to gamble their lives.

## THE LIZARD'S ADAPTIVE WISDOM: A STARK CONTRAST TO HUMAN FOLLY

Lizards, through eons of evolution, have developed a sophisticated and adaptive interplay between their physiology and behavior to ensure optimal vitamin D homeostasis. They actively modulate their sun-basking behavior not only to thermoregulate but also to maintain serum vitamin D levels essential for their overall health and fitness. This "vitamin D intelligence" is a beautiful example of an organism living in harmony with its solar environment, utilizing its resources efficiently and adaptively.

Now, contrast this innate wisdom with the behavior of modern Western humans. Unlike the vitamin D–intelligent lizard, which instinctively seeks the sun when its internal stores are low, humans in developed societies have largely lost, or willfully suppressed, this adaptive capability. Driven by a pervasive and often exaggerated fear of skin cancer and bombarded with public health messages promoting aggressive sun avoidance and constant sunscreen use, we have purposefully isolated ourselves from the very source of this essential hormone.[11]

The consequences of this deliberate estrangement are profound and devastating.

The avoidance of the sun, and the consequent widespread Vitamin D deficiency, has hampered our immune regulation, fueled chronic inflammation, and created a permissive environment for the development of these debilitating and life-shortening conditions. As HHS Secretary Kennedy said on September 4, 2025, the CDC estimates that 80 percent of Americans now have a chronic disease; in the early 1960s it was 11 percent.[12, 13] Humans in the developed world are literally overthinking themselves to death. The lizard, in its simple wisdom, offers a profound lesson that we have tragically failed to heed.

## RECLAIMING OUR SOLAR BIRTHRIGHT—LEARNING FROM THE LIZARD

The sun-basking lizard, often viewed as a simple creature driven by basic instincts, is, in reality, a sophisticated physiological marvel, demonstrating an innate intelligence in regulating its vitamin D status through precise behavioral adaptations. Its life is a continuous dialogue with the sun, a testament to the vital importance of UVB radiation for health and survival. The lizard understands, at a deep biological level, what modern humans have forgotten or chosen to ignore: that sunlight is not an enemy to be feared, but an essential elixir, a life-giving force that fuels critical physiological processes.

It is time to humbly learn from the lizard, to shed our culturally ingrained heliophobia, and to reclaim our solar birthright. Sensible, non-burning sun exposure is not a reckless indulgence but a fundamental biological necessity, a prerequisite for a robust immune system, balanced adaptive inflammation, and the prevention of a vast array of chronic diseases. The path to reversing the chronic disease epidemic begins with stepping back into the light.

## CHAPTER 4

# BEYOND VITAMIN D: THE SUN-FORGED ANTIMICROBIAL SHIELD

While the previous chapter firmly established the profound significance of vitamin D, synthesized in our skin under the influence of sunlight, it is important to understand that the sun's impact on our innate defenses extends far beyond this single hormone. Our evolutionary dance with sunlight has endowed us with a sophisticated, multilayered protective system. Key players in this arsenal are remarkable sunlight and vitamin D–dependent antimicrobial peptides, particularly the well-studied cathelicidins and the equally important defensins. This chapter will illuminate the discovery, function, and critical importance of these peptides, particularly their sun-dependent production in the skin and their role as frontline defenders against a hostile microbial world. We will see that the modern, fear-driven avoidance of the sun and the ubiquitous overuse of sunscreens not only interferes with our vitamin D synthesis but also dangerously compromise the production and efficacy of this vital antimicrobial shield, leaving us more vulnerable to a host of infectious and inflammatory conditions. The idea that sun avoidance is solely about vitamin D is a gross oversimplification; it is about crippling a fundamental component of our innate immunity of antimicrobial peptides.

### THE DISCOVERY OF OUR INNATE ANTIBIOTICS: UNVEILING AN ANCIENT DEFENSE

The story of our endogenous antibiotics begins with the broader scientific exploration of antimicrobial peptides, which are ancient, evolutionarily conserved molecules that form a critical part of the innate immune system across diverse species, from insects to mammals.[1] These peptides, nature's own antibiotics, are broadly classified into families, with the two most prominent in humans being the defensins and the cathelicidins. Both provide rapid, broad-spectrum defense against bacteria, fungi, and many viruses.

The specific identification of the cathelicidin family can be traced back to the late 1980s and early 1990s through the work of several research groups. Pioneering studies on neutrophils, the frontline warrior cells of our innate immune system, revealed the presence of potent antimicrobial proteins within their granules. Zanetti and colleagues were instrumental in isolating and characterizing a precursor protein from bovine neutrophils that, upon processing, yielded an antimicrobial peptide.[2]

Scientists quickly found similar cathelicidin proteins in many mammals, including humans. In humans, the gene for cathelicidin is called CAMP. This gene creates a protein called hCAP18. When enzymes, like those from neutrophils or epithelial cells, cut hCAP18, it releases an active piece called LL-37.[3] LL-37 is a 37-amino acid peptide, rich in leucine, and is the main human cathelicidin. Its discovery was very important for understanding how our bodies defend against infections.

The initial applications stemming from this discovery were primarily focused on understanding LL-37's role in fighting infections. It was quickly recognized that LL-37 possessed potent bactericidal activity against a broad spectrum of bacteria.[4] This sparked interest in its potential as a novel antibiotic, especially in an era of rising antibiotic resistance. However, as research progressed, it became clear that cathelicidin's functions were far more diverse and intricate than initially imagined, extending beyond direct microbial killing to encompass important roles in immune modulation, wound healing, and inflammation.

## A UBIQUITOUS SHIELD: DISTRIBUTION OF ANTIMICROBIAL PEPTIDES ON SKIN AND BARRIER SURFACES

Cathelicidin and defensins are not just confined to neutrophils; they are strategically deployed at the body's critical interfaces with the external environment—the very barriers that are constantly challenged by microbes. Their distribution underscores their role as a first line of defense.

**The Skin: Our Primary Armor.** The skin is a major site of antimicrobial peptide production and activity. Keratinocytes, the predominant cell type in the epidermis, are potent producers of hCAP18/LL-37 and various beta-defensins, especially in response to injury, infection, and, importantly, sunlight exposure.[5] These peptides are found in sweat and on the surface of the skin, creating an antimicrobial barrier that helps to control the skin microbiota and protect against invading pathogens. Their presence is vital for preventing skin infections and maintaining skin homeostasis.

**Respiratory Epithelium.** The lining of the respiratory tract is another key location for antimicrobial peptide expression. Epithelial cells here produce both LL-37 and beta-defensins, which play a critical role in defending against inhaled bacteria and viruses.[6] Their activity is essential for preventing respiratory infections like influenza, pneumonia, and bronchitis.

**Gastrointestinal Tract.** The epithelial cells lining the gut also produce antimicrobial peptides. Here, cathelicidin, alongside various defensins (e.g., human defensin 5 and 6), contributes to the regulation of the gut microbiome and provides defense against gastrointestinal pathogens.[7] Given the gut's constant exposure to a vast array of microbes, the presence of these peptides is vital for intestinal health.

**Urogenital Tract.** Cathelicidin is also expressed in the epithelial lining of the urogenital tract, where it, along with defensins, provides protection against urinary tract infections and sexually transmitted pathogens.[8]

**Eyes and Oral Cavity.** The surfaces of the eyes and the oral cavity also express both cathelicidin and defensins, offering localized protection against microbial invasion in these vulnerable areas.[9]

This widespread distribution highlights the fundamental importance of these peptides as a ubiquitous component of our innate immune defenses, guarding virtually every portal of entry for potential pathogens by creating an antimicrobial force field all dependent on adequate sunlight.

## THE HEALTH IMPACT OF CATHELICIDIN: MORE THAN JUST BUG KILLING

The impact of cathelicidin on human health is profound and multifaceted, extending well beyond its direct antimicrobial properties.

- **Direct Antimicrobial Action:** LL-37 can directly kill a wide range of bacteria, fungi, and even some enveloped viruses by disrupting their cell membranes.[10]
- **Neutralization of Endotoxins:** LL-37 can bind to and neutralize lipopolysaccharide (LPS), a potent inflammatory component of gram-negative bacteria, thereby dampening excessive inflammation that can lead to sepsis.[11]
- **Immune Cell Recruitment:** LL-37 acts as a chemoattractant, recruiting neutrophils, monocytes, and T cells to sites of infection or injury, thus orchestrating a broader immune response.[12]
- **Modulation of Inflammation:** Cathelicidin has complex immunomodulatory roles, both promoting inflammation to fight infection and helping to resolve it to promote tissue repair.[13]

- **Promotion of Wound Healing and Angiogenesis:** LL-37 stimulates keratinocyte proliferation and the formation of new blood vessels, which are essential for tissue repair.[14]
- **Barrier Function Enhancement:** Cathelicidin can strengthen epithelial barrier integrity, for example, in the gut, helping to prevent the translocation of bacteria into the bloodstream.[15]

Deficiencies or dysregulation in cathelicidin or defensin production have been linked to increased susceptibility to infections, chronic inflammatory conditions like rosacea and atopic dermatitis, and impaired wound healing.[16] These peptides are unequivocally vital molecules for maintaining health.

## SUNLIGHT'S ANTIMICROBIAL EMBRACE: THE VITAMIN D–ANTIMICROBIAL PEPTIDE CONNECTION

The historical recognition of sunlight as a disinfectant is not folklore; it has a solid scientific basis, and both cathelicidin and defensins are key players. It is now irrefutably established that sunlight, specifically UVB radiation, is a potent inducer of antimicrobial peptide production in the skin. The synthesis of hCAP18/LL-37 and key defensins in keratinocytes is significantly upregulated by vitamin D.[17, 18] This process links the innate immune system's first alert signal—the activation of toll-like receptors by microbes—directly to the vitamin D pathway, culminating in the production of these protective peptides.[19]

Therefore, sun exposure directly leads to increased local production of these critical antimicrobial peptides. This provides an immediate, sun-activated antimicrobial shield—nature's own topical antiseptic. The empirical use of heliotherapy (sun therapy) in the pre-antibiotic era for treating cutaneous tuberculosis (lupus vulgaris), for which Niels Finsen received the Nobel Prize in 1903, can now be explained by this sun-induced antimicrobial peptide production.[20] The "goodness" of sunlight was, in part, its ability to arm our skin with its own antimicrobial weapons.

## THE SHADOWS OF DEFICIENCY: CONSEQUENCES OF SUN AVOIDANCE AND SUNSCREEN OVERUSE

The modern dogma of aggressive sun avoidance and the indiscriminate overuse of sunscreens have had a profoundly negative and largely unacknowledged consequence: the suppression of cutaneous cathelicidin and defensin production. Sunscreens, particularly those with high sun protection factors (SPFs), are designed to block UVB radiation—the very wavelengths required for both vitamin D synthesis and the subsequent vitamin D–dependent induction of these antimicrobial peptides.[21] In essence, we are disarming our skin's first line of defense. This self-inflicted weakening can lead to:

- **Increased Susceptibility to Skin Infections:** Reduced antimicrobial peptide levels can leave the skin more vulnerable to bacterial and fungal infections.
- **Dysregulation of Skin Microbiota:** Antimicrobial peptides help shape the skin's microbial community, and altered levels could lead to dysbiosis, which is implicated in various skin conditions.[22]
- **Impaired Wound Healing:** Given LL-37's role in promoting wound healing, reduced production could lead to slower repair of skin injuries.[23]
- **Exacerbation of Inflammatory Skin Conditions:** While complex, optimal antimicrobial peptide levels are important for regulating skin inflammation. Chronic suppression through sun avoidance might exacerbate conditions like atopic dermatitis or rosacea in the long term.[24]

## RECLAIMING THE SUN'S ANTIMICROBIAL POWER

The discovery of cathelicidin and defensins and the elucidation of their sun-dependent production, provide profound insights into our coevolution with our environment. Sunlight is an activator of our innate immune defenses, a trigger for the production of potent antimicrobial peptides that stand guard at our primary barriers. The current societal trend of aggressive sun avoidance, while intended to mitigate one risk, has inadvertently created many others by suppressing this vital defense mechanism. It is time to move beyond a simplistic, fear-based narrative and embrace a more balanced understanding of the sun's complex and essential role in human health. Restoring sensible sun exposure is not just about vitamin D; it is about rearming our bodies with the natural antimicrobial shield that evolution has provided—a shield that is more critical than ever in our ongoing interaction with the microbial world.

## CHAPTER 5

# THE SUN'S GIFT: YOUR SKIN'S VITAMIN D FACTORY AND THE GREAT US RDA DISCONNECT

Humankind evolved under the full, unfiltered light of the sun. For millennia, this celestial body was not merely a source of warmth and light but the primary driver of a critical biochemical process in our skin: the synthesis of vitamin D. This elegant, self-regulating system is capable of producing vast quantities of this essential prohormone, amounts that dwarf the recommendations set forth by modern public health authorities. To understand the profound disconnect between our physiology and current medical advice, we must first appreciate the magnificent efficiency of our own biology.

Although we've briefly covered this before, this chapter will discuss, in more detail, the mechanics of cutaneous vitamin D production, quantify its output, examine the factors that impede it, and expose the dangerous gap between what our bodies are designed to have, what they actually use, and the startlingly inadequate official dietary recommendations. The evidence, when viewed dispassionately, points to a conclusion that is as disturbing as it is inescapable: Our modern guidelines are not only failing us, they are based on a demonstrable statistical error that has never been corrected, leaving the populace vulnerable to the very diseases vitamin D deficiency promotes.

## THE CUTANEOUS VITAMIN D SYNTHESIS ENGINE

The production of vitamin D in the skin is a testament to evolutionary brilliance. It is a process that begins with one of the most fundamental molecules in our biology: cholesterol. A derivative of cholesterol, called 7-dehydrocholesterol (7-DHC), is present in high concentrations in the epidermal layers of human skin, specifically the stratum basale and stratum spinosum.[1, 2] This is our raw material, the substrate waiting for its catalyst.

When full-spectrum sunlight, specifically ultraviolet B (UVB) radiation in the wavelength range of 290–315 nanometers, strikes the skin, these photons are absorbed by 7-DHC. The energy from a UVB photon cleaves a specific bond in the 7-DHC molecule, transforming it into a new, unstable compound known as pre-vitamin D3.[3] This initial step is purely photochemical; it requires light and nothing more.

What happens next is a subtle, yet important, temperature-dependent process. The pre-vitamin D3 formed in the epidermis slowly rearranges its molecular structure over several hours, converting into the stable form we know as vitamin D3, or cholecalciferol. This thermal transformation process uses the body's own heat, ensuring a slow, steady conversion.[4] This two-step process has an ingenious, built-in safety mechanism. If sun exposure is prolonged, the buildup of pre-vitamin D3 leads to its degradation into biologically inert byproducts like lumisterol and tachysterol, while existing vitamin D3 is also broken down. This feedback loop makes it impossible to generate toxic levels of vitamin D from sun exposure, a natural safeguard that oral supplementation does not possess.[5, 6] Nature, it seems, has already solved the problem of vitamin D overdose.

Once formed, vitamin D3 is released from the skin cells into the bloodstream, where it is primarily transported by the vitamin D–binding protein on its journey through the body.[7]

## PHARMACOKINETICS: THE JOURNEY AND TRANSFORMATION OF VITAMIN D

The vitamin D3 produced in the skin (or ingested) is not yet biologically active; it is a prohormone. Its activation is a two-step process. First, vitamin D–binding protein carries vitamin D3 to the liver. There, the enzyme 25-hydroxylase converts it to 25-hydroxyvitamin D [25(OH)D].[8, 9] This is the major circulating form of vitamin D and the metabolite that is measured in blood tests currently used to determine a person's vitamin D status. It has a relatively long half-life of about two to three weeks, making it an excellent biomarker of overall vitamin D availability.[10]

From the liver, 25(OH)D travels, again via vitamin D–binding protein, to the kidneys. Here, the enzyme 1-alpha-hydroxylase creates the biologically active hormone 1,25-dihydroxyvitamin D [1,25(OH)2D], also known as calcitriol.[11, 12] Calcitriol is the potent steroid hormone that interacts with the vitamin D receptor present in the nucleus of cells in virtually every tissue in the body, from bones and intestines to the brain and immune cells. This interaction regulates the expression of hundreds of genes, profoundly influencing calcium metabolism, immune function, cell proliferation, and much more.[13] It is important to note that while the kidneys are the primary site of calcitriol production for regulating blood calcium, many other tissues, including immune cells and muscle, can produce their own calcitriol from 25(OH)D for local, or "autocrine," use, highlighting its critical role in localized immune responses.[14]

## QUANTIFYING THE SUN'S BOUNTY AND THE BODY'S DEMAND

So, how much vitamin D can the skin actually make? The amounts are staggering when compared to official government recommendations embodied in US Recommended Dietary Allowances (RDA). Landmark research has demonstrated that exposing the full body of a light-skinned young adult to one minimal erythemal dose (MED) of sun—the amount that causes a slight pinkness of the skin twenty-four hours later—is equivalent to taking an oral dose of between 10,000 and 25,000 IU of vitamin D.[15] For a fair-skinned person in the midday summer sun, one MED might be achieved in just fifteen to twenty minutes. The body is designed to generate a massive amount of vitamin D in a very short period of time.

Now, let's compare this production capacity with the body's daily consumption rate. Groundbreaking work by leading vitamin D researchers like Bruce Hollis and Michael Holick has established that the human body catabolizes, or "uses," a significant amount of vitamin D each day to maintain its physiological functions. Studies on normal populations and those with high metabolic demands, such as pregnant and lactating women, indicate that the daily turnover is approximately 3,000 to 5,000 IU per day, a figure often averaged to about 4,000 IU per day to maintain stable blood levels.[16, 17] This is the baseline physiological demand that must be met, day in and day out, simply to keep the system running.

## THE INEVITABLE DECLINE: THE IMPACT OF AGING AND SKIN COLOR

Two key factors dramatically reduce the skin's ability to perform this vital function: age and skin pigmentation.

**Aging.** The decline in vitamin D synthesis with age is not a minor adjustment; it is a catastrophic drop. The primary reason is a sharp decrease in the concentration of the precursor molecule, 7-DHC, in the epidermis. By the age of seventy, an individual has only about 25 percent of the 7-DHC in their skin that a twenty-year-old does.[18] This means that a seventy-year-old exposed to the exact same amount of sunlight as a twenty-year-old will produce approximately 75 percent less vitamin D. This is a physiological certainty, a built-in feature of aging.[19]

**Skin Color.** Melanin, the pigment that determines skin color, is a highly effective natural sunblock. It absorbs the same UVB photons that are needed to initiate vitamin D synthesis. While this provides excellent protection against sun damage, it comes at a cost to vitamin D production. Individuals with darker skin pigmentation require significantly more sun exposure to produce the same amount of vitamin D as a fair-skinned person, with some studies suggesting the required increase in exposure time can be anywhere from three to five times longer, or even more.[20] This places dark-skinned individuals living in temperate latitudes at a uniquely high risk for profound vitamin D deficiency.

## WHY ARE WE SO VITAMIN D DEFICIENT?

Here we arrive at the heart of the matter. We have a built-in system designed to produce over 10,000 IU of vitamin D in minutes. We have a body that consumes at least 4,000 IU per day.[21] And we have a US RDA for most adults of 600 IU, and 800 IU for those over seventy.[22] These recommendations, first established in 2010, were reviewed and reaffirmed without change in 2024 by the National Academy of Medicine (a name change from Institute of Medicine but the same body), locking in these same figures despite a decade of mounting contradictory evidence. The disparity is not just large; it is nonsensical. How could the official recommendation be so profoundly out of sync with human physiology?

The answer is found in a shocking statistical error made by the Institute of Medicine (IOM), now perpetuated by the National Academy of Medicine (NAM), when they formulated their 2010 recommendations. An RDA is defined as the average daily intake level sufficient to meet the nutrient requirements of nearly all (97.5 percent) healthy individuals. However, as Paul Veugelers and John Paul Ekwaru pointed out in a blistering 2014 paper published in the peer-reviewed journal *Nutrients*, the IOM made a fundamental statistical mistake.[23] They intended to calculate the dose of vitamin D required to get 97.5 percent of the population above their target serum level of 20 ng/mL (50 nmol/L). Instead, they calculated the average requirement—the dose that would only bring 50 percent of the population to that level. Their own data, when analyzed correctly, showed that to achieve the stated goal for 97.5 percent of the population, a daily intake of at least 8,895 IU would be required.[24] The IOM's RDA of 600 IU was not just an underestimate; it was a blunder of epic proportions that guaranteed a majority of the population would remain deficient or insufficient by their own stated target.

This finding is independently corroborated by the work of the late Dr. Robert Heaney, who, in a sharp critique of the IOM report, found that for 97.5 percent of individuals to reach a serum 25(OH)D level of just 20 ng/mL, a daily intake of approximately 7,000 IU was necessary.[25] The scientific evidence is overwhelming and consistent.

Why has this glaring error, published in a peer-reviewed journal and confirmed by independent researchers, never been addressed or remedied by the IOM/NAM? One can only speculate, but several factors are likely at play. First, institutional inertia and the profound difficulty a prestigious body has in admitting a foundational error. Second, a pervasive and largely unfounded fear of vitamin D toxicity, a fear that ignores the body's own ability to safely generate and regulate massive amounts from the sun. Third, a historical focus on vitamin D's role in bone health (for which low doses prevent rickets) to the exclusion of its far more complex and dose-dependent role in immunity, cancer prevention, and cardiovascular health. It is far simpler to recommend a small, "safe" number than to grapple with the paradigm-shifting implications that optimal health requires intake levels ten times higher. And, finally, fourth, and most disturbing, it is not an error at all but a deliberate attempt to keep the population vitamin D deficient.

The disturbing scenario detailed above has been outdone by yet an even more nonsensical recommendation by The Endocrine Society to doctors: Do not routinely test vitamin D status in patients![26] This directive is based on a meta-analysis that found that vitamin D status was okey dokey in the population, so testing vitamin D status was not necessary. That's a first: a medical test that doctors are advised not to administer![27]

Here's what's happening. The flawed target of 20 ng/mL is creating an artificial target based on the IOM's flawed methodology. The target of 20 ng/mL is not just deficient, it is starvation-level deficiency, and basing advice on that number is fundamentally flawed. This bad information is being magnified throughout the medical community by the additional bad advice not to test for vitamin D status because it is presumed to be likely above starvation level. Of course, if a test is ordered by your doctor, insurance will usually pay for it. However, if your doctor is convinced by propaganda that the test is not necessary, then it must be paid for by you, if you insist on getting the test.

So what's worse? The systematic destruction of people's health by lulling them into a false sense of security by telling them starvation levels of vitamin D are healthy? Or, lying to them by saying that knowing how deficient they are through testing is not necessary? Together, the two approaches suggest a coordinated effort to keep people vitamin D deficient and prevent them from knowing the true extent of that deficiency.

## THE SUNSET OF LIFE: VITAMIN D DEFICIENCY AS A BUILT-IN DEATH MECHANISM

Let us now synthesize these facts into the sobering reality. Vitamin D is not a vitamin; it is a master steroid hormone essential for the proper functioning of the immune system.[28, 29] It is required for warding off infections, suppressing autoimmunity, and conducting surveillance against malignant cells. Our primary and most potent source of this hormone is the sun.

As we age, our ability to produce this critical hormone plummets by 75 percent or more.[30, 31] This is not a random occurrence; it is a programmed aspect of senescence. In an ancestral environment, this decline would be a significant liability, increasing susceptibility to the infectious diseases and cancers that are more common in old age. The biggest risk factor for most diseases is age. In the modern world, where we compound this biological decline with indoor lifestyles, sun avoidance, and tragically flawed public health recommendations, the situation becomes dire.

This age-related collapse in cutaneous vitamin D production, coupled with an inadequate intake, effectively cripples the immune system at the very time it is most needed. It is akin to a built-in obsolescence, a preprogrammed vulnerability that accelerates the decline of the organism. The decline in vitamin D synthesis is a harbinger of the sunset of life, a key mechanism through which an aging body loses its ability to defend itself. It is not an intentional "death switch" in a conspiratorial sense, but an evolutionary reality that we are now capable of understanding and, more importantly, correcting. To continue to recommend 800 IU per day to a seventy-year-old whose body uses at least 4,000 IU and whose skin can no longer effectively produce it, is not just a scientific failure—it is a public health tragedy. Get your vitamin D level checked, get in the sun, and supplement with vitamin D if necessary.

## MEASUREMENT UNITS FOR VITAMIN D

Vitamin D content in blood and pills is measured in the nanoscale range, this means very small as in a gram divided up into a billion equal parts. Vitamin D levels are typically measured in blood as serum 25-hydroxyvitamin D [25(OH) D], expressed in nanograms per milliliter (ng/mL) or nanomoles per liter (nmol/L). Vitamin D supplement amounts are expressed in one-millionth of a gram (micrograms, µg) or international units (IU).[32]

- ng/mL (nanograms per milliliter): Widely used in the United States and some clinical laboratories.
- nmol/L (nanomoles per liter): The SI (international) standard unit, used in Europe and global research settings.
- µg (micrograms): Refers to vitamin D dose rather than blood concentration, typically when describing dietary intake or supplement content.[33]

Throughout this book we'll refer to serum levels and dosage amounts of vitamin D. For the sake of consistency, we will convert and display all measurements for serum levels as ng/mL and all dosage amounts in IUs. There may be instances in your outside reading where you want to compare vitamin D studies that use different measures. Here is how to convert:

1 ng/mL = 2.5 nmol/L
1 nmol/L = 0.4 ng/mL

To interconvert:
From ng/mL to nmol/L:
nmol/L = ng/mL multiplied by 2.5, e.g. 50 ng/mL = 125 nmol/L (50 x 2.5 = 125)

From nmol/L to ng/mL:
ng/mL = nmol/L multiplied by 0.4, e.g. 125 nmol/L = 50 ng/mL (125 x 0.4 = 50)

Example serum level calculation:
A blood vitamin D level of 30 ng/mL equals 75 nmol/L, while 50 nmol/L corresponds to 20 ng/mL.

For supplement labeling:
1 µg vitamin D = 40 IU
So, for example, 25 µg = 1000 IU of vitamin D, 100 µg = 4000 IU of vitamin D and so on.

These relationships allow consistent comparison of vitamin D results and dosage across research, clinical, and public health contexts. Also, be aware that the use of IU in standard vitamin D supplement measurement appears to engage an interesting psychological perceptual phenomenon known as the illusion of magnitude or numerosity.[34] Generally speaking, when evaluating the difference between two attribute levels, more attention is paid to the number of units rather than the type of units. In our example, which seems greater, 100 µg or 4000 IU? As we'll discuss later, this ploy is used against the public as a scare tactic to maintain the status quo of vitamin D deficiency.

## CHAPTER 6

# THE SHIFTING SANDS OF SERUM VITAMIN D: POPULATION VALUES AND THE QUEST FOR OPTIMAL HEALTH

Understanding the true vitamin D status of a population is critical for public health, and the most reliable measure we have is the serum concentration of 25-hydroxyvitamin D [25(OH)D]. This chapter delves into the fascinating and concerning trends of 25(OH)D levels in the United States, tracing its historical trajectory, highlighting stark demographic disparities, and ultimately making the case for a significant reevaluation of current recommended daily allowances. It's important to note that serum 25(OH)D measurements are a relatively recent development, with widespread availability and understanding only emerging in the 1970s with the discovery of vitamin D metabolites. Therefore, our historical data is limited to the period following this scientific breakthrough.

## DECADES OF DATA: A LOOK AT US POPULATION TRENDS

The average serum 25(OH)D level in the United States has been a moving target, primarily tracked through the National Health and Nutrition Examination Surveys (NHANES). These surveys offer a decadal snapshot, revealing both concerning declines and more recent, albeit modest, increases. Let's examine the key periods:

- 1988–1994 (NHANES III) 30 ng/mL, range 28–32 by age/sex; higher than later years.[1]
- 2001–2004 24 ng/mL, Drop of ~6 ng/mL from prior decade; differences by age and sex nearly equalized.[2]
- 2001–2002 26.3 ng/mL.[3]
- 2017–2018 29.5 ng/mL. Significant increase among elderly and women; 20–39-yr group saw a decrease.[4]

## 1988-1994: A HIGHER BASELINE

During the NHANES III survey (1988–1994), the mean serum 25(OH)D level was 30 ng/mL. While this average appears respectable by some standards, it's important to acknowledge that there were already variations, with older adults averaging 28 ng/mL and younger individuals around 32 ng/mL.

A persistent and stark reality even then was the pronounced racial and ethnic disparities, with non-Hispanic Blacks exhibiting significantly lower average levels compared to non-Hispanic Whites.[5] This early data point serves as a critical benchmark, representing a period before the more dramatic declines observed in the subsequent decades.

## 2001-2004: THE ALARMING DECLINE

The turn of the millennium brought a concerning shift. By 2001–2004, overall serum 25(OH)D levels plummeted to an average of 24 ng/mL, representing a substantial 6 ng/mL drop from the previous decade. While differences in levels between age and sex groups largely disappeared during this period, the deeply entrenched ethnic disparities remained, an unsettling constant in the data. This decline was accompanied by a sharp rise in the prevalence of vitamin D insufficiency, impacting a majority of demographic groups across the nation. This period marked a low point, underscoring a widespread and worsening public health concern.

## 2001-2018: A MODEST REBOUND, WITH CAVEATS

Following the low point of the early 2000s, a modest upward trend in average serum 25(OH)D levels has been observed. Data from 2001–2002 showed an average of 26.3 ng/mL, which increased to 29.5 ng/mL by 2017–2018 for adults. However, a troubling countertrend emerged among young adults aged 20–39 years, who actually experienced a decrease in their serum vitamin D levels. For some low-income subgroups within this demographic, deficiency rates soared above 80 percent, highlighting persistent vulnerabilities despite the overall population increase.[6]

Summarizing these values across groups, it has been determined that 77 percent of the US population is deficient in serum vitamin D level with deficiency being defined as below 30 ng/mL.[7]

## DEMOGRAPHIC DISPARITIES: A PERSISTENT CHALLENGE

One undeniable and consistent finding throughout all these periods is the marked disparity in vitamin D levels among different racial and ethnic groups. Non-Hispanic Blacks consistently register lower serum 25(OH)D levels than other ethnic groups, with average serum levels of 16 ng/mL and estimates of 76 percent of the population severely deficient.[8] This persistent pattern demands a closer examination, moving beyond generalized population averages to understand the unique challenges faced by specific communities.

## BEYOND US AVERAGES: A COMPARISON OF BLACK AMERICANS AND EQUATORIAL BLACK AFRICANS

While examining US population trends provides valuable insights, it's equally important to consider how these levels compare internationally, especially when trying to understand the full impact of environmental and lifestyle factors on vitamin D status. A particularly insightful comparison involves Black Americans living in the United States and Black Africans living near the equator. This comparison of populations with similar skin pigmentation can help us isolate the effects of factors like sunlight exposure and urbanization, which may be masked when solely focusing on diverse populations within a single country.

The data reveals a stark contrast: Black Africans living near the equator typically exhibit significantly higher serum vitamin D levels than African Americans in the United States—often double or more.

Let's delve into the details of this comparison:

- African Americans (US) ~16 ng/mL. Urban lifestyle, high latitude, limited sun exposure, higher prevalence of deficiency.[9, 10, 11]
- Africans (Equatorial) 29–46 ng/mL. Rural/labor-intensive, high sun exposure; can reach 43–59 ng/mL in traditional groups.[12, 13]

## AFRICAN AMERICANS: A DEFICIT ROOTED IN ENVIRONMENT AND LIFESTYLE

For African Americans, average vitamin D levels hover around 16 ng/mL, with some studies reporting even lower figures.[14] This significantly lower average is a complex issue, primarily driven by a combination of factors:

- **Greater Skin Pigmentation:** Melanin, which provides protection from UV radiation, also reduces the skin's ability to synthesize vitamin D from sunlight.
- **Reduced Sunlight Exposure:** Urban living and residence at higher latitudes in the United States significantly limit the amount of effective sun exposure, especially during colder months. Modern indoor lifestyles further exacerbate this.
- **Lower Supplement Use and Fortified Food Intake:** Studies indicate that African Americans often have lower rates of vitamin D supplement use and consume fewer vitamin D–fortified foods, such as dairy products.

These factors contribute to a much higher prevalence of vitamin D deficiency among African Americans, often cited as 15 to 20 times greater than that observed in White Americans.[15]

## AFRICANS NEAR THE EQUATOR: THE POWER OF TRADITIONAL LIFESTYLES

In stark contrast, populations in equatorial Africa, such as the Maasai and Hadzabe, who often maintain traditional, labor-intensive, and outdoor lifestyles, routinely exhibit much higher serum 25(OH)D levels, typically ranging from 29 to 46 ng/mL. In some traditional groups with extensive sun exposure, these levels can even reach 43–59 ng/mL.[16] Even among urbanized equatorial Africans, average serum levels tend to be higher than those of African Americans, though not as high as their rural counterparts who experience constant sun exposure. Consequently, vitamin D deficiency is rarely reported in these populations, except among those who have adopted more urbanized, sun-avoiding cultural practices.

This direct comparison highlights two critical points:

- **Environmental Dominance:** Lifestyle and environmental factors, particularly sunlight exposure, play a profound role in determining vitamin D status, even for individuals with highly pigmented skin.
- **Beyond Measured Levels:** It's important to consider that lower measured 25(OH)D levels in African Americans may not always correlate directly with functional deficiency in the same way they do in other populations. Differences in vitamin D binding proteins and bioavailable vitamin D can influence how the body utilizes what it has.[17]

The dramatic difference in vitamin D levels between these two groups underscores the immense impact of latitude, sun exposure, and lifestyle on vitamin D status. It reveals a concerning deficit in vitamin D for many Black Americans, primarily due to factors related to modern living rather than an inherent biological inability to produce sufficient vitamin D.

## RETHINKING THE RDA: AIMING FOR OPTIMAL SERUM LEVELS

The preceding discussions on population vitamin D levels in the United States and the stark contrast with equatorial African populations lead to an inescapable conclusion: Current vitamin D recommendations are woefully inadequate for achieving optimal health outcomes for the vast majority of people, especially in a population that is advised to avoid sunlight. The current Recommended Dietary Allowance (RDA) for vitamin D, set by the Institute of Medicine (IOM, now the National Academy of Medicine or NAM) at 600 IU, is based on a foundational statistical error that effectively guaranteed widespread insufficiency.

As discussed in the previous chapter, the IOM's 2010 recommendations were meant to establish an average daily intake sufficient to meet the nutrient requirements of nearly all (97.5 percent) healthy individuals. However, a groundbreaking paper by Paul Veugelers and John Paul Ekwaru[18] exposed a critical flaw: The IOM calculated the average requirement—the dose that would only bring 50 percent of the population to their target serum level of 20 ng/mL (50 nmol/L)—instead of the dose needed for 97.5 percent of the population. When Veugelers and Ekwaru correctly reanalyzed the IOM's own data, they found that an intake of at least 8,895 IU per day was required to get 97.5 percent of the population above 20 ng/mL. This brings us to a critical question: If 8,895 IU per day is needed to get 97.5 percent of the population to merely 20 ng/mL, what daily intake is required to achieve genuinely optimal serum levels, generally considered to be between 60 and 80 ng/mL? While the precise dose to achieve this higher target for 97.5 percent of the population will vary based on individual factors like body weight, skin pigmentation, and sun exposure, we can estimate based on existing dose-response data.

Studies have consistently shown that higher daily intakes of vitamin D are required to significantly elevate serum 25(OH)D levels. For instance, research by Kimball et al. (2017)[19] demonstrated that daily intakes of up to 15,000 IU of vitamin D3 could lead to serum 25(OH)D concentrations up to 300 nmol/L (approximately 120 ng/mL) without adverse effects on calcium metabolism in a community setting. Given that 8,895 IU raises 97.5 percent of the population to 20 ng/mL, and knowing that there is a generally linear relationship between vitamin D intake and serum levels at these lower ranges, a significant increase in daily intake is clearly necessary to reach 60–80 ng/mL. To reach 60 ng/mL, which is three times the IOM's target of 20 ng/mL, it is reasonable to expect that the daily intake would need to be at least triple the 8,895 IU figure, perhaps even higher to account for individual variability and to ensure the 97.5 percent threshold.

This may seem like an extraordinarily high dose compared to current official recommendations, but it is important to reiterate two critical points:

1. **Safety of Higher Doses:** Numerous studies, including the aforementioned work by Kimball et al., have established the safety of long-term vitamin D3 intakes far exceeding the current RDA. Intakes of 10,000 IU/day and even up to 15,000 IU/day have been shown to be well-tolerated and without adverse effects on calcium metabolism in healthy individuals. True vitamin D toxicity (hypercalcemia) is

extremely rare and typically only occurs with much higher, often accidental, megadoses over prolonged periods, usually above 40,000 IU to 50,000 IU daily.[20]

2. **The Goal of Optimal Health:** The aim is not merely to avoid frank deficiency, but to achieve optimal vitamin D status that supports a wide array of physiological functions, from bone health and immune function to mood regulation and chronic disease prevention. This goal requires a fundamental shift in our understanding of what constitutes an adequate daily intake.

## THE VITAMIN D SAFETY VALVE: STORED VITAMIN D RESERVES

Vitamin D3 is classified as a fat-soluble vitamin, which means it dissolves in fats rather than water and is absorbed and transported in the body along with dietary fats.[21] Fat-soluble vitamins can be stored for extended periods in the body's tissues, unlike water-soluble vitamins, which are readily excreted if not used.[22]

Vitamin D3 is primarily stored in adipose tissue (body fat). Smaller amounts may also be stored in the liver, where it can be converted to its active form as needed. The stored form in adipose tissue serves as a reserve that can be gradually released and activated when the body requires it, helping maintain levels during periods of low dietary intake or reduced sunlight exposure.[23] The body uses circulating vitamin D first, but shifts to stored vitamin D in muscle and adipose tissue when circulating levels drop due to insufficient solar generation or dietary intake. The transition is regulated and not simply a passive process—the body relies on hormonal signals (especially parathyroid hormone, PTH) and nutrient status to control mobilization and activation of vitamin D reserves.[24]

## WHAT DETERMINES USAGE OF STORED VS. CIRCULATING VITAMIN D?

The body always first utilizes circulating vitamin D, primarily 25(OH)D, derived from recent skin synthesis (sunlight) and dietary intake. When circulating levels decline (for example, during winter or lack of UVB exposure), stored vitamin D is gradually released from adipose and muscle tissue into the blood, replenishing serum 25(OH)D.[25]

The body relies on circulating vitamin D when available, then taps into stored reserves during deficiency or low sunlight, regulated by hormonal signals and physiologic demand. Generally, once sun exposure becomes insufficient for cutaneously generated vitamin D (which happens in temperate climates during winter), the body starts relying on its stored vitamin D. These stores can last anywhere from a few weeks to a month for someone who is already deficient. This means that in the United States the vitamin D "winter" period, when the sun's angle is too low for effective vitamin D synthesis, generally occurs during from about October 15th to March 15th above the 37th parallel.[26] Those that are deficient going into the winter are essentially on empty by December 1st.

In conclusion, the current RDA for vitamin D is fundamentally flawed and inadequate. To genuinely achieve serum 25(OH)D levels between 60 and 80 ng/mL for 97.5 percent of the population—levels increasingly recognized as optimal for overall health—daily total vitamin D intakes in the range of 15,000 to 20,000 IU are likely necessary. We are not suggesting or advocating for that dramatic an increase in oral intake of daily vitamin D. However, the figure of 8895 IU calculated by Veugelers and Ekwaru is a starting point to the minimal 20 ng/mL level. While over-supplementation with extreme oral doses (50,000 IU/day) can lead to hypercalcemia and other issues, there is no such risk of overdosing on solar-generated vitamin D (have you ever seen a sickly-looking lifeguard?) Therefore, a reasonable plan would be to use both oral and solar-generated vitamin D to achieve an ideal and safe vitamin D serum level. For example, 5,000 to 10,000 IU vitamin D3 per day by mouth to achieve 20 ng/mL combined with sensible sun exposure should generate the aggregate 10,000–15,000 IU functional equivalent to reach the optimal 60–80 ng/mL status. It is important to involve your medical professional to monitor your progress, obtain vitamin D measurements and adjust your plan based on your own specific situation.

I personally take 10,000 IU vitamin D3 per day and get plenty of sunlight year-round. I have taken this amount for more than twenty years with nothing but exceptional health and wellness as a side effect. Recall that since I initially used vitamin D to eradicate my psoriasis, I adjusted and arrived at that amount to maintain clear skin. Your situation may be different.

This revised perspective, grounded in corrected statistical analysis and supported by safety data, is essential for truly addressing the widespread vitamin D insufficiency and deficiency that plagues modern populations.

# CHAPTER 7

# SUNLIGHT'S PROCREATIVE POWER: VITAMIN D, CATHELICIDIN, AND DEFENSINS—A TRIO FOR FERTILITY

The profound and often underappreciated influence of sunlight on human health extends far beyond bone metabolism. Our solar benefactor orchestrates an intricate and powerful system to support human reproduction, a system built upon a triumvirate of key biological actors: the steroid hormone vitamin D and two families of antimicrobial peptides (AMPs) it commands, cathelicidins and defensins.

This chapter will explain how these three sun-dependent components work in synergy, acting as master regulators, versatile defenders, and epithelial guardians of fertility. We will show that vitamin D is not merely a "vitamin" but a fundamental steroid hormone with direct, receptor-mediated actions across the entire reproductive axis in both men and women. We will explore how vitamin D directs the synthesis of cathelicidin and defensins in key reproductive tissues, deploying them as sentinels against infection and modulators of the delicate immune balance required for successful conception and pregnancy.[1, 2]

## VITAMIN D—THE MASTER REGULATOR OF REPRODUCTIVE FITNESS

Before examining its role as a commander of antimicrobial peptides, it is important to understand Vitamin D's direct and profound influence on the machinery of reproduction. Far from being a passive nutrient, the active form of Vitamin D, 1,25-dihydroxyvitamin D3, 1,25$(OH)_2$D, functions as a potent steroid hormone that modulates gene expression. As we've learned, it achieves this by binding to the vitamin D receptor (VDR), a nuclear receptor found in the cells of virtually every major organ, including those of the male and female reproductive systems.[3] The strategic expression of VDR and the enzymes that activate vitamin D throughout the reproductive tract is definitive evidence of its integral role.

## VITAMIN D IN MALE FERTILITY

The male reproductive system is a key target for vitamin D action. VDRs are densely expressed in the testes, specifically in the Sertoli cells (which nurture developing sperm), Leydig cells (which produce testosterone), and even on mature spermatozoa themselves.[4, 5]

This widespread presence translates into direct physiological effects:

- **Hormone Regulation:** Vitamin D is positively correlated with total testosterone levels in men. By regulating the expression of genes involved in steroid synthesis, it plays a role in maintaining the androgenic environment essential for robust spermatogenesis.
- **Spermatogenesis and Sperm Quality:** Studies have consistently demonstrated a strong association between sufficient Vitamin D status and superior sperm quality. Men with adequate Vitamin D levels exhibit significantly better sperm motility, morphology (normal shape), and higher total sperm counts compared to their deficient counterparts.[6] Vitamin D also influences calcium signaling within sperm, which is critical for motility and the reaction required to fertilize an egg.

## VITAMIN D IN FEMALE FERTILITY

In the female reproductive system, vitamin D acts as a master regulator of ovarian function, uterine receptivity, and pregnancy maintenance. VDR is expressed in the ovaries, uterus (endometrium), fallopian tubes, and placenta, signaling its involvement at every stage.[7, 8]

- **Ovarian Function and Follicle Development:** Vitamin D modulates the production of progesterone, estradiol, and estrone in the ovaries. It also regulates anti-Müllerian hormone gene expression, a key marker of ovarian reserve. In conditions like polycystic ovary syndrome (PCOS), a leading cause of infertility, vitamin D deficiency is highly prevalent and is linked to worsened metabolic and hormonal profiles. Supplementation has been shown to improve follicular development and menstrual regularity in some women with PCOS.[9]
- **Endometrial Receptivity and Implantation:** For an embryo to successfully implant, the uterine lining (endometrium) must become "receptive." Vitamin D plays an important role in this process by regulating the expression of key implantation genes, such as HOXA10, within the endometrium. An adequate vitamin D level helps create the optimal immunological and structural environment for the embryo to attach and thrive. Studies of women undergoing in vitro fertilization

(IVF) have found that those with sufficient vitamin D levels have significantly higher rates of becoming pregnant compared to women who are deficient.[10]

- **Pregnancy Outcomes:** Maternal vitamin D status is a powerful predictor of pregnancy success. Deficiency is strongly linked to an increased risk of major pregnancy complications, including preeclampsia (a dangerous hypertensive disorder), gestational diabetes, and bacterial vaginosis, all of which threaten both mother and child.[11] Most significantly, low vitamin D is a major risk factor for preterm birth, the leading cause of infant mortality.

Altogether, this evidence unequivocally establishes vitamin D as a frontline hormone in reproductive health. Its deficiency directly compromises the core biological processes of fertility, independent of its role in immunity.

## CATHELICIDIN—THE VERSATILE DEFENDER OF REPRODUCTIVE SUCCESS

With vitamin D established as the master regulator, we now turn to the sentinels it commands. The human cathelicidin peptide, LL-37, was first recognized for its potent antimicrobial properties against bacteria, viruses, and fungi.[12, 13] The gene for cathelicidin contains a vitamin D response element (VDRE), meaning its production is initiated by the active form of vitamin D. This directly links sunlight exposure to the production of a key defender in the reproductive tract. Its role, however, extends far beyond simply killing microbes; it is a critical modulator of the reproductive environment.[14]

## STRATEGIC DEPLOYMENT: CATHELICIDIN'S PRESENCE IN THE REPRODUCTIVE ARENA

Nature has strategically positioned cathelicidin at the most critical junctures within both male and female reproductive systems, underscoring its integral role in the choreography of conception and gestation.

**The Male Reproductive Tract:** Cathelicidin is robustly expressed in the testes (Sertoli and Leydig cells) and epididymis, providing an antimicrobial shield that protects sperm production and maturation from infection. Furthermore, LL-37 is a significant component of seminal plasma, where it protects sperm from vaginal microbes during their journey.[15, 16]

**The Female Reproductive Tract:** The ovaries, fallopian tubes, and especially the uterine endometrium exhibit dynamic, hormonally regulated expression of cathelicidin.[17] As primary barrier sites, the cervix and vagina are also major producers, creating a formidable, sun-influenced chemical shield against pathogens.[18] During pregnancy, the placenta and amniotic fluid become rich sources of cathelicidin, which is absolutely critical for shielding the fetus from intrauterine infections.[19]

## CATHELICIDIN'S MULTIFACETED IMPACT ON REPRODUCTION

- **Antimicrobial Defense:** This is its most obvious role. By defending against pathogens that cause conditions like epididymitis or pelvic inflammatory disease, cathelicidin directly prevents infection-related infertility.[20]
- **Optimizing Sperm Function:** Research suggests cathelicidin may directly influence sperm motility and viability, prerequisites for male fertility.[21]
- **Orchestrating Implantation:** Successful implantation requires a precisely tuned local immune environment. Cathelicidin helps modulate this environment, fostering tolerance toward the semi-allogeneic (immunologically foreign/semi-not-of-the-self) embryo while maintaining defense against infection.[22]
- **Maintaining Maternal-Fetal Tolerance:** Pregnancy is a unique immunological state. Placental cathelicidin is a key contributor to maternal-fetal tolerance, helping to prevent the mother's immune system from rejecting the fetus.[23]

## DEFENSINS—THE EPITHELIAL GUARDIANS OF REPRODUCTIVE INTEGRITY

Complementing cathelicidin, the defensins are another formidable family of sun-influenced antimicrobial peptides. Discovered in the mid-1980s,[24] these peptides are potent microbial killers.[25] The epithelial-derived beta-defensins (hBDs) are of particular relevance to reproduction, and like cathelicidin, the gene for a key defensin, hBD-2, is also directly induced by vitamin D.[26, 27]

## STRATEGIC FORTIFICATIONS: DEFENSINS IN THE REPRODUCTIVE TRACTS

**The Male Reproductive Fortress:** Beta-defensins are abundantly expressed in the epididymis, protecting maturing sperm.[28] Specific defensins, such as DEFB126, coat the sperm, playing a non-antimicrobial role in motility and the ability to penetrate cervical mucus.[29]

**The Female Reproductive Citadel:** The vagina and cervix are major sites of beta-defensin production, creating an effective barrier against sexually transmitted pathogens.[30] The uterus, fallopian tubes, and placenta also express defensins, contributing to the antimicrobial shield that protects the embryo and fetus.[31, 32, 33, 34]

## DEFENSINS AT WORK: ROLES IN FERTILITY AND FECUNDITY

- **Guardian of Gametes and Tract:** By creating an antimicrobial shield, defensins protect sperm, oocytes, and the developing embryo from pathogens, thereby directly safeguarding fertility.[35, 36]
- **Enhancing Sperm Function:** Beyond protection, certain defensins are essential for sperm maturation and function. Defects in the DEFB126 gene, for example, are a known cause of male infertility in some populations.[37]
- **Modulating Implantation:** Similar to cathelicidins, defensins contribute to the finely balanced immune environment in the endometrium that is required for successful embryo implantation.[38]

## THE RHYTHM OF LIFE: HOW SUNLIGHT AND VITAMIN D DRIVE SEASONAL FERTILITY

For centuries, it has been known that human life has a rhythm that follows the seasons. In locations with distinct summers and winters, like North America and Europe, birth rates have consistently peaked in the spring and early summer. This is not a coincidence. A spring birth peak means that conceptions—the very beginning of life—were most likely to happen in the late summer and early autumn months.[39] In the past, experts credited this pattern to social factors like holiday schedules or environmental triggers like temperature. But a far more powerful and precise explanation has come into focus. The evidence is now clear that vitamin D, the "sunshine vitamin," acts as a master conductor of this seasonal fertility. It works largely by fine-tuning the immune system of the reproductive tract, ensuring the body is perfectly prepared to begin a pregnancy.

## THE ANCIENT PATTERN OF HUMAN REPRODUCTION

The seasonal spike in conceptions is a remarkably stable phenomenon, observed in diverse cultures and across different eras. Even in our modern, climate-controlled world, the pattern holds, which tells us that a powerful biological force is at work.[40] The most logical candidate for a biological signal that perfectly tracks the seasons is vitamin D. Our bodies produce vitamin D when our skin is exposed to the sun's ultraviolet B (UVB) rays. This means our vitamin D levels naturally rise throughout the sunny months and hit their annual peak in late summer—precisely when conception rates have historically begun to climb.[41]

This timing is too perfect to ignore. The deep connection between sunlight, vitamin D, and fertility is so strong that we can start to see its effects fade as our lifestyles change. A landmark study from Spain provides a stunning historical record of this shift. Researchers analyzed an incredible 33 million births over sixty years, from 1941 to 2000.[42] Their findings were profound. In the earlier decades, they saw the classic, predictable peak in births every spring, which resulted from conceptions the previous summer. But as the decades passed, the pattern began to fade. By the year 2000, the sharp seasonal peak had flattened into a barely noticeable wave. The researchers concluded that modern life—with its urbanization, indoor jobs, artificial light, and air-conditioning—had insulated us from the environmental signals that once governed our biology.

This "blunting" of our natural reproductive rhythm also runs parallel to the modern epidemic of vitamin D deficiency. As we have moved our lives indoors, vilified the sun, and adopted near universal sunscreen use, we have severed our primary connection to the sun, the source of over 90 percent of our vitamin D.[43] The disappearance of the summer conception peak is powerful, large-scale evidence of how our modern environment has altered our fundamental reproductive biology.

## THE TRIPLE-EDGED SWORD: HOW SUN AVOIDANCE CRIPPLES FERTILITY

The central idea of this chapter is that widespread sun avoidance inflicts a devastating triple assault on human reproductive potential by systematically dismantling the sun-dependent fertility mechanisms.

- First, sun deprivation starves the body of vitamin D, the master hormonal regulator. As detailed earlier, this deficiency directly compromises gonadal steroid hormone production, impairs spermatogenesis, disrupts ovarian function, and renders the uterus less receptive to implantation.
- Second, this same vitamin D deficiency disarms our reproductive tissues of cathelicidin. Chronically low levels of this peptide leave the male and female tracts vulnerable to fertility-damaging infections, compromise the immune modulation necessary for implantation, and weaken the placental barrier, increasing the risk of preterm birth.
- Third, the lack of vitamin D simultaneously suppresses the production of epithelial beta-defensins. This further degrades the antimicrobial shield of the reproductive mucosa, impairs sperm function, and contributes to an immunological environment hostile to pregnancy.

The epidemiological data aligns with this biological data. Developed, wealthier nations—precisely those where sun avoidance and sunscreen use are most deeply ingrained—are experiencing a precipitous fertility decline.[44] To attribute this solely to socioeconomic factors is to ignore the profound biological consequences of chronically suppressing an entire physiological system dependent on the sun and vitamin D that is essential for reproduction.

While oral vitamin D supplementation is beneficial and often necessary, it cannot fully replicate the intricate, localized, and systemic benefits conferred by sunlight. Cutaneous sunlight exposure remains the evolutionarily ordained and most comprehensive method to co-stimulate vitamin D hormone synthesis and the localized production of its antimicrobial peptide agents. Reclaiming sensible sun exposure is not about reckless tanning; it is about restoring a fundamental biological prerequisite for the continuation of our species—the sun-forged power to procreate. The ancient rhythm of human life is not a myth. It is a biological reality orchestrated by the sun. By ensuring our bodies have optimal levels of vitamin D, we are not just supporting our bones or general health; we are reconnecting with a fundamental cycle that has guided human reproduction for millennia.

# CHAPTER 8

# THE SUN'S EMBRACE: SUNLIGHT, LIBIDO, AND THE FORGOTTEN APHRODISIAC

Continuing with the theme of the previous chapter regarding effects of sun avoidance on fertility, another factor influencing fertility is frequency. In our sun-starved existence, maybe we're just not having enough sex? Successful procreation requires many things to operate correctly all at once, in addition to the mechanisms that affect fertility and fertilization. The insane avoidance of the sun has even more insidious effects as sunlight also affects mood, sexual performance, and libido in both subtle and dramatic ways. Living a virtually sun-free life has unintended consequences of generally less feelings of well-being, lower libido, and likely less satisfying and rewarding sexual experiences.

While the implications for vitamin D synthesis and its downstream effects on immunity and chronic disease are profound, this chapter will show that the consequences of our collective sun-shunning extend even further, into the deeply personal and fundamental realm of human sexual desire, behavior, and, ultimately, reproductive success. We will show that sunlight, far from being solely a source of a vital vitamin, acts as a potent, albeit largely unrecognized, natural aphrodisiac, influencing mood, hormonal balance, and overall well-being in ways that directly impact libido and sexual activity. The current fertility crisis plaguing many developed, sun-avoidant nations may not only be a consequence of compromised physiological fertility due to chronic sunlight deficiency but also, in part, a reflection of diminished sexual desire and frequency, as another casualty of our estrangement from the sun. It is time to boldly reexamine sunlight's role, not just as a biological necessity, but as an essential spark for human connection and procreation.

## A HISTORICAL GLOW: SUNLIGHT, VITALITY, AND ANCIENT UNDERSTANDINGS OF VIRILITY

Throughout human history, across diverse cultures, the sun has been revered as a symbol of life, vitality, and power. While ancient civilizations may not have understood the precise biochemical pathways, they intuitively recognized the life-sustaining and invigorating properties of sunlight. This reverence often extended to notions of fertility and virility.

**Ancient Deities and Solar Potency:** Many ancient cultures worshipped sun gods and goddesses who were often associated with fertility, creation, and life force. Think of Ra in ancient Egypt, Apollo in Greek mythology, and Inti in Incan culture. These deities embodied the sun's power to nurture growth and ensure abundance, themes intrinsically linked to procreation.[1]

**Folk Wisdom and Seasonal Rhythms:** Traditional societies often observed seasonal patterns in both animal and human behavior, including mating and birth rates, which often correlated with periods of increased sunlight. Spring, with its lengthening days and returning warmth, has long been associated with renewal, romance, and heightened vitality—a time when life, in all its forms, seems to reawaken. This intuitive understanding, though not "scientific" in the modern sense, reflected an underlying biological reality.

**Literary and Artistic Echoes:** Literature and art throughout the ages have frequently used sunlight as a metaphor for passion, desire, and life's vibrant energy. From the sun-drenched landscapes of Renaissance paintings to the fervent poetry of Romantic writers, sunlight has often been depicted as an elemental force that stirs the senses and ignites the spirit. Consider D. H. Lawrence's evocative, sun-infused prose in works like *Lady Chatterley's Lover*, in which nature and sunlight are almost characters themselves, fueling passion and a return to primal instincts.[2] While metaphorical, these artistic expressions tap into a deep-seated human association between sunlight and vitality, including sexual vitality.

While these historical and cultural associations do not constitute scientific proof, they provide a compelling backdrop, suggesting a long-held, intuitive understanding of sunlight's profound influence on human energy, mood, and by extension, sexual desire.

## THE SUN'S BIOLOGICAL CARESS: MECHANISMS INFLUENCING SEXUAL DESIRE AND BEHAVIOR

Modern science is now beginning to unravel the specific biological pathways through which sunlight exposure can directly and indirectly influence sexual desire and behavior. The effects are not singular but rather a complex interplay of hormonal and neurochemical responses.

**Testosterone:** Vitamin D plays an important role in male reproductive health, and studies have shown a positive correlation between vitamin D levels and testosterone levels in men.[3] Testosterone is the primary male sex hormone, essential for libido, sexual function, and sperm production. Sunlight exposure, by boosting vitamin D, can therefore indirectly support healthy testosterone levels.[4]

**Estrogen and Progesterone:** In women, vitamin D receptors are present in the ovaries and uterus, suggesting a role in ovarian function and the regulation of female sex hormones like estrogen and progesterone. Balanced hormonal profiles are critical for female libido and reproductive health.

**Serotonin and Mood Enhancement:** Sunlight exposure is known to increase the production of serotonin, a neurotransmitter often referred to as the "feel-good" hormone.[5] Serotonin plays a significant role in regulating mood, reducing anxiety, and promoting feelings of well-being. A positive mood and reduced stress are undeniably conducive to healthy sexual desire and intimacy. The gloom of sun-deprived winters, often associated with seasonal affective disorder (SAD) and lowered mood, frequently correlates with a dip in libido for many individuals.

**Oxytocin, Orgasms, and Warm Fuzzies:** Oxytocin is commonly known as the cuddling hormone but it has much more racy effects as well. The "big O" could stand for oxytocin since there is a surge of oxytocin during orgasm and ejaculation that precedes the warm afterglow and urge to cuddle afterwards. Proper oxytocin levels are highly dependent on vitamin D.[6]

**Melatonin Regulation and Circadian Rhythms:** Sunlight helps to regulate the production of melatonin, the hormone that governs our sleep-wake cycles.[7] Proper melatonin regulation and healthy circadian rhythms are essential for overall energy levels, mood stability, and hormonal balance, all of which can impact sexual desire. Disruptions in sleep and circadian rhythms, often exacerbated by insufficient daytime sun exposure, can negatively affect libido.

**Endorphins and Pleasure:** Exposure to UV radiation from sunlight can also stimulate the release of β-endorphins, natural opioid peptides that can induce feelings of pleasure and well-being.[8] The mood-enhancing effects of endorphins certainly contribute to a more positive disposition toward sexual activity.

**Nitric Oxide and Vascular Health:** Sunlight exposure, particularly UVA radiation, can stimulate the release of nitric oxide (NO) from skin stores into the bloodstream.[9] Nitric oxide is a potent vasodilator, meaning it relaxes and widens blood vessels, improving circulation. Healthy blood flow is required for sexual arousal and function in both men (erectile function) and women (clitoral and vaginal engorgement). Vitamin D–deficient men are more likely to experience erectile dysfunction while vitamin D supplementation can sometimes correct it.[10] While this effect is often discussed in the context of cardiovascular health, its implications for sexual physiology are direct and significant.

**General Well-Being and Energy Levels:** Beyond specific hormones and neurotransmitters, adequate sun exposure contributes to a general sense of vitality, increased energy levels, and reduced fatigue. When individuals feel physically and mentally well, their interest in and capacity for sexual activity is naturally enhanced. Chronic sun deprivation, leading to vitamin D deficiency and disrupted circadian rhythms, can create a state of lethargy and malaise that is antithetical to a healthy libido.

It is not one single mechanism, but rather this symphony of hormonal, neurochemical, and physiological responses triggered by sunlight that collectively contributes to its aphrodisiac qualities. Sunlight is not just "good for you"; it actively primes the body and mind for connection and intimacy.

## THE SHADOW OF SUN AVOIDANCE: DAMPENING DESIRE IN DEVELOPED NATIONS

If sunlight is indeed a natural stimulant of sexual desire and function, then the widespread sun avoidance practices and the obsessive use of sunscreens that have characterized developed nations since the 1970s must have had a discernible impact on sexual behavior and, consequently, on fertility rates. The public health campaigns of that era extending into today, driven by the fear of melanoma, effectively demonized the sun, leading to a significant reduction in natural UVB exposure for vast segments of the population.[11]

## EPIDEMIOLOGICAL EVIDENCE OF CHANGING SEXUAL BEHAVIOR

**Declining Frequency of Intercourse:** Numerous sociological and health surveys in developed countries have reported a trend toward declining frequency of sexual intercourse, particularly among younger generations, over the past few decades.[12] While multiple factors contribute to this trend (e.g., stress, economic pressures, digital distractions), the potential role of widespread vitamin D deficiency and chronically suppressed sun-dependent neurochemical pathways cannot be ignored.

**Rising Reports of Low Libido:** Clinical reports and surveys also indicate an increasing prevalence of low libido or hypoactive sexual desire disorder (HSDD) in both men and women in these same sun-shunning societies.[13]

## THE FERTILITY CRISIS CORRELATION

As discussed in the previous chapter, developed, sun-avoidant nations are facing a significant fertility crisis, with plummeting birth rates.[14] While compromised physiological fertility (sperm quality, ovulation issues, etc.) due to lack of cathelicidin and direct vitamin D effects is a major factor, an often-unrecognized contributor to lower birth rates is simply a lower rate of intercourse. If desire is diminished, opportunities for conception naturally decrease. It is a fundamental, yet often overlooked, part of the fertility equation.

## SUN-DRENCHED NATIONS: A CONTRAST IN FECUNDITY AND (POTENTIALLY) DESIRE

Contrast this with many sun-drenched, often poorer, nations. While detailed comparative data on sexual desire across such diverse cultures is complex and often lacking, these populations generally exhibit significantly higher fertility rates.[15] It is a reasonable and scientifically plausible hypothesis that consistent, lifelong exposure to abundant sunlight contributes not only to better physiological fertility (via vitamin D and cathelicidin impacting gametes and reproductive tracts) but also to a more robust baseline of sexual desire due to optimized hormonal and neurochemical environments. The "rampant fecundity" observed is likely a confluence of cultural factors, socioeconomic realities, and fundamental biological drivers enhanced by an abundance of sunlight.

## SUNLIGHT—THE NEGLECTED APHRODISIAC ESSENTIAL FOR LIBIDO, BEHAVIOR, AND PROCREATION

The central thesis of this chapter is bold and unequivocal: The avoidance of the sun, a cornerstone of modern health advice in developed nations, affects far more than cutaneously synthesized vitamin D and cathelicidin. It directly and consequentially undermines multiple biological pathways essential for healthy sexual desire, behavior, and ultimately, fecundity and fertility. Solar-generated vitamin D and other sun-induced biological products and processes act as direct or indirect aphrodisiacs, influencing mood, hormonal balance, energy levels, and vascular health in ways that are fundamental to human libido and sexual function. In a world currently grappling with a widespread fertility crisis, particularly in sun-shunning wealthy countries, disabling the effectiveness of this natural, evolutionarily ancient stimulant by systematically avoiding the sun is not merely unhelpful; it is profoundly maladaptive.

There is currently no pill or pharmaceutical intervention that can holistically and safely replicate the complex cascade of beneficial physiological responses triggered by full-spectrum sunlight exposure—from vitamin D and cathelicidin synthesis to serotonin and endorphin release, and nitric oxide production, plus likely many other substances yet to be discovered. These are interconnected systems that have evolved to respond to the natural stimulus of the sun.

## REIGNITING THE SPARK: PRACTICAL STRATEGIES TO ENHANCE SEXUAL DESIRE THROUGH SENSIBLE SUN EXPOSURE

If sun deprivation is indeed a contributing factor to diminished libido and the current fertility crisis, then a logical and empowering step is to consciously and sensibly reintroduce full-spectrum sunlight into our lives. This is not a call for a return to reckless tanning but for an intelligent embrace of our biological need for the sun.

## SENSIBLE FULL-SPECTRUM SUN EXPOSURE

**Aim for Non-Burning Exposure:** The goal is to achieve sufficient UVB exposure to stimulate vitamin D and related pathways without causing sunburn. Short, regular exposures (e.g., 10–30 minutes, depending on skin type, time of day, season, and latitude) to a significant portion of the skin (arms, legs, torso) are more effective and safer than infrequent, prolonged exposures.

**Midday Sun for Efficiency:** UVB rays, responsible for vitamin D synthesis, are most intense during midday hours (roughly 10 a.m. to 3 p.m.). While caution is needed to avoid burning, short exposures during this window can be highly efficient.

**Gradual Acclimatization:** For individuals unaccustomed to sun exposure, it's wise to start slowly and gradually increase exposure time to allow the skin to adapt and build a natural tolerance (mild, non-burning tanning is a sign of this adaptation).

**Listen to Your Body:** Pay attention to your skin's response. If you feel any signs of burning, seek shade or cover up.

## THE ACT OF SUN EXPOSURE ITSELF: AN APHRODISIAC?

Beyond the biochemical effects, the very act of engaging in nearly full-body sun exposure can, for many healthy individuals, be an inherently pleasurable and even aphrodisiac experience. The warmth of the sun on the skin, the connection with nature, the sense of freedom and relaxation—these can all contribute to a positive mood, reduced stress, and an enhanced sense of well-being that is conducive to intimacy. This is an often-underestimated psychological and sensory component of sunlight's benefits.[16]

Feeling more attractive and confident due to a healthy, sun-kissed glow (not a deep tan from overexposure) can also positively impact libido and sexual self-esteem for some individuals.[17] Plus, who doesn't love tan lines?

## RECLAIMING THE SUN'S VITAL EMBRACE FOR DESIRE AND PROCREATION

The modern world has, in its quest to mitigate one risk (skin cancer), inadvertently created a host of others by fostering an unnatural and biologically detrimental fear of the sun. The evidence strongly suggests that this sun-shunning has far-reaching consequences, extending beyond vitamin D deficiency to impact our innate antimicrobial defenses (cathelicidin) and our fundamental sexual desire and reproductive capacity.

Solar-generated vitamin D and the cascade of other beneficial biological processes stimulated by sunlight are not mere luxuries; they are integral to our hormonal balance, mood regulation, and overall vitality—all critical components of a healthy libido and successful procreation. To disable these natural mechanisms by systematically avoiding the sun is to fight against our own evolutionary heritage and to contribute to the very fertility crisis we are now facing.

There is no pharmaceutical quick fix that can replicate the holistic benefits of sensible, full-spectrum sunlight. Reengaging with the sun intelligently and respectfully is not just a path to better physical health; it is a path to rediscovering a natural, potent aphrodisiac that can reignite desire, enhance intimacy, and support the fundamental human drive to procreate. It is time to step out of the shadows and reclaim the sun's vital embrace, not just for our bones and our immunity, but for the spark of life itself.

## CHAPTER 9

# THE SUN'S COMMAND: VITAMIN D AS THE MASTER REGULATOR OF IMMUNITY AND INFLAMMATION

The human immune system is a marvel of biological engineering, a complex and dynamic network of cells, tissues, and molecules designed to defend us against a relentless barrage of pathogens and to maintain internal order by eliminating damaged or cancerous cells. For too long, the prevailing understanding of immunity has focused primarily on pathogen recognition and effector responses, often overlooking the profound regulatory influences that govern its delicate balance. This chapter will show that vitamin D, the "sunshine hormone" synthesized in our skin, is not merely a supportive nutrient for immunity but a master regulator, a signaling molecule that orchestrates both the innate and adaptive components of our immune defenses. We will explore in detail how vitamin D directly and indirectly commands a vast array of immune cells and processes, ensuring appropriate activation, preventing excessive inflammation, and maintaining the critical equilibrium between robust defense and self-tolerance.

The widespread vitamin D deficiency that plagues modern, sun-shunning societies, a direct consequence of shortsighted public health guidance, has unequivocally crippled this master regulatory system, leaving populations vulnerable to a spectrum of immune dysfunctions, from heightened susceptibility to infections to the escalating crisis of chronic inflammation, autoimmune disease, cancer, and avoidable diseases of aging. Understanding vitamin D's reign over the immune system is paramount to reclaiming our health.

## THE TWO ARMS OF DEFENSE: INNATE AND ADAPTIVE IMMUNITY UNVEILED

Before delving into vitamin D's regulatory prowess, it is essential to distinguish between the two fundamental branches of our immune system: innate immunity and adaptive immunity. These two systems, while distinct in their mechanisms and timing, work in intricate coordination to provide comprehensive protection against disease causing pathogens.

## INNATE IMMUNITY

**The First Responders:** The innate immune system is our ancient, hard-wired, first line of defense. It is characterized by its rapid, nonspecific response to invading pathogens or tissue damage.[1]

Key players in innate immunity include:

- **Physical Barriers:** The skin and mucous membranes (both rich in vitamin D–dependent antimicrobial peptides), and the acidic environment of the stomach provide initial physical and chemical barriers against microbial entry.
- **Phagocytic Cells:** Macrophages, neutrophils, and dendritic cells are "eating cells" that engulf and destroy invading microbes and cellular debris. They recognize broad patterns associated with pathogens (pathogen-associated molecular patterns or PAMPs) via pattern recognition receptors like toll-like receptors (TLRs).[2]
- **Natural Killer (NK) Cells:** These cells are specialized in recognizing and killing virus-infected cells and certain tumor cells without prior sensitization.
- **Antimicrobial Peptides:** Molecules like defensins and cathelicidins (like LL-37 in humans), are directly toxic to a wide range of microbes, acting as the body's own natural antibiotic defense shield.[3]

**The Complement System:** A cascade of plasma proteins that, when activated, can directly kill pathogens, enhance phagocytosis, and promote inflammation. Inflammation is the hallmark of the innate response, characterized by redness, swelling, heat, and pain, which serves to recruit immune cells to the site of infection or injury and to contain the threat. While essential acutely, chronic inflammation is detrimental over the long term.

The innate immune system provides immediate defense, buying time for the more specialized adaptive immune response to develop. It is a system of rapid recognition and immediate action of outside threats in the form of bacteria, viruses, some parasites, and fungi.

## ADAPTIVE IMMUNITY

**The Specialized Forces:** The adaptive (or acquired) immune system is a more sophisticated and highly specific defense mechanism that develops over days to weeks following initial exposure to a pathogen or antigen (a molecule that can trigger an immune response). Its key characteristics are specificity, memory, and the ability to distinguish self from nonself.[4]

The adaptive immune system relies on several specialized cells that work together to identify and destroy specific threats. Here are the main players:

Lymphocytes are a type of white blood cell that do most of the heavy lifting in the adaptive immune response. There are two main types: B cells and T cells:

- **B Lymphocytes (B Cells):** B cells are responsible for making antibodies—proteins that act like a "wanted poster" system for the immune system. Antibodies latch onto specific germs or foreign substances (called antigens), which either neutralizes them directly or flags them for destruction by other immune cells. When a B cell encounters a threat, it can transform into two important cell types: plasma cells, which are essentially antibody factories churning out large amounts of antibodies, and memory B cells, which stick around long after the infection is gone and allow your body to respond faster if the same threat shows up again. This is the basis of long-term immunity.[5]
- **T Lymphocytes (T Cells):** T cells are a more diverse group that mature in an organ called the thymus (that's where the "T" comes from). They take on several different roles depending on their type.

  **Helper T Cells (CD4+ T Cells):** Helper T cells act like conductors of an orchestra, coordinating the overall immune response. They read signals from other immune cells and then direct different parts of the immune system to respond appropriately—for example, calling for more antibody production or signaling other cells to hunt down infected cells inside the body.[6]

  **Cytotoxic T Cells (CD8+ T Cells):** Cytotoxic T cells are the immune system's assassins. They scan the body for cells that have been infected by viruses, parasites or that have turned cancerous. Once they find a target, they kill it directly—either by punching holes in the cell's outer membrane or by triggering a self-destruct sequence inside the target cell (a process called programmed cell death).[7]

  **Regulatory T Cells (Tregs):** Regulatory T cells act as the immune system's referees. Their job is to keep everything in check and prevent the immune system from overreacting or mistakenly attacking the body's own healthy tissue. Without them, the immune system could cause serious damage to the body itself—which is what happens in autoimmune diseases.[8]
- **Antigen-Presenting Cells (The Scouts):** Before T cells can respond to a threat, they need to be shown what to look for. That's the job of

antigen-presenting cells, which include dendritic cells, macrophages, and B cells. These cells capture germs or foreign particles, break them down, and then display pieces of them (the antigens) on their surface—almost like holding up a "most wanted" flyer for T cells to examine. Dendritic cells are considered the best at this job, particularly when it comes to activating T cells that have never encountered a threat before.[9]

**Immunological Memory:** A hallmark of adaptive immunity is the generation of immunological memory. After an initial encounter with a pathogen, memory B cells and memory T cells are formed, allowing for a faster, stronger, and more effective response upon subsequent exposure to the same pathogen. This is the rationale underpinning vaccination.

If your head is spinning from the cast of characters and their roles in the immune response, you're not alone. To add to the complexity, the innate and adaptive immune systems are not independent entities but are intricately interconnected, constantly communicating and influencing each other to mount an effective and coordinated defense against a vast array of threats. Fortunately, the executive and controlling genius of this complex system is vitamin D.

## VITAMIN D'S COMMAND: REGULATING THE IMMUNE SYMPHONY

The discovery that vitamin D receptors are expressed not just in bone, muscle, and intestinal cells but are, in fact, widely distributed throughout the immune system, including on macrophages, dendritic cells, T cells, and B cells, was a watershed moment.[10] It unequivocally signaled that vitamin D was far more than a calcium-regulating hormone; it was a potent immunomodulator with direct and profound effects on nearly every facet of immune function.

Furthermore, many immune cells themselves possess the enzyme 1α-hydroxylase (CYP27B1), enabling them to convert the circulating precursor 25-hydroxyvitamin D, 25(OH)D, into the active hormonal form, 1,25-dihydroxyvitamin D, 1,25(OH)2D or calcitriol, on the spot, allowing for local, autocrine, and paracrine regulation of immune responses within specific tissues.[11] This local production is a critical aspect of vitamin D's immunoregulatory role, allowing for tailored responses at sites of inflammation or infection.

Vitamin D exerts its influence by binding to the VDR, which then forms a complex with the retinoid X receptor (RXR). This VDR-RXR complex moves to the cell nucleus and binds to specific DNA sequences called vitamin D response elements (VDREs) in the relevant regions of target genes.[12] This binding can either activate or repress gene transcription, leading to changes in protein expression and ultimately altering cellular function. Thousands of genes are now known to be directly or indirectly regulated by vitamin D, many of which are centrally involved in immune responses. It is this sophisticated orchestration of the immune system by vitamin D that maintains the balance necessary for proper immune function.

## VITAMIN D'S DOMINION OVER INNATE IMMUNITY

Vitamin D significantly shapes the first line of defense provided by the innate immune system, playing a powerful role in helping your immune system fight off bacteria, viruses, and fungi. Here's how it works on the front lines of your body's defenses.

- **Cathelicidin (LL-37) Production:** One of the body's own natural infection-fighters—a protein that acts almost like a built-in antibiotic. As discussed in a previous chapter, vitamin D directly triggers the production of this protein in several key immune and barrier cells, including macrophages (cells that engulf and destroy germs), neutrophils (the immune system's first responders), and the epithelial cells that line your skin and airways.[13, 14] LL-37 is remarkably versatile, able to attack bacteria, viruses, and fungi. Because this entire defense mechanism depends on having adequate vitamin D, habits that chronically reduce sun exposure—like staying indoors or routinely applying heavy sunscreen—can meaningfully weaken this pathway, potentially making the body more vulnerable to infections.
- **β-Defensin Production:** Beta-defensins are another category of natural antimicrobial proteins that vitamin D helps activate. Specifically, it increases production of β-defensin 2 in epithelial cells, adding another weapon to the body's frontline chemical defenses against invading microbes.[15]
- **Supercharging Macrophage Function:** Macrophages are the immune system's all-purpose cleanup crew—they engulf and destroy pathogens, and they also help alert the rest of the immune system to threats. Vitamin D influences how these cells develop and how well they function in several important ways.
- **Enhanced Phagocytosis and Microbial Killing:** When it comes to killing pathogens, vitamin D enhances the ability of macrophages to swallow and destroy harmful microorganisms. This has been studied specifically in the context of mycobacterium tuberculosis, the bacterium responsible for tuberculosis, where vitamin D was shown to help macrophages destroy the pathogen more effectively—partly through the cathelicidin pathway described above.[16]

- **Regulation of Cytokine Production:** Vitamin D also shapes how macrophages communicate with the rest of the immune system through chemical signals called cytokines. In general, it steers macrophages toward a calmer, less-inflammatory mode—dialing down the production of cytokines that drive inflammation (like TNF-α and IL-6) while turning up the production of cytokines that reduce inflammation (like IL-10). This balancing act helps prevent the immune system from overreacting and causing collateral damage to healthy tissue.[17]
- **Keeping Dendritic Cells (DC) in Check:** Dendritic cells are the immune system's scouts and messengers—they detect threats and then instruct T cells on how to respond, bridging the gap between the innate and adaptive immune systems. Vitamin D influences their maturation and ability to activate T cells.

  **Inhibition of DC Maturation:** Vitamin D plays a subtle but important role here by slowing down the full maturation of dendritic cells. While that might sound counterproductive, it actually serves an important purpose: Less fully matured dendritic cells are less likely to trigger aggressive, inflammatory immune responses. Instead, they help foster the development of regulatory T cells (the immune system's referees, as discussed in the previous section), which keeps the immune response measured and prevents the body from mistakenly attacking its own healthy tissue. This is one of the ways vitamin D helps protect against autoimmune conditions.[18]
- **Supporting Neutrophil Activity:** Neutrophils—the immune system's first responders—are also influenced by vitamin D. It affects both their production of antimicrobial proteins and their ability to migrate toward sites of infection, ensuring these critical cells are well-equipped and properly directed when the body comes under attack.[19]

It is unequivocally clear that adequate vitamin D is essential for the robust and appropriate functioning of our innate immune defenses. Deficiency leaves this first line of defense significantly weakened and without command.

## HOW VITAMIN D SHAPES YOUR ADAPTIVE IMMUNE SYSTEM

While vitamin D's role in the innate immune system is impressive on its own, its influence reaches even deeper into the adaptive immune system—the more specialized branch that mounts targeted attacks against specific threats. Vitamin D helps fine-tune both T cell and B cell responses, acting less like an on/off switch and more like a careful volume knob, turning certain responses up or down to keep the immune system balanced.

- **Regulating T Cells:** Vitamin D exerts profound effects on T lymphocyte development, differentiation, and function.
- **Calming of Pro-inflammatory T Cell Subsets:** Two of the most inflammation-promoting types of T cells are Th1 and Th17 cells, and vitamin D puts the brakes on both.[20]
- **Th1 Cells:** Th1 cells are important for fighting infections that hide inside your body's own cells—but when they become overactive, they can contribute to autoimmune diseases, where the immune system starts attacking healthy tissue. Vitamin D directly reduces the inflammatory signals that Th1 cells produce, helping to keep their activity within safe limits.
- **Th17 Cells:** Th17 cells are similarly double-edged. They help fight certain infections, but excessive Th17 activity has been linked to a range of autoimmune and inflammatory conditions. Vitamin D suppresses the development of Th17 cells and dials down the inflammatory proteins they produce, reducing the risk of this type of immune overreach.

## PROMOTING THE IMMUNE SYSTEM'S REFEREES

Perhaps vitamin D's most important role in adaptive immunity is its ability to encourage the growth and activity of regulatory T cells, or Tregs—the immune system's referees that were introduced in the previous section. Tregs prevent the immune system from mistakenly attacking the body's own healthy tissues. Vitamin D supports Tregs both directly, by acting on T cells themselves, and indirectly, by influencing dendritic cells to steer T cell development toward the regulatory rather than the inflammatory path. This pro-Treg effect is considered one of the key reasons adequate vitamin D levels appear to be protective against autoimmune diseases.[21, 22]

- **Modulation of Cytotoxic T Cell (CTL) Activity:** Vitamin D's effects on cytotoxic T cells—the immune system's assassins that directly kill infected or cancerous cells—are more nuanced and still being studied. Evidence suggests it can adjust both their killing power and the inflammatory signals they send out, though exactly how this plays out likely depends on the specific context and disease environment.
- **B Cell Regulation:** Vitamin D doesn't stop at T cells—it also directly influences B cells, the antibody-producing arm of the adaptive immune system.
- **Inhibition of Antibody Production:** Vitamin D can slow down B cell multiplication and reduce the amount of antibodies that plasma cells (the B cell's antibody-factory form) churn out. At first glance, this

might seem like a bad thing—don't we want more antibodies? But in the context of autoimmune diseases like lupus, the problem is actually too many antibodies being made against the body's own tissues. By putting a check on this process, vitamin D helps prevent the kind of antibody overproduction that drives these conditions.[23]

- **Encouraging Regulatory B Cells (B-regs):** Emerging research suggests that vitamin D may also promote the development of regulatory B cells—a lesser-known but important cell type that, much like regulatory T cells, helps calm inflammatory responses. They do this largely by releasing an anti-inflammatory signal called IL-10, adding yet another layer to vitamin D's role as a moderating force within the immune system.[24]

The overarching effect of vitamin D on adaptive immunity is one of promoting a more balanced and tolerogenic (not attacking healthy tissue) state, preventing excessive inflammation and autoimmunity while still allowing for effective pathogen clearance. It is not a simple "on" or "off" switch but a sophisticated rheostat, fine-tuning the immune response to meet the specific challenge. If you understand that vitamin D's role is to balance the immune system response between protective immunity and pathological inflammation, and that when the immune system is in balance there is health, and that when it is imbalanced there is disease, you have a great grasp on why vitamin D is critical for good health.

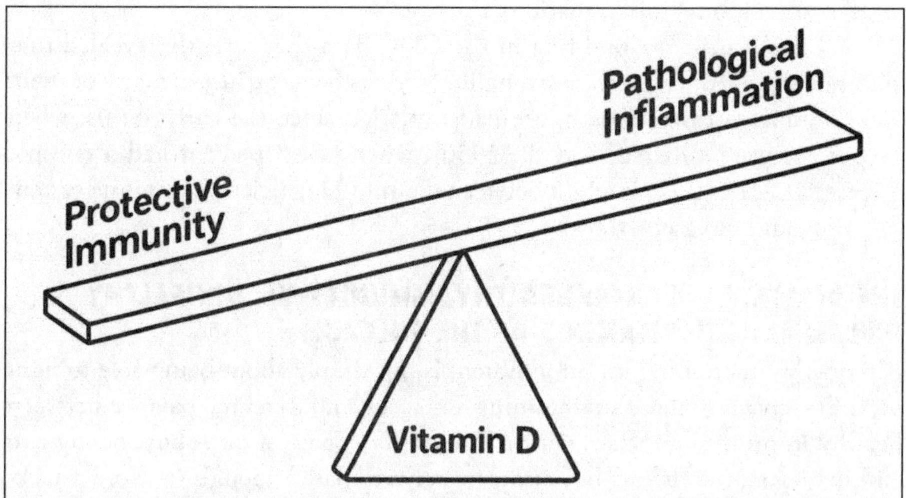


A functioning and balanced immune system creates a picture of health. If your immune system is broken, so is your health. The immune system is really like a dictionary of disease, in that, when the immune system dysfunctions, all the immune-system-related diseases in that dictionary can become expressed. When your immune system is humming along, greased and balanced by optimal vitamin D, that book of disease stays on the shelf where it belongs.

## THE UNWAVERING CONCLUSION: IMMUNE DYSFUNCTION IN THE SHADOW OF VITAMIN D DEFICIENCY

Given the pervasive regulatory roles of vitamin D across both innate and adaptive immunity, the conclusion is inescapable: Without adequate vitamin D, the immune system cannot function effectively or appropriately. A deficiency in this master regulator leads to a state of immune dysregulation, characterized by weakened innate defenses and impaired adaptive immune control.

The failure to adequately suppress pro-inflammatory pathways and promote anti-inflammatory responses due to vitamin D deficiency can lead to a state of chronic, low-grade inflammation. This smoldering inflammation is now recognized as a common underlying factor in a vast array of chronic diseases, including cardiovascular disease, type 2 diabetes, neurodegenerative disorders, aging, and many types of cancer.[25]

An immune system operating without sufficient vitamin D is like an orchestra without its conductor—capable of making noise, but lacking the harmony, precision, and control necessary for an effective and appropriate performance. It becomes prone to both underreacting to genuine threats (increased susceptibility to infections) and overreacting or misdirecting its power (autoimmunity and chronic inflammation).[26]

The proof is in the pudding in the CDC data that recently revealed that 76.4 percent of Americans are struggling with a chronic disease, many of them autoimmune diseases. This figure had exploded since the early 1960s, when 11 percent were afflicted, and the 1950s, when just 3 percent had a chronic disease.[27] Clearly there is a link between vitamin D deficiency, immune system function, and disease.

## THE DELICATE BALANCE: HEALTHY IMMUNITY VS. UNHEALTHY INFLAMMATION–VITAMIN D AS THE FULCRUM

A properly functioning immune system is not simply about being able to fight off infections; it is about maintaining a delicate and dynamic balance between healthy immunity and harmful inflammation. It must be robust enough to eliminate genuine threats but also precisely regulated enough to avoid attacking self-tissues (autoimmunity) and to resolve inflammation once a threat has been neutralized. Chronic, unresolved inflammation is now recognized as a common soil in which many chronic diseases take root.[28]

Vitamin D, as we have seen, acts as a fulcrum in this balancing act.

- **Promoting Anti-Inflammatory Pathways:** Vitamin D actively promotes anti-inflammatory responses. It stimulates the production of anti-inflammatory cytokines like IL-10 and TGF-β. It supports the function of Tregs, which are key players in suppressing excessive inflammation and maintaining immune tolerance.
- **Dampening Pro-Inflammatory Pathways:** Conversely, vitamin D works to dampen excessive pro-inflammatory responses. It can inhibit the production of pro-inflammatory cytokines like TNF-α, IL-1, IL-6, and IL-17. It guides dendritic cells toward a more tolerogenic state, preventing them from over-stimulating inflammatory T cell responses.
- **Maintaining Homeostasis:** By orchestrating these opposing forces, vitamin D helps to maintain immune homeostasis—a state of equilibrium where the immune system is vigilant but not hyperactive, responsive but not self-destructive.

When vitamin D levels are chronically insufficient, this delicate balance is disrupted. The immune system can become skewed toward a pro-inflammatory state. The brakes (Tregs, anti-inflammatory cytokines) are weakened, and the accelerators (pro-inflammatory T cells and cytokines) are less controlled. This creates a fertile ground for chronic inflammation to smolder throughout the body.

The prevention of chronic inflammation is the mechanism through which vitamin D and its regulation of the immune system is at the root of good health while the induction of chronic inflammation, through chronic vitamin D deficiency, is at the root of poor health and disease.

## THE PRECURSOR TO AUTOIMMUNITY: VITAMIN D DEFICIENCY, CHRONIC INFLAMMATION, AND THE ATTACK ON SELF

This state of chronic vitamin D deficiency-induced immune dysregulation and persistent inflammation is not merely a theoretical concern; it is, as this book strongly asserts, a critical precursor to the development of autoimmune diseases. This will be the central focus of the next chapter, where we will explore in detail how the crippling of our sun-dependent immune regulation opens the door for the immune system to turn against the body's own tissues, leading to the devastating array of autoimmune conditions that now afflict an alarming number of individuals in modern society. The path from sun avoidance to vitamin D deficiency, to immune dysregulation, to chronic inflammation, and finally to autoimmunity is a direct and scientifically plausible cascade, a cascade that we have, in large part, brought upon ourselves through our misguided estrangement from the sun.

It is time to dismantle the fear-based narrative surrounding sunlight and to recognize its profound and essential role in forging a robust and well-regulated immune system. Restoring optimal vitamin D levels through sensible sun exposure, and supplementation where necessary, is not just a matter of bone health; it is a fundamental prerequisite for reclaiming our immune sovereignty and reversing the rising tide of chronic inflammatory and autoimmune diseases.

# CHAPTER 10

# THE SUN-STARVED IMMUNE SYSTEM: AUTOIMMUNE DISEASE AND THE VITAMIN D CONNECTION

The human immune system is designed to distinguish "self" from "nonself." Its primary directive is to identify and eliminate foreign invaders like bacteria, viruses, and fungi while leaving the body's own tissues unharmed. In autoimmune disease, this fundamental instruction breaks down. The immune system, in a tragic case of mistaken identity, turns on the very body it is meant to protect. This attack of healthy tissue by a dysfunctional immune system causes chronic inflammation, leading to progressive tissue breakdown and organ malfunction, manifesting as a wide range of debilitating conditions known as autoimmune diseases.

This chapter will explore a compelling and increasingly supported observation: that the dramatic rise in autoimmune diseases over the past half-century is not a coincidence, but is strongly linked to a parallel, silent epidemic of chronic vitamin D deficiency driven by modern, sun-avoidant lifestyles. We will examine the evidence, from large-scale population studies to the intricate molecular dance within our cells, that positions vitamin D not as a minor player, but as a master conductor of immune harmony. We will show that many modern, powerful pharmaceuticals are, in effect, treating the downstream symptoms of an immune system that is fundamentally starved of this critical vitamin D hormone.

## THE RISING TIDE: AN EPIDEMIC OF AUTOIMMUNITY

A striking and alarming trend has emerged in industrialized nations since the mid-twentieth century: a dramatic and sustained increase in the incidence of autoimmune diseases. As HHS Secretary Kennedy recently said, "I got the latest numbers from the CDC that 76.4 percent of Americans now have a chronic disease. This is stunning. When my uncle was president, it was eleven percent and in 1950, it was three percent."[1, 2] These numbers cannot be explained by genetics alone, as our gene pool does not change this rapidly. The evidence points squarely toward environmental and lifestyle factors, with changes in sun exposure habits and resulting vitamin D status being a prime suspect.

**Multiple Sclerosis (MS):** This demyelinating disease of the central nervous system shows a clear geographical gradient, with prevalence increasing significantly at higher latitudes where sun exposure is lower.[3, 4] More telling, multiple studies have confirmed a genuine rise in incidence over time. A comprehensive Danish study found the incidence of MS doubled between 1970 and 2005.[5] Similarly, studies in Canada and Norway have shown a steady increase, particularly among women.[6] This rise coincides with public health campaigns promoting sun avoidance and the shift to more indoor-centric occupations and recreation.

**Type 1 Diabetes (T1D):** The autoimmune destruction of insulin-producing beta cells in the pancreas, type 1 diabetes was once a relatively rare disease. Today, its incidence is increasing by a staggering 3 to 4 percent per year globally, with some European countries seeing a doubling of cases every twenty years.[7] This rapid increase points away from purely genetic causes and toward environmental triggers, with low vitamin D levels in pregnancy and early childhood being strongly implicated as a major risk factor.[8]

**Inflammatory Bowel Disease (IBD):** This category, including Crohn's disease and ulcerative colitis, has also seen its incidence skyrocket. In North America, prevalence has risen sharply since the 1960s, and the disease is now rapidly emerging in newly industrialized nations in Asia and South America as they adopt Western lifestyles.[9] This geographical and temporal pattern strongly mirrors the latitude gradient and lifestyle changes associated with vitamin D deficiency.

**Rheumatoid Arthritis (RA):** While the data for RA is more complex, several long-term studies show a notable increase in incidence, particularly in women, after 1995.[10] This increase has been linked to lower vitamin D levels, which are consistently observed in patients with active RA compared to healthy controls.

**Celiac Disease:** This autoimmune reaction to gluten has seen a true increase in incidence, not just an increase in diagnosis. A study analyzing stored blood samples from US Air Force recruits between 1948 and 1954 found a fourfold lower prevalence compared to modern-day populations, confirming a genuine rise in the disease.[11]

**Systemic Lupus Erythematosus (SLE) and Thyroid Autoimmunity (Hashimoto's and Graves' Disease):** While historical data is harder to track, these conditions also appear to be increasing in prevalence.[12] Patients with SLE and autoimmune thyroid disease almost universally exhibit lower levels of vitamin D compared to the general population, and low levels are associated with more severe disease activity.[13, 14]

This collective evidence paints a clear picture. Across a spectrum of autoimmune diseases with different target tissues, the common thread is a dysfunctional immune system. The parallel timeline of their rise with the increase in sun-avoidant behavior and documented widespread vitamin D deficiency is too strong to be a mere coincidence.

## THE IMMUNE SYSTEM UNDER SIEGE: CELLULAR MECHANISMS OF AUTOIMMUNITY

To understand how vitamin D can influence these diseases, we must first understand the specific immune cells and signaling molecules (cytokines) that go awry in each of the above conditions.

- **T-Helper Cells (The Generals of the Immune Army):** A critical imbalance in autoimmune disease occurs within a subset of T lymphocytes called T helper (Th) cells.
- **Th1 cells:** Produce pro-inflammatory cytokines like interferon-gamma (IFN-γ) and are important for fighting intracellular pathogens. In autoimmunity, overactive Th1 cells drive cellular damage.
- **Th17 cells:** A more recently discovered subset, these are potent drivers of inflammation and tissue destruction, primarily through their production of the cytokine Interleukin-17 (IL-17). They are now considered central players in many autoimmune conditions.
- **T regulatory cells (Tregs):** These are the peacekeepers. They actively suppress other immune cells and produce anti-inflammatory cytokines like Interleukin-10 (IL-10) to prevent excessive reactions and maintain self-tolerance. A deficiency or dysfunction of Tregs is a hallmark of autoimmunity.

Here is how these cells contribute to specific diseases:

- **Rheumatoid Arthritis:** The synovial joint lining is infiltrated by aggressive Th1 and Th17 cells. They release a storm of cytokines, including tumor necrosis factor-alpha (TNF-α), interleukin-1 (IL-1), interleukin-6 (IL-6), and IL-17. These signals cause cartilage and bone erosion. B cells also play a role by producing autoantibodies (rheumatoid factor, anti-CCP).[15]

- **Psoriasis:** This is now understood as a classic Th17-driven disease. Overactive Th17 cells migrate to the skin and release vast amounts of IL-17 and other cytokines, causing the characteristic rapid skin cell proliferation, inflammation, and plaque formation.[16]
- **Multiple Sclerosis:** In MS, Th1 and Th17 cells cross the blood-brain barrier. They attack the myelin sheath that insulates nerve fibers, with IL-17 and IFN-γ being key mediators of the neural damage.[17]
- **Type 1 Diabetes:** The destruction of pancreatic beta cells is driven primarily by Th1 cells and cytotoxic T lymphocytes.
- **Ulcerative Colitis and Crohn's Disease (IBD)**: Crohn's disease is often characterized as a Th1/Th17-mediated condition, while ulcerative colitis has historically been seen as more Th2-driven, although recent evidence shows significant Th17 involvement as well. An overactive response to gut microbiota is a key feature.[18]
- **Systemic Lupus Erythematosus (SLE):** Lupus is a complex disease involving multiple immune branches. It features hyperactive B cells producing a wide array of autoantibodies, dysfunction in Tregs, and an overproduction of Type I interferons and other pro-inflammatory cytokines from Th1 and Th17 cells.[19]
- **Hashimoto's Thyroiditis and Graves' Disease:** In Hashimoto's thyroiditis, the thyroid is destroyed by a Th1-dominant cellular attack. In Graves' disease, B cells produce antibodies that mimic thyroid-stimulating hormone (TSH), leading to hyperthyroidism, a process often supported by Th2 cells.[20]

The common theme is a dangerous imbalance: too many pro-inflammatory Th1 and Th17 cells and not enough immune system–tolerant Treg cells. If you or a loved one has an autoimmune-based disease, it is important to understand the players so that you'll understand the immune imbalance causing the disease, how vitamin D corrects it, and how most pharmaceuticals are designed to replicate what vitamin D already does.

## VITAMIN D: THE MASTER REGULATOR OF IMMUNE TOLERANCE

The connection between vitamin D and autoimmunity becomes crystal clear when we examine its profound effects on the very immune cells and pathways implicated above. Immune cells—including T cells, B cells, macrophages, and dendritic cells—are equipped with the vitamin D receptor. When the active form of vitamin D (calcitriol) binds to this receptor, it directly influences the expression of hundreds of genes, effectively acting as a master switch to restore immune balance.[21]

Here is how vitamin D orchestrates the immune system, correcting the very defects seen in autoimmune disease:

1. **It Suppresses Pro-Inflammatory T Cells:** Vitamin D directly inhibits the proliferation and differentiation of the aggressive Th1 and Th17 cells. It reduces their production of damaging cytokines like IFN-γ (from Th1 cells) and, IL-17 (from Th17 cells).[22]
2. **It Promotes Regulatory T Cells (Tregs):** This may be its most critical function. Vitamin D powerfully promotes the development of the "peacekeeper" Treg cells. These cells then produce the anti-inflammatory cytokine IL-10, which actively shuts down autoimmune responses.
3. **It Regulates Cytokine Production:** Beyond its effect on T cells, vitamin D broadly shifts the cytokine environment from pro-inflammatory to anti-inflammatory. It directly suppresses the production of major inflammatory molecules like TNF-α, IL-1, and IL-6 by immune cells like macrophages.[23]
4. **It Modulates B Cell Function:** Vitamin D inhibits B cell proliferation and their differentiation into plasma cells that produce autoantibodies, a key mechanism in diseases like lupus and RA.[24]

In essence, vitamin D reestablishes immune tolerance. It strikes a balance between healthy immunity and harmful inflammation and dials down the aggressive, self-attacking components of the immune system while simultaneously dialing up the regulatory, self-preserving components. A chronic deficiency of vitamin D removes this essential "brake" and "tuner," allowing the immune system to spiral into a state of chronic self-attack. It is also important to realize that good old vitamin D performs all of these actions on the immune system simultaneously and expertly, just like it was designed to do.

## MODERN DRUGS: A MAN-MADE PHARMACOLOGICAL ECHO OF VITAMIN D'S FUNCTIONS

The last two decades have seen a revolution in the treatment of autoimmune disease with the development of "biologic" drugs. These are highly specific, engineered antibodies that target single molecules in the inflammatory cascade. While often effective, they are also extremely expensive and come with significant side effects, including an increased risk of serious infections.

What is fascinating is that these modern marvels of pharmacology are designed to affect the same pathways that vitamin D naturally regulates. They are, in a very real sense, a man-made, single-target solution to a problem that nature intended to solve with a broad, multi-target regulator, vitamin D.

Let's examine the parallels:

For Rheumatoid Arthritis, Psoriasis, and IBD:

- **Drugs:** TNF-α inhibitors like adalimumab (Humira), infliximab (Remicade), and etanercept (Enbrel).
- **Mechanism:** These drugs bind to and neutralize TNF-α, a master inflammatory cytokine.
- **Vitamin D's Role:** Vitamin D deficiency leads to increased TNF-α production. Adequate vitamin D, by binding to the VDR in macrophages, suppresses the gene that produces TNF-α.[25]

The drugs are a highly targeted intervention to correct a problem that sufficient vitamin D prevents at its source.

For Psoriasis, Psoriatic Arthritis, and Ankylosing Spondylitis:

- **Drugs:** IL-17 inhibitors like secukinumab (Cosentyx) and ixekizumab (Taltz).
- **Mechanism:** These drugs specifically block the action of IL-17, the key cytokine produced by Th17 cells.
- **Vitamin D's Role:** Vitamin D is a potent natural inhibitor of Th17 cell development and directly suppresses their production of IL-17.[26]

The drugs are a direct pharmacological replacement for one of vitamin D's most important immunomodulatory functions.

For multiple sclerosis and some forms of lupus:

- **Drugs:** B cell–depleting therapies like rituximab (Rituxan) and ocrelizumab (Ocrevus).
- **Mechanism:** These drugs target and destroy B cells, preventing them from producing autoantibodies and presenting antigens.
- **Vitamin D's Role:** Vitamin D naturally regulates B cell proliferation and maturation, inhibiting the very hyperactivity seen in these diseases.[27]

This pattern is undeniable. The pharmaceutical industry has spent billions of dollars developing sophisticated tools to block individual pathological pathways. Yet, vitamin D, when present in sufficient amounts, regulates all of these pathways simultaneously and harmoniously just as nature intended, without the cost or side effects of targeted immunosuppression. The sophisticated balanced approach that vitamin D uses to govern the immune system cannot be replicated by drugs, which is why there are no side effects with vitamin D compared to many with unbalanced immune-system-manipulating drugs.

Biologic drugs are simply treating a symptom of chronic vitamin D deficiency. Adequate vitamin D prevents the disease from occurring and eradicates the disease when immune system balance is restored through vitamin D therapy.

## AUTOIMMUNE DISEASE AS A SYMPTOM OF CHRONIC VITAMIN D DEFICIENCY

Integrating all of the preceding evidence leads to a powerful and comprehensive conclusion: The dramatic increase in the incidence of autoimmune disease is a direct consequence of a population-wide, chronic vitamin D deficiency driven by our modern, indoor, sun-avoidant lifestyle.

From this perspective, modern biologic drugs, while life-changing for many, are treating a symptom, not the root cause. Blocking IL-17 in a psoriasis patient is like taking a highly specific cough suppressant for a cough caused by pneumonia. It alleviates the most obvious symptom but does nothing to address the underlying infection causing the pneumonia. The drug just temporarily quiets one rogue instrument in an unruly immune orchestra.

Therefore, we must reframe our understanding of what autoimmune disease actually is. Many cases of autoimmune disease are not an inescapable fate written in our genes, but rather a preventable, and perhaps even reversible, state of immune dysfunction characterized by an immune system imbalance caused by an easily correctable vitamin D deficiency. The evidence strongly suggests vitamin D, whether it be from the sun or supplements, should be a foundational and nonnegotiable part of the prevention and management strategy for all autoimmune diseases.

# CHAPTER 11

# SUNSHINE, VITAMIN D, AND YOUR HEART: UNRAVELING THE TRUE CAUSE OF CARDIOVASCULAR DISEASE

In our preceding chapters, we established a compelling case for the widespread, chronic vitamin D deficiency that plagues modern society—a direct consequence of our collective retreat from the sun. This shift in behavior, driven by well-intentioned but perhaps misguided public health campaigns, has had far-reaching consequences. As we will explore in this chapter, the epidemic of cardiovascular disease (CVD), the leading cause of death globally, is not an isolated phenomenon. It is deeply intertwined with our sun-avoidant lifestyles, not only through the loss of vitamin D but also through the absence of other sun-dependent physiological processes, like the production of nitric oxide, which are critical for a healthy heart and vascular system.

## WHAT IS CARDIOVASCULAR DISEASE? THE FIRE WITHIN YOUR ARTERIES

When we hear the term "cardiovascular disease," we often picture a plumbing problem: a clogged pipe (artery) leading to a catastrophic failure (heart attack or stroke). While this analogy is simple, it is dangerously incomplete. The reality of CVD is not a passive accumulation of sludge in an inert tube; it is a dynamic, aggressive biological process rooted in chronic inflammation at the most fundamental level of our blood vessels: the endothelium.

The endothelium is a delicate, single-cell-thick layer that lines the interior of all our blood vessels, from the mighty aorta to the tiniest capillaries. Far from being a simple barrier, it is a highly active and intelligent organ. A healthy endothelium orchestrates blood flow, prevents unwanted clotting, and regulates the passage of substances and cells into and out of the bloodstream.

It is the gatekeeper of vascular health. Cardiovascular disease begins when this gatekeeper becomes dysfunctional.[1]

The primary culprit in endothelial dysfunction is chronic, low-grade inflammation.[2] As we've learned, while acute inflammation is a necessary and lifesaving healing response to injury or infection, chronic inflammation is a persistent, smoldering fire that damages the very tissues it is supposed to protect. In the context of our arteries, this process unfolds in several key stages:

1. **Initial Insult:** The process is triggered by various stressors, including high blood pressure, toxins from smoking, high blood sugar, and a state of immune dysregulation caused by chronic vitamin D deficiency.
2. **Endothelial Activation:** These stressors "activate" the endothelial cells. They begin to express adhesion molecules on their surface, acting like molecular Velcro that snags passing white blood cells (immune cells).
3. **Immune Cell Infiltration:** Monocytes, a type of white blood cell, stick to the activated endothelium and squeeze through it into the artery wall (a space called the intima). Once inside, they transform into aggressive macrophages.
4. **Lipid Accumulation and Foam Cell Formation:** These macrophages begin to gobble up low-density lipoprotein (LDL, or "bad") cholesterol that has also become trapped and oxidized within the inflamed artery wall. As the macrophages become engorged with these lipids, they transform into "foam cells," a hallmark of early atherosclerosis.
5. **Plaque Formation:** A cascade of inflammatory signals (cytokines) is released, attracting more immune cells, promoting the proliferation of smooth muscle cells, and laying down a fibrous cap over the growing lesion. This combination of foam cells, cellular debris, cholesterol, and calcium from the blood forms an atherosclerotic plaque.[3, 4]

This plaque is not a stable, inert blockage. It is a volatile, inflamed lesion. The inflammatory processes within the plaque can degrade the fibrous cap that holds it in place. If the cap ruptures, the highly thrombogenic (clot-promoting) core is exposed to the blood, causing a clot (thrombus) to form rapidly. If this clot blocks the artery, it cuts off oxygen to the tissue downstream, resulting in a heart attack (myocardial infarction) or an ischemic stroke. This entire pathological cascade is driven and sustained by inflammation. It is the fire of chronic inflammation of the artery, not the cholesterol "smoke," that is the fundamental problem in atherosclerosis.

## THE RISING TIDE OF HEART DISEASE: AN EPIDEMIOLOGICAL SNAPSHOT

The narrative of the twentieth century is one of remarkable medical progress, yet it is also the story of the meteoric rise of cardiovascular disease. Since the 1960s, despite advancements in treatment, CVD has become the principal cause of morbidity and mortality in the developed world.

- **Coronary Artery Disease (CAD) and Heart Attack:** The incidence of heart attacks surged through the mid-twentieth century, becoming the quintessential modern disease.
- **Hypertension (High Blood Pressure):** The prevalence of hypertension has dramatically increased, with now nearly half of adults in the United States meeting the criteria for this condition.[5] Hypertension is a primary driver of endothelial damage and a major risk factor for heart attack, stroke, and heart failure.
- **Heart Failure:** This condition, where the heart cannot pump blood effectively, is a growing epidemic, particularly among the elderly.
- **Stroke:** While mortality rates from stroke have decreased due to better acute care, the incidence remains alarmingly high.

This timeline of rising CVD incidence runs in stunning parallel with the timeline of increasing vitamin D deficiency. The public health campaigns that began in earnest in the latter half of the twentieth century, urging people to cover up, seek shade, and slather on sunscreen, have been extraordinarily successful in changing public behavior. As sun exposure plummeted, so did average population-wide vitamin D levels.

The correlation is more than circumstantial. Numerous large-scale observational studies have demonstrated a powerful link between low serum vitamin D levels and an increased incidence of virtually every form of CVD:

- **Hypertension:** Individuals with lower vitamin D levels are significantly more likely to have high blood pressure.
- **Coronary Artery Disease:** Vitamin D deficiency is a well-established independent risk factor for the development and severity of CAD.
- **Heart Attack:** Low vitamin D status is associated with a higher risk of suffering a fatal or nonfatal heart attack.
- **Stroke and Heart Failure:** Deficiency is linked to an increased risk of both ischemic stroke and chronic heart failure.[6, 7]

While correlation does not prove causation, the sheer consistency and strength of this association across different populations and disease types demand a deeper look at the underlying mechanisms. The evidence strongly suggests that our retreat from the sun has left our cardiovascular systems uniquely vulnerable.

## SUNLIGHT, VITAMIN D, AND CVD: MECHANISMS OF PROTECTION

The link between sun avoidance and CVD is not a simple statistical correlation; it is a story of deep biological mechanisms. As we have seen, the dysfunction of the endothelium is the common denominator of hypertension, stroke, and heart failure—the very diseases where vitamin D deficiency is most prevalent. To understand the connection, we must look at the cellular and molecular level.

## NANOMEDICINE REVEALS THAT VITAMIN D IS A POWERFUL HEALER: THE MALINSKY STUDY

A groundbreaking 2018 study by Khan, Dawoud, and Malinski provided a stunning demonstration of vitamin D's power to heal the cardiovascular system.[8] Using highly advanced nanomedical technology, they were able to measure, in real time, the health of individual human endothelial cells. The key metric of a healthy endothelial cell is its ability to produce nitric oxide (NO), a critical signaling molecule that relaxes blood vessels (vasodilation), lowers blood pressure, and prevents inflammation and clotting. The main threat to NO is a highly destructive free radical called peroxynitrite ($ONOO^-$). In a state of inflammation and disease, NO production plummets while peroxynitrite production soars. A high $NO/ONOO^-$ ratio signifies health; a low ratio signifies severe dysfunction.

The researchers conducted a brilliantly designed series of experiments:

1. **Baseline Measurement:** Using nanosensors 1,000 times smaller than a human hair, they measured the $NO/ONOO^-$ ratio in healthy, cultured human endothelial cells, confirming a high, healthy ratio.
2. **Inducing Disease:** They then exposed these healthy cells to tumor necrosis factor-alpha (TNF-α), a potent inflammatory cytokine known to be involved in the pathology of atherosclerosis, hypertension, and diabetes. As expected, the cells quickly became dysfunctional: NO production crashed, and peroxynitrite levels skyrocketed, mimicking the cellular state of cardiovascular disease.
3. **The Vitamin D Intervention:** The critical step was next. They treated these "sick," dysfunctional endothelial cells with 1,25-dihydroxyvitamin D3, the active form of vitamin D. The results were remarkable. Within hours, vitamin D treatment completely restored the healthy balance. It dramatically boosted the production of nitric oxide and simultaneously quenched the production of

> destructive peroxynitrite. The vitamin D had, in effect, cured the diseased cells at a molecular level.

The authors' conclusions from this elegant work are profound. They state that vitamin D is a powerful agent not only for preventing cardiovascular diseases from developing but also for repairing the vascular damage that has already occurred. This has staggering clinical implications for reversing the endothelial damage caused by heart attacks, strokes, hypertension, atherosclerosis, and diabetes. It suggests that by ensuring vitamin D sufficiency, we can directly combat the root cellular pathology of cardiovascular disease. Vitamin D can indeed mend a broken heart.

## CHRONIC INFLAMMATION: THE TRUE ARSONIST IN ATHEROSCLEROSIS

With the findings of the Malinsky study in mind, the role of inflammation in atherosclerosis becomes crystal clear. As we've learned, chronic vitamin D deficiency leads to a state of chronic immune dysregulation and inflammation. As supported by Malinsky et al., this state cripples the endothelium's ability to produce protective nitric oxide and increases its production of damaging peroxynitrite. This inflamed, dysfunctional endothelium becomes "sticky," allowing LDL cholesterol and calcium to infiltrate the artery wall and become trapped, creating a plaque. This process reframes the entire cholesterol debate.

## REVISITING CHOLESTEROL: A MISLABELED VILLAIN?

For decades, dietary fat and cholesterol have been vilified as the primary causes of atherosclerosis. The evidence now points to a different culprit. Cholesterol is not the cause of the fiery crash; it is simply part of the wreckage found at the scene.[9] It is a component of the "plaque" that forms over the underlying inflammatory lesion. Without the initial inflammatory damage to the endothelium—damage promoted by vitamin D deficiency—cholesterol would largely circulate harmlessly—as it is designed to do—without accumulating in the artery wall.

Consider the relationship between vitamin D and lipid profiles. While studies vary, a common finding is that low vitamin D levels are associated with higher LDL and lower high-density lipoprotein (HDL, or "good") cholesterol.[10] This is likely a symptom of the same underlying inflammatory state, not the cause of it. In a very interesting study reported by the American College of Cardiology, an analysis of the lipid profiles of 227,359 individuals found that their cholesterol levels varied with the changing seasons. Specifically, LDL cholesterol rose in the winter by 7 mg/dL compared to summer.[11] Again, whenever there is a seasonal effect on any measured biological variable we have to ask, what is the connection to vitamin D?

The protective effect of estrogen in premenopausal women provides another compelling example regarding the relationship between vitamin D, cholesterol, and CVD. Women have a much lower risk of heart disease than men until menopause. Estrogen appears to synergize with vitamin D, promoting vascular health and directing calcium into the bones.[12] After menopause, as estrogen levels plummet, this selective protection of the female is lost. In a vitamin D–deficient woman, the situation is exacerbated. Calcium that was once preferentially deposited in her skeleton is now more likely to be deposited in her inflamed, damaged arteries, accelerating atherosclerosis.[13] This disturbed process, caused by chronic vitamin D deficiency and a dysfunctional immune system, allows her to "catch up" to the CVD risk of men after menopause. The problem isn't the calcium or the cholesterol; it's the inflamed state of the blood vessel that allows both of them to accumulate as a result of chronic vitamin D deficiency.

## THE SUN'S DIRECT GIFT: NITRIC OXIDE AND BLOOD PRESSURE

Vitamin D is not the only cardiovascular benefit we get from the sun. The sun's UVA rays, which are distinct from the UVB rays that produce vitamin D, have a direct and immediate effect on blood pressure. When UVA light strikes the skin, it triggers the release of massive stores of nitric oxide (NO) into the bloodstream.[14] As we learned from the Malinsky study, NO is a potent vasodilator. It relaxes the smooth muscle in the artery walls, causing them to widen, which immediately lowers blood pressure.

The effect is not trivial. A 2014 study published in the *Journal of Investigative Dermatology* found that exposing skin to the equivalent of thirty minutes of summer sunlight, without burning, could lower blood pressure by an average of 2.8/3.4 mmHg within an hour.[15] This reduction is comparable to the effect of some common antihypertensive medications and is associated with a significant reduction in heart attack and stroke risk.[16] This suggests that for many, sensible, regular sun exposure could be a safe, free, and effective strategy for blood pressure control, addressing the problem at its source rather than merely managing a symptom.

## THE IMMUNE SYSTEM'S FOOT SOLDIERS: ANTIMICROBIAL PEPTIDES

The benefits of the sun don't stop there. Vitamin D is essential for the production of potent antimicrobial peptides (AMPs), most notably cathelicidin and LL-37. While their primary role is to kill invading pathogens, they are also powerful modulators of the immune system. In the cardiovascular system, these AMPs have protective effects that go beyond fighting infection. They can help regulate the inflammatory response within the artery wall, potentially reducing the risk of plaque formation and helping to stabilize existing plaques, making them less likely to rupture.[17]

## THE ORAL-SYSTEMIC CONNECTION: YOUR MOUTH AND YOUR HEART

The role of AMPs highlights an important link between oral health and cardiovascular health. It is well-established that bacteria from the mouth, particularly from gum disease (periodontitis), can enter the bloodstream during dental procedures or even vigorous brushing. These bacteria can seed inflammation in the arteries, contributing directly to atherosclerosis.[18] An individual with robust vitamin D levels will have a stronger defense system, with higher levels of cathelicidin and other AMPs ready to neutralize these pathogens in the bloodstream. Conversely, a vitamin D–deficient person has a compromised defense, making them more susceptible to the vascular inflammation triggered by these oral bacteria.

## SYMPTOM MANAGEMENT VS. CURING THE DISEASE: A PARADIGM SHIFT

This brings us to a critical assessment of modern cardiovascular pharmacology. Most of our blockbuster drugs for CVD—statins, blood pressure medications, beta-blockers—are brilliant at managing symptoms. They lower cholesterol, force blood vessels to relax, and reduce the workload on the heart. However, they do not address the fundamental, underlying cause of the disease: chronic inflammation and endothelial dysfunction rooted in a sun-deficient lifestyle.

In contrast, restoring vitamin D sufficiency through sensible sun exposure and, when necessary, supplementation, targets the disease at its origin. It heals the endothelium, restores nitric oxide balance, quells inflammation, and bolsters the immune system's defenses.

Worse yet, some treatments intended to help CVD may be counterproductive. Statins, for example, work by inhibiting an enzyme (HMG-CoA reductase) that is essential for producing cholesterol. While this lowers blood cholesterol, it also interferes with the body's ability to synthesize the precursor molecule, 7-dehydrocholesterol.[19] This is the very molecule in the skin that is converted to pre-vitamin D3 by UVB sunlight. Therefore, it is biologically plausible that by aggressively lowering cholesterol, statins may inadvertently hinder the body's natural, sun-driven pathway for producing the very vitamin that is essential for preventing the underlying inflammation that causes heart disease in the first place.

Furthermore, our previous discussion on endothelial inflammation and plaque formation indicates that cholesterol is not the culprit in atherosclerosis. Inflammation is the cause.

## REFRAMING CARDIOVASCULAR DISEASE AS AN IMMUNE DISORDER OF DARKNESS

The evidence presented in this chapter converges on a single, transformative conclusion: Cardiovascular disease, in its many forms, is not primarily a disease of cholesterol, fat, or old age. It is, at its core, a disease of immune dysfunction, driven by chronic inflammation, which is itself a direct consequence of chronic vitamin D deficiency and a lack of sunlight exposure. Of course this does not mean that all CVD is caused by these mechanisms. But given the epidemic vitamin D crisis in the Western world, it surely plays a huge, yet currently, unappreciated role.

In a report just issued by the Journal of the American College of Cardiology, the authors said that the high-sensitivity C-reactive protein (hsCRP) blood test that measures CRP, a known inflammatory marker that increases in response to inflammation in the body, can determine whether a person is at risk of developing cardiovascular disease.[20] This is essentially what we have been claiming here regarding vitamin D, inflammation, and CVD. Of course, the American College of Cardiology may not like the solution to most CVD at all, which is safe, inexpensive (mostly free) vitamin D. For my personal situation for more than twenty years I have requested a CRP test to determine if there is inflammation anywhere. There isn't, so I don't worry about heart disease. How long will it be that routine CRP tests are deemed superfluous and unnecessary by some medical trade group entity?

Our modern, indoor, sun-avoidant lifestyle has inadvertently created the perfect storm for heart disease. By depriving our bodies of UVB for vitamin D synthesis and UVA for nitric oxide release, we have sabotaged our cardiovascular system's primary defense and repair mechanisms. This leaves our endothelium vulnerable to a state of constant, low-grade inflammation. This inflammation is the true cause of atherosclerosis and hypertension and their devastating consequences. Cholesterol and calcium are merely secondary players, accumulating at the site of this inflammatory damage. Returning to our auto accident analogy, cholesterol and calcium are at the scene of the accident while the cause of the accident, inflammation, is covered up.

Effectively treating the CVD epidemic requires a fundamental paradigm shift. We must move beyond simply managing symptoms with pharmaceuticals and start addressing the root cause. The solution is not necessarily a new pill, but a return to a more biologically appropriate relationship with our environment. By embracing sensible sun exposure and ensuring vitamin D sufficiency for all, we can reengage our body's innate, powerful systems for preventing, and even reversing, the fire of inflammation within our arteries. The path to a healthy heart may be as simple, and as profound, as stepping back into the light.

# CHAPTER 12

# THE SUNSHINE SHIELD: VITAMIN D, THE IMMUNE SYSTEM, AND THE BATTLE AGAINST CANCER

The story of cancer in the modern world is a tale of paradox. As we have conquered many infectious diseases and extended lifespans, we have witnessed a relentless rise in the incidence of various cancers. This surge, particularly since the mid-twentieth century, cannot be explained by genetics or aging alone. A very concerning development is a dramatic increase in cancers that usually plague the elderly in a much younger group in the prime of their life.[1] It points toward profound changes in our environment and lifestyle. This chapter will explore a compelling and increasingly supported hypothesis: that a significant portion of this increase is also linked to a widespread, silent epidemic of vitamin D deficiency, driven primarily by a societal shift away from sun exposure.

We will journey through the epidemiological evidence linking low vitamin D status to higher cancer risk. We will then delve into the intricate dance between our immune system and cancer, exploring how a healthy immune response prevents cancer and how a dysfunctional one, often characterized by chronic inflammation, can actively promote it. The central idea of this chapter is that vitamin D is not merely a vitamin but a master regulator of the immune system. Its deficiency cripples our natural defenses, creating a fertile ground for cancer to develop. Finally, we will examine the cutting edge of oncology—immunotherapy—and reveal a stunning irony: These revolutionary, multibillion-dollar drugs often work by pharmacologically mimicking the very immune-regulating functions that sufficient vitamin D naturally provides. This chapter will show that many cancers may be, in part, diseases of vitamin D deficiency, and that restoring our natural "sunshine shield" is a critical, yet overlooked, strategy in cancer prevention.

## THE RISING TIDE OF CANCER: AN EPIDEMIOLOGICAL PUZZLE

Since the 1960s, a clear and disturbing trend has emerged: The incidence of many types of cancer has significantly increased in industrialized nations. While improved diagnostics account for some of this rise, the magnitude and pattern of the increase point to underlying environmental and lifestyle factors.[2, 3, 4] One such environmental factor is sun exposure and vitamin D. Reduced sun exposure and low serum 25(OH)D concentrations are associated with increased risk for twelve types of cancer, including melanoma.[5]

**Colorectal Cancer:** Incidence rates for colorectal cancer have been rising, particularly in younger adults under fifty, a group for whom screening is not routine.[6] Epidemiological studies have long suggested a strong link between vitamin D status and colorectal cancer risk. Landmark research by Garland and Garland in the 1980s first proposed that vitamin D from sun exposure could reduce the risk of colon cancer, an observation supported by decades of subsequent research showing a 30 to 50 percent reduction in risk in individuals with the highest vitamin D levels compared to the lowest.[7, 8] They found that those with serum 25(OH)D levels between 27 and 32 ng/mL had a 75 percent lower risk of colon cancer, and those with levels between 33 and 41 ng/mL enjoyed an 80 percent lower risk compared to those with low concentrations of 25(OH)D (4 to 19 ng/mL).[9]

**Breast Cancer:** Breast cancer is the most common cancer in women worldwide. Its incidence has risen steadily over the past several decades. Numerous studies have shown an inverse correlation between vitamin D levels and breast cancer risk. Women with higher blood levels of 25-hydroxyvitamin D, 25(OH)D, the marker for vitamin D status, have a significantly lower risk of developing breast cancer, with some studies suggesting up to a 50 percent risk reduction.[10, 11] Specifically, an analysis of 1,760 women found that those with serum 25(OH)D concentrations of 52 ng/mL had a 50 percent lower risk of developing breast cancer compared to women with levels below 13 ng/mL.[12]

**Prostate Cancer:** While mortality has decreased due to better treatments, the incidence of prostate cancer remains high and has increased over the past fifty years. It is particularly aggressive in men of African descent (who are in the West), who are also more likely to be vitamin D deficient due to darker skin pigmentation, which reduces vitamin D synthesis from sunlight.[13] Studies indicate that men with vitamin D deficiency have a higher risk of being diagnosed with more aggressive forms of prostate cancer.[14]

**Melanoma and Other Skin Cancers:** This one presents a paradox. While excessive, burning sun exposure is a known risk factor for melanoma, studies suggest that chronic, non-burning sun exposure, which leads to higher vitamin D levels, is associated with increased survival from melanoma.[15] This suggests that while UV radiation can initiate skin cancer, vitamin D produced by that same UV exposure may equip the immune system to better control the disease once it appears. For nonmelanoma skin cancers like basal cell and squamous cell carcinoma, occupational sun exposure, as would be obtained by those that work outdoors, appears protective against melanoma, hinting at the complex, dose-dependent role of sunlight and vitamin D.[16]

**Lung Cancer:** In individuals with lung cancer, a significant impairment of vitamin D metabolism occurs, largely due to the upregulation of the enzyme CYP24A1, also known as 24-hydroxylase. This enzyme is frequently overexpressed in lung tumor tissues.[17] When CYP24A1 is upregulated, its increased catalytic activity rapidly converts the bioactive form of vitamin D, 1,25(OH)2D3, into its inactive metabolite, 24,25-(OH)2D3. This accelerated metabolism of vitamin D leads to a reduction in circulating levels of active vitamin D. In essence the cancer is attacking vitamin D, which implies that vitamin D is destructive to the cancer. Studies have also shown that serum 25-(OH) D levels progressively decline in cancer patients as lung tumor stages advance, further highlighting this metabolic abnormality. The implication of this impairment is that lung cancer patients may benefit from therapeutic strategies that incorporate vitamin D. And that devising methods to block the increased CYP24A1 in lung cancer may be a fruitful area of research.

This parallel rise of cancer incidence and vitamin D deficiency is not a coincidence. It is the first clue that a fundamental biological system, governed by vitamin D, has been compromised. That system is our immune system.

## THE SUNSCREEN PARADOX: WHY MELANOMA KEEPS RISING IN THE AGE OF SUN AVOIDANCE AND SUNSCREEN PROTECTION

For more than four decades, the public has been given a clear message: Wear sunscreen, avoid the sun, and you will lower your risk of skin cancer. It is a message that has been repeated by doctors, cancer charities, and government health agencies around the world. And the public has listened. Sunscreen use has increased dramatically since the 1970s, and sun protection is now a routine part of daily life for millions of people. Yet despite all of this, the most dangerous form of skin cancer—malignant melanoma—has not declined. It has risen sharply, and continues to rise today.

This is not a minor statistical footnote. It is a full-scale paradox, and it is beginning to attract serious scientific scrutiny. Two important recent studies have now formalized what epidemiologists have quietly noticed for years: Sunscreen use is simply not associated with a reduction in melanoma risk. What neither study fully addresses, however, is the most biologically plausible explanation for why this might be true—one that is hiding in plain sight.

Before exploring the science, it helps to understand the scale of the problem. Melanoma is the fifth-most-common cancer in the United States, and it is the most lethal form of skin cancer. When caught early, it can be cured with surgery. When it spreads, it is notoriously difficult to treat, with historically poor survival rates at the metastatic stage.

The incidence of melanoma has been increasing since at least 1975, the year the US National Cancer Institute began systematic tracking through its SEER (Surveillance, Epidemiology, and End Results) database.[18] This upward trend has unfolded alongside—and despite—a massive expansion in sunscreen use, sun avoidance messaging, and UV protection clothing. The two curves, rising sunscreen adoption and rising melanoma incidence, have moved in the same direction for half a century.

## WHAT THE RESEARCH ACTUALLY SHOWS: NO PROTECTIVE EFFECT

A major 2025 systematic review and meta-analysis published in *Anticancer Research* by Brunner, Haddad, and colleagues at Saarland University Medical Center in Germany analyzed twenty-three published studies examining the relationship between sunscreen use and melanoma risk.[19] The findings are striking in their clarity.

Pooled analysis of the twenty-three studies found that there is no meaningful statistical association between sunscreen use and melanoma risk, in either direction. People who regularly used sunscreen were no less likely to develop melanoma than people who rarely or never used it.

This is not a fringe finding. It is the result of the most comprehensive analysis of this specific question to date, conducted by mainstream academic dermatologists and published in a peer-reviewed oncology journal. A population advised to apply sunscreen since the 1970s got zero benefit in terms of the major reason for using sunscreen: lowered risk of melanoma!

## FIVE EXPLANATIONS—BUT ONE IS MISSING

Researchers at Harvard Medical School and Massachusetts General Hospital tackled the same paradox in a 2023 paper published in *Cancers*. Lapides and colleagues reviewed the available literature and generated five hypotheses to explain why melanoma incidence continues to rise despite increased sunscreen use.[20]

Their five proposed explanations were:

1. **Increased Awareness and Reporting:** Better detection and diagnostic technology may be identifying more melanomas that would previously have gone unnoticed or been misclassified.
2. **Longer Time in the Sun:** People who use sunscreen may feel protected and therefore spend significantly more time outdoors in strong sunlight, potentially canceling out any biological benefit.

3. **Lack of Broad-Spectrum Protection:** Older sunscreens primarily blocked UVB rays but allowed UVA rays to penetrate. UVA is now understood to play a role in melanoma development, and early sunscreens may have given people false confidence while leaving them vulnerable.
4. **Reactive Oxygen Species (ROS) Formation:** Some sunscreen chemicals, when activated by UV light, may actually generate harmful free radicals—reactive molecules that can damage DNA. This is particularly true of the ingredient avobenzone and some others when they degrade in sunlight.
5. **Climate Change and Changing Vacation Habits:** More warm days and the growing trend of high-UV winter travel destinations expose people—including children—to intense sunlight for which they are unprepared.

These are all reasonable hypotheses, and some are supported by meaningful evidence. But a careful reader will immediately notice what is absent from this list. Not one of the five hypotheses considers what sunscreen does to the body's ability to maintain its own natural cancer defenses.

## THE MISSING HYPOTHESIS: WHAT SUNSCREEN TAKES AWAY

Sunscreen works by blocking UV radiation from reaching the skin. That is, of course, exactly what it is designed to do. But UV radiation, specifically UVB, is also the primary way the human body produces vitamin D. When sunscreen effectively blocks UVB, it also dramatically reduces vitamin D synthesis in the skin.

This is not a controversial point. It is basic physiology, acknowledged by dermatologists and vitamin D researchers alike. The question that the Lapides paper, the Brunner et al. meta-analysis, and most of the mainstream sunscreen-and-melanoma literature conspicuously fail to ask is this: What happens to melanoma risk when circulating vitamin D levels fall?

The answer, it turns out, is deeply relevant—and it may be the most biologically plausible explanation for the sunscreen paradox that nobody in the mainstream discussion is naming.

## VITAMIN D'S DOCUMENTED ANTICANCER PROPERTIES IN MELANOMA

The relationship between vitamin D and melanoma has been examined in a second major 2025 paper from the same group that published the sunscreen meta-analysis. Haddad, Weise, and Reichrath, writing in *Anticancer Research*, conducted a systematic review and nine separate meta-analyses on vitamin

D status as a risk and prognostic factor in melanoma.[21] Their findings are significant.

Patients diagnosed with melanoma had significantly lower mean circulating vitamin D levels compared to healthy control subjects. There was also a clear trend, consistent across multiple analyses, toward worsened melanoma prognosis in patients with true vitamin D deficiency, measured by all recognized prognostic factors including tumor thickness, mitotic rate, stage, and ulceration.

The mechanisms behind this association are well established at the cellular level. The vitamin D receptor (VDR) is expressed in melanocytes—the very skin cells that give rise to melanoma—and VDR has been described as functioning as a tumor suppressor in the skin.[22] When vitamin D activates VDR, it triggers a cascade of anticancer responses.

Specifically, active vitamin D has been shown to: inhibit the proliferation of melanoma cells; suppress tumor invasion and angiogenesis (the process by which tumors grow new blood vessels to feed themselves) through an IL-8-regulated pathway; induce differentiation of melanoma cells (pushing them toward normal cell behavior); stimulate apoptosis—programmed cancer cell death—by repressing survival proteins and inducing pro-death proteins; and enhance the activity of DNA repair mechanisms including p53, the genome's primary guardian against mutations.[23]

A comprehensive 2024 review in *Cancers* by Slominski and colleagues concluded explicitly that active forms of vitamin D can prevent or inhibit melanoma development and progression, and proposed that vitamin D biology offers real solutions for the prevention and therapy of melanoma.

As early as 1981, Colston and colleagues found vitamin D receptors in malignant melanoma tissue and showed that vitamin D's inhibitory effects on melanoma cells were dose-related. The science here is not new.[24] It has simply been ignored in the sunscreen-and-melanoma debate.

## THE IRONY AT THE HEART OF THE PARADOX

When these two bodies of evidence are placed side by side, the irony is difficult to escape. Sunscreen is applied specifically to block UV radiation. Blocking UV radiation substantially reduces the body's ability to produce vitamin D. Vitamin D has well-documented, dose-related anticancer effects on the exact cells that give rise to melanoma. Melanoma incidence has risen continuously and in parallel with increased sunscreen use. And the most thorough analysis of this relationship to date finds no protective association between sunscreen use and melanoma risk.

What is perhaps most remarkable is that the Lapides paper—the most focused published effort to explain this paradox—examined five possible reasons for it and did not mention vitamin D once.[25] There is no discussion in the paper of the possibility that sunscreen's mechanism of blocking UV might simultaneously eliminate the body's primary anticancer hormonal defense against the very cancer under discussion. It should be noted that the authors of the Lapides paper were all dermatologists.

This is not a minor oversight. Vitamin D's anticancer properties in melanocytes are not obscure findings from a handful of cell culture experiments. They are supported by multiple systematic reviews, meta-analyses, and decades of experimental evidence across in vitro, animal, and human epidemiological studies. The omission represents a significant gap in the academic conversation.

This does not mean that UV radiation is harmless, or that sunburn is safe. UV exposure is a genuine risk factor for skin cancer, particularly for squamous cell carcinoma and for melanoma caused by intermittent, intense, burning exposures. The goal is not to abandon all sun protection, but to stop treating blanket sun avoidance and chemical sunscreen use as a proven strategy against melanoma when the evidence does not support that conclusion—and when that strategy may be eliminating a critical line of biological defense.

The major justification given since the 1970s for avoiding the sun and slathering on sunscreen is to reduce the risk of melanoma. Clearly, that goal has not been achieved as melanoma incidence continues to increase despite those behaviors. What has been achieved is a vitamin D–starved population that is suffering the wrath of that misguided advice in the form of epidemic levels of autoimmune disease, cardiovascular disease, cancer, neurological disease and accelerated aging.

## THE GUARDIAN WITHIN: THE IMMUNE SYSTEM'S WAR ON CANCER

Our immune system is our body's department of defense. Its best-known role is fighting off external invaders like bacteria and viruses. However, it has an equally critical, though less appreciated, function: immunosurveillance. This is the process by which immune cells patrol the body, identifying and eliminating nascent cancer cells before they can form a clinically relevant tumor.[26]

The development of cancer is often a story of immune escape. A tumor succeeds not just by growing fast, but by learning to hide from, suppress, or even co-opt the immune system. A key mechanism in this process is inflammation.

## CHRONIC INFLAMMATION: THE BETRAYAL OF A HEALING RESPONSE

Inflammation is a double-edged sword. Acute inflammation is a lifesaving response to injury or infection, marshaling immune cells to clear debris and pathogens and initiate healing. However, when this process fails to resolve, it becomes chronic inflammation, a smoldering, low-grade state that, instead of healing, inflicts persistent damage. As the foundational work by Medzhitov explains, the very mechanisms designed for defense and repair can, when chronically activated, contribute to pathology.[27]

Chronic inflammation promotes cancer in several ways:[28]

- **Genomic Instability:** Inflammatory cells release reactive oxygen species, which can directly damage the DNA of nearby cells, leading to cancer-causing mutations.
- **Cell Proliferation:** To repair damage, inflammation releases growth factors that encourage cells to divide. In a chronic state, this constant signal to "grow" can fuel the uncontrolled proliferation of mutated cells.
- **Angiogenesis:** Tumors need a blood supply to grow. Chronic inflammation promotes the formation of new blood vessels (angiogenesis), which a tumor can hijack to nourish itself.
- **Immune Evasion:** A chronically inflamed environment can actively suppress the antitumor immune response, creating a safe haven for cancer cells to hide and thrive.

The link is now undeniable: Chronic inflammation is not just a bystander but a key driver of cancer development, progression, and metastasis. And at the heart of controlling inflammation lies vitamin D.

## HOW VITAMIN D SUPPORTS A CANCER-RESISTANT IMMUNE SYSTEM

Vitamin D's classic role is in calcium metabolism and bone health, but this is only a fraction of its true function. The active form of vitamin D, calcitriol [1,25(OH)D], acts as a potent steroid hormone that regulates the expression of hundreds of genes. The vitamin D receptor (VDR) and the enzyme that converts circulating 25(OH)D to active calcitriol are present in nearly all major immune cells, including T cells, B cells, macrophages, and dendritic cells.[29] This means the immune system is exquisitely designed to be modulated by vitamin D.[30]

The immune system is supposed to detect and destroy cancer cells just as it does bacteria or viruses—but this only works when the immune system is functioning properly. Vitamin D plays an important and underappreciated role in keeping that cancer-surveillance system sharp. Here's how it supports each of the key players involved:

**Dendritic Cells (DCs):** As discussed earlier, dendritic cells act as the immune system's scouts, capturing suspicious material—whether from a pathogen or a cancer cell—and presenting it to T cells to trigger a targeted response. Vitamin D supports dendritic cell maturation in a way that keeps the immune response effective without tipping into excessive inflammation.

When vitamin D levels are low, dendritic cells can become sluggish and less effective at sounding the alarm, which means cancer cells are more likely to go undetected and unchallenged.

- **T Lymphocytes (T Cells):** T cells carry out the actual immune attack once the scouts have identified a threat, and vitamin D influences several different types.
- **Helper T Cells (CD4+):** Coordinate the overall immune response, and as discussed in the previous section, vitamin D helps balance their activity—dampening the most aggressively inflammatory subtypes (Th1 and Th17) while encouraging the development of regulatory T cells (Tregs). It's worth noting that in the context of an already-established tumor, Tregs can actually work against the body by suppressing the very immune response needed to destroy cancer cells. However, vitamin D–supported Tregs play a more important preventative role—helping to keep the kind of chronic, low-grade inflammation in check that, over time, creates the conditions in which cancer is more likely to develop in the first place. In other words, vitamin D helps prevent the fire from starting, rather than fanning it.[31]
- **Cytotoxic T Cells (CD8+):** These are the immune system's primary cancer-killers, directly identifying and destroying tumor cells. Vitamin D's role here is about maintaining a healthy immune environment overall. While it moderates some aspects of T cell activation to prevent dangerous levels of inflammation, it also supports the ability of these cells to do their jobs effectively. When vitamin D is deficient, the resulting dysfunction across the immune system weakens these cells' ability to recognize tumor cells and carry out the kill—giving cancer a meaningful advantage.
- **Macrophages, the Heavy Infantry:** Macrophages are powerful, versatile immune cells that can behave in very different ways depending on their environment. In their M1 state, they are aggressive inflammation-promoting cancer fighters. In their M2 state, they shift into a tissue-repair and anti-inflammatory mode. Both states serve legitimate purposes in the right context—but tumors are remarkably good at hijacking M2 macrophages and reprogramming them to assist with their own growth and spread, essentially turning a defensive cell into an accomplice.

  Vitamin D helps regulate this balance by guiding macrophages toward a more flexible, middle-ground state—one that is capable of fighting genuine threats without locking into the chronic inflammatory mode that damages healthy tissue or the passive M2 mode that tumors exploit. When vitamin D levels are adequate, macrophages are better equipped to respond appropriately to what the situation actually demands. When deficiency is present, this balance breaks down, and the immune environment becomes easier for tumors to manipulate.[32]

In short, a vitamin D–sufficient state is one of immune balance between phasic, healthy immunity and chronic, harmful inflammation. This vitamin D–mediated balance allows for a strong, targeted attack against legitimate threats like cancer cells while simultaneously holding in check the chronic, smoldering inflammation that helps cancer grow. Vitamin D deficiency removes this master regulator, leading to an immune system that is both ineffective against tumor formation and prone to the very chronic inflammation that fuels tumors.

## MODERN IMMUNOTHERAPY: A PHARMACOLOGICAL MIMIC OF VITAMIN D'S FUNCTION

Some of the most celebrated advances in modern cancer treatment involve a class of drugs called immune checkpoint inhibitors. These drugs work by releasing the brakes that tumors apply to the immune system, freeing T cells to recognize and destroy cancer cells. What is remarkable—and largely underappreciated—is how closely these drugs mirror what vitamin D does naturally in the body. Understanding this connection reframes vitamin D deficiency not just as a health inconvenience, but as a potentially serious gap in the body's built-in cancer defenses.

The two most important immune checkpoints are CTLA-4 and PD-1.

- **CTLA-4 (Cytotoxic T-Lymphocyte-Associated Protein 4):** Acts as an early "brake" on T cell activation, preventing an overexuberant initial immune response.
- **PD-1 (Programmed Cell Death Protein 1):** Acts as a later "brake" on T cells that are already activated. Many tumor cells have an affinity for the receptor, PD-L1, which allows them to directly engage the PD-1 brake on T cells and shut them down just as they are about to attack.

Let's examine the leading immunotherapy drugs and their striking connection to the functions of vitamin D:

## ANTI-PD-1 DRUGS: RELEASING THE BRAKE ON T CELLS

Pembrolizumab (Keytruda) and nivolumab (Opdivo) are among the most widely used cancer immunotherapy drugs in the world, approved for treating melanoma, lung cancer, kidney cancer, head and neck cancers, and more. They work by blocking a receptor on T cells called PD-1. Under normal circumstances, tumor cells exploit this receptor by displaying a molecule called PD-L1 on their surface—essentially flashing a "stand down" signal that tricks T cells into going dormant instead of attacking. These drugs block that interaction, stripping the tumor of its ability to silence the immune response.

Vitamin D does something remarkably similar. Research has shown that adequate vitamin D levels directly suppress the expression of PD-L1 on cancer cells and on inflammatory immune cells. In other words, vitamin D naturally reduces the tumor's ability to hijack and display that "stand down" signal in the first place. Keytruda and Opdivo are powerful, pharmaceutical ways of achieving an outcome that sufficient vitamin D levels help bring about on their own.[33, 34]

## ANTI-CTLA-4 DRUGS: STRENGTHENING THE INITIAL IMMUNE ATTACK

Ipilimumab (Yervoy), used to treat melanoma, kidney cancer, and colorectal cancer, works through a different but related mechanism. It blocks a checkpoint called CTLA-4, which normally puts a cap on T cell activation early in the immune response. By blocking it, ipilimumab allows T cells to mount a stronger, more aggressive initial attack against tumor cells.[35] The CTLA-4 pathway is deeply intertwined with the balance between active, attacking T cells and regulatory T cells—the immune system's referees that prevent overreaction. As discussed in previous sections, vitamin D is a master regulator of exactly this balance. By promoting healthy Treg function and maintaining overall immune equilibrium, vitamin D helps ensure the immune system doesn't become so dysregulated that these checkpoint pathways have to work overtime in the first place. Chronic vitamin D deficiency, by contrast, can tip the immune system out of balance in ways that allow these checkpoints to become overly dominant—making it easier for tumors to exploit them.

## ANTI-PD-L1 DRUGS: TARGETING THE TUMOR'S SILENCING MOLECULE DIRECTLY

A third category of checkpoint inhibitors—including atezolizumab (Tecentriq) and avelumab (Bavencio), used for bladder cancer, lung cancer, and breast cancer—represents the flip side of the anti-PD-1 approach. Rather than blocking the PD-1 receptor on the T cell, these drugs block the PD-L1 molecule on the tumor cell itself. The end result is the same: The tumor loses its ability to flash that "stand down" signal at approaching T cells.[36]

Once again, this is a function that vitamin D naturally supports. By directly suppressing PD-L1 expression on tumor cells, adequate vitamin D levels reduce the tumor's silencing power through the same mechanism these drugs are specifically engineered to replicate. The fact that multiple billion-dollar drug classes are essentially doing pharmacologically what vitamin D does biologically should give serious pause to anyone who views vitamin D as a minor nutritional footnote. It is, in this light, one of the body's own built-in checkpoint regulators—and deficiency in it represents a meaningful and largely preventable weakening of that system.

Consistent with all of the above, patients with higher vitamin D levels have been shown to have better responses to ICI therapy.[37] Some emerging clinical trial data suggest systematic vitamin D repletion during immunotherapy enhances efficacy and immune activation while maintaining safety.[38] In a very exciting finding, doctors in China have found that vitamin D acts synergistically with immune checkpoint inhibitor drugs to enhance the efficacy of those drugs in treating lung cancer and melanoma.[39, 40] The findings were that patients with higher serum vitamin D levels had better responses and outcomes to the ICI cancer treatments.

This evidence leads to a powerful and provocative conclusion. The cancer immunotherapy industry is, in large part, built upon creating drugs that correct an immune dysfunction—over-expression of immune checkpoints like PD-L1—that is exacerbated or even caused by chronic inflammation and a lack of the immune system's master regulator, vitamin D. This is not to say that these drugs are clones of vitamin D. There are subtleties in function and outcome that distinguish this class of drugs from the effects of vitamin D on immune regulation. One of the differences is the incidence of side effects. There are no side effects with vitamin D. As apparently brilliant as these drugs appear, they suffer a fatal flaw: lack of specificity. Disrupting the built-in safety mechanisms with ICI drugs affects not only cancer cells but healthy cells as well. This defect results in the immune system unleashing hell on both the cancer cells and the patient's healthy cells, causing devastating and sometimes fatal outcomes.

## CANCER AS A DISEASE OF IMMUNE DYSFUNCTION DRIVEN BY VITAMIN D DEFICIENCY

Let us integrate these threads into a single, cohesive thought regarding vitamin D, the immune system, and cancer:

1. **The Cause:** For much of human history, we lived outdoors, and our bodies evolved under the expectation of ample sun exposure and, consequently, sufficient vitamin D. The modern shift to an indoor lifestyle, coupled with aggressive sun avoidance messaging, has created a population-wide state of chronic vitamin D deficiency.

2. **The Consequence:** This deficiency cripples the immune system's regulatory capacity. Without its hormonal guide, the immune system becomes prone to chronic, low-grade inflammation. It loses the balance between aggressive action and tolerant self-control.
3. **The Mechanism:** This chronic inflammation, as detailed by modern cancer biology, directly fuels cancer. It damages DNA, promotes cell proliferation, and builds a supportive microenvironment for tumors. Simultaneously, the dysregulated immune system fails at its job of immunosurveillance, allowing mutated cells to survive and thrive. The tumor itself then learns to exploit the dysregulation, for example by upregulating PD-L1 to shut down any remaining T cell response, among several other immune evasion strategies.
4. **The Treatment:** After decades of this process culminating in a cancer diagnosis, the patient is treated with revolutionary immunotherapeutic drugs. These drugs, such as anti-PD-1/PD-L1 inhibitors, work spectacularly in some patients by blocking the very "off switch" manipulation that the tumor is using to protect itself.
5. **The Irony:** The fundamental irony is that the immune dysfunction being treated—an exhausted T cell response suppressed by checkpoints like PD-1/PD-L1—is a hallmark of a chronically inflamed, dysregulated state that vitamin D is physiologically programmed to prevent. We are using highly advanced, expensive pharmaceuticals to fix a problem that should never have occurred, or would have been far less severe,[41] if the person had maintained the vitamin D status our species evolved to maintain for millennia.

It is not an overstatement to propose that many modern cancers are, at their core, diseases of a dysfunctional immune system,[42] and that this dysfunction is significantly driven by the chronic inflammation resulting from vitamin D deficiency. We are again treating the downstream symptoms of this deficiency with brilliant yet side-effect-ridden pharmacology, while largely ignoring the upstream cause.

## VITAMIN D BLOCKS A MAJOR SIDE EFFECT OF ICI DRUGS

As an example of the cross talk between vitamin D and immune checkpoint inhibitors consider the major side effect of colitis from ICI drugs. In particular, immune-related colitis is among the most frequent and severe adverse reactions often leading to treatment interruption, immunosuppression that may negatively impact tumor immune response, and ICI discontinuation. It was found that melanoma cancer patients taking vitamin D at the time their first ICI treatment was initiated had significantly reduced odds of developing ICI colitis over the course of their immunotherapy regimen.[43] These results suggest benefit in prophylactic use of vitamin D supplementation to prevent ICI colitis. For the purposes of our discussion, it shows that ICI drugs and vitamin D appear to be operating in the same and complementary immunological spaces.

Furthermore, the studies mentioned earlier that found that vitamin D status of lung cancer and melanoma patients greatly influenced the effectiveness of ICI drugs, indicates an interesting synergistic effect between the ICI drugs and vitamin D on cancer.

## REENGAGING OUR NATURAL DEFENSES

This chapter does not claim that vitamin D is a "cure" for cancer, although others have suggested that vitamin D be repurposed as a cancer treatment.[44] Exciting new cancer cures using safe repurposed drugs including the antiparasitic fenbendazole, are the subject of intense research.[45, 46] Through its regulation and optimization of the immune system vitamin D is better thought of as a potent preventative for the development of cancer.[47] Cancer is a complex, multifactorial disease. However, the evidence is overwhelming that vitamin D is a foundational pillar of a healthy immune system capable of resisting cancer getting a foothold. In fact, a recent review article on vitamin D and cancer suggests that achieving a population-wide serum 25(OH)D concentration of 80 ng/mL would reduce cancer incidence rates by 70 percent.[48] Its role as a systemic immune regulator, a suppressor of chronic inflammation, and a direct modulator of cancer-relevant pathways like PD-L1 expression places it at the center of cancer prevention.

The modern immunotherapy revolution is a testament to the power of our own immune system. But it also serves as a stark warning. The very success of these drugs highlights the profound immune failure they are designed to correct. The great irony is that we may be paying billions to pharmacologically correct a deficiency that could be largely avoided by sensible sun exposure, and when necessary, simple supplementation. Restoring physiological vitamin D sufficiency across the population represents one of the most cost-effective, evidence-based, and profound public health strategies available for reducing the burden of cancer.

# CHAPTER 13

# VITAMIN D: A MASTER REGULATOR OF METABOLIC HEALTH, OBESITY, AND CANCER

The modern world is facing a collision of epidemics. Obesity, metabolic disorders like type 2 diabetes, and cancer are not separate crises but deeply interconnected public health challenges. With over a billion people worldwide now living with obesity, the downstream consequences are becoming devastatingly clear.[1] Not so long ago it used to be that there was one fat kid in a group, now there is one skinny kid in a group of fat kids. Obesity is not a passive state of excess weight; it is a metabolically disruptive force that creates systemic inflammation, insulin resistance, and hormonal chaos—a perfect storm that significantly increases the risk for both type 2 diabetes and numerous cancers.

In this complex landscape, vitamin D emerges as a critical modifying factor. We now understand that vitamin D is a powerful steroid hormone that exerts profound regulatory control over immunity, inflammation, and cellular growth. This chapter will first illuminate the role of vitamin D in maintaining metabolic health and how its deficiency contributes to obesity and diabetes. We will then explore the mechanisms by which this metabolic dysfunction drives cancer, detail how obesity itself compromises vitamin D status, and demonstrate how restoring vitamin D sufficiency can serve as a powerful biological countermeasure to the pro-carcinogenic environment created by metabolic disease.

## VITAMIN D AND THE METABOLIC CRISIS: A FOCUS ON OBESITY AND DIABETES

The link between low vitamin D levels and metabolic disorders is exceptionally strong and consistent. Large-scale analyses have shown that individuals with the lowest vitamin D levels have a significantly higher risk of developing type

2 diabetes compared to those with the highest levels.[2] While this is an observation, a deeper look at physiology reveals clear mechanisms by which vitamin D actively protects metabolic health. This is not a simple correlation; it is a matter of biological cause and effect.

The role of vitamin D in preventing and managing diabetes unfolds through several key actions:

**Supporting Pancreatic Beta-Cell Function:** The very cells in the pancreas responsible for producing and secreting insulin—known as beta cells—are equipped with vitamin D receptors (VDRs). When vitamin D binds to these receptors, it helps protect the beta cells from inflammatory damage and improves their ability to release insulin in response to blood sugar.[3] In a state of vitamin D deficiency, these critical cells become less efficient and more vulnerable, impairing the body's primary defense against high blood sugar.

**Improving Insulin Sensitivity:** Type 2 diabetes is defined by insulin resistance, a condition where the body's cells no longer respond properly to insulin's signal to absorb glucose from the blood. Vitamin D directly combats this in two ways. First, it powerfully suppresses the chronic inflammation that is a primary driver of insulin resistance.[4] Second, it appears to directly enhance the expression and function of the insulin receptor on cells, making them more receptive to insulin's signal.

**Quelling Adipose Tissue Inflammation:** In obesity, adipose (fat) tissue is not a passive storage site. It becomes an active, inflamed endocrine organ, churning out pro-inflammatory cytokines like tumor necrosis factor-alpha (TNF-$\alpha$) and interleukin-6 (IL-6). These inflammatory molecules spill into the bloodstream and are a major cause of the systemic insulin resistance seen in obesity.[5] Vitamin D acts as a master regulator of inflammation, directly inhibiting the pathways that produce these harmful cytokines, thereby calming the metabolic fire stoked by excess fat. This creates a dangerous feedback loop. Obesity itself leads to lower vitamin D levels, and those lower levels, in turn, exacerbate the metabolic dysfunction caused by obesity. This is the vitamin D paradox: The very condition that most needs its protective effects is the one that actively depletes it.

## VITAMIN D, GUT BACTERIA, AND GUT HEALTH

In contrast to these "anti-synergistic" effects of obesity on vitamin D availability, vitamin D is associated with an increase in the abundance of Bifidobacterium species—including *B. bifidum*—in the gut, supporting a mutually beneficial relationship between vitamin D and these key probiotic bacteria.[6]

Vitamin D supplementation has been shown in multiple clinical trials to significantly increase the relative abundance of Bifidobacterium in the human gut microbiota.[7] This shift is considered beneficial, as Bifidobacterium species play important roles in gut health, immune modulation, and maintenance of the intestinal barrier.

Studies indicate that not only does vitamin D favor the growth of Bifidobacterium, but also that certain Bifidobacterium strains (such as *B. longum*) can enhance vitamin D metabolism and upregulate expression of the vitamin D receptor (VDR) in intestinal cells.[8] The interaction is bidirectional: Vitamin D increases Bifidobacterium abundance, and Bifidobacterium can potentially amplify the biological effects of vitamin D. Increases in Bifidobacterium linked with vitamin D are correlated with improved gut barrier integrity, reduced inflammation, enhanced folate and amino acid production, and potential protection against gut dysbiosis and bowel inflammation.[9] Additionally, probiotic strains such as *B. longum* have been found to increase blood levels of bioactive vitamin D metabolites, suggesting a reinforcing loop between vitamin D and bifidobacterial activity.[10]

This mutual relationship highlights the importance of adequate vitamin D levels for supporting a beneficial gut microbiome, particularly populations of Bifidobacterium, which in turn may optimize the actions of vitamin D within the body.

## FROM METABOLIC DYSFUNCTION TO MALIGNANCY: OBESITY AS A CARCINOGENIC FORCE

The state of chronic inflammation and insulin resistance that defines obesity and type 2 diabetes does more than disrupt blood sugar; it creates fertile ground for cancer. The evidence is now unequivocal: Excess body fat is a major risk factor for at least seventeen different types of cancer, including colorectal, postmenopausal breast, endometrial, and pancreatic cancers.[11] Obesity is estimated to be a direct contributor to 4 to 8 percent of all cancer cases globally[12], and being obese at the time of diagnosis is associated with a 17 percent increased risk of dying from the disease.[13] This link is driven by the same biological disruptions that cause metabolic disease, now amplified to the point of promoting malignancy.

Comprehensive reviews by Avgerinos et al. (2019)[14] and Martinez & Grant (2025)[15] identified several key mechanisms:

### CHRONIC INFLAMMATION AND OXIDATIVE STRESS

As discussed, obese adipose tissue secretes a storm of pro-inflammatory cytokines. This constant inflammation promotes genetic instability and drives uncontrolled cell division. At the same time, dysfunctional mitochondria in fat cells produce an excess of reactive oxygen species (ROS), which inflict direct damage on DNA, leading to cancer-causing mutations.[16]

- **Insulin Resistance and Hyperinsulinemia:** Obesity-induced insulin resistance forces the pancreas to pump out excessive amounts of insulin. Both insulin and the related insulin-like growth factor 1 (IGF-1) are potent growth factors that command cells to divide and prevent them from dying—precisely the signals that fuel tumor growth.[17]
- **Sex Hormone Dysregulation:** Excess fat tissue contains the enzyme aromatase, which converts androgens into estrogens. In postmenopausal women, this results in high estrogen levels, a primary driver of breast and endometrial cancers.[18]
- **Adipokine Imbalance:** Obese adipose tissue secretes high levels of leptin, which promotes cell proliferation, and low levels of adiponectin, which is anti-inflammatory and tumor-suppressing.[19]
- **Activation of the Renin-Angiotensin System (RAS):** Known for regulating blood pressure, the RAS is overactivated in obesity. Its primary product, angiotensin II, is a powerful promoter of cell proliferation, inflammation, and angiogenesis (the growth of new blood vessels that feed tumors).[20]

## THE VITAMIN D PARADOX: COMPROMISED BY THE VERY CONDITION IT CAN HELP

A critical consequence of obesity is its profoundly negative impact on vitamin D status. A major meta-analysis established that individuals with obesity have a 35 percent higher prevalence of vitamin D deficiency compared to their normal-weight counterparts.[21] This is a direct physiological consequence driven by two primary mechanisms:

1. **Sequestration in Adipose Tissue:** As a fat-soluble hormone, vitamin D is eagerly taken up and stored by fat tissue. In an individual with obesity, the massive reservoir of body fat acts like a sponge, trapping vitamin D and preventing its release into the circulation where it is needed.[22]
2. **Volumetric Dilution:** The larger body and blood volume of an obese individual means that any given amount of vitamin D becomes more diluted, resulting in a lower serum concentration.[23] This creates the ultimate paradox: The very condition that elevates cancer risk through metabolic chaos simultaneously depletes the body of a key hormone that can restore order.

## VITAMIN D'S COUNTEROFFENSIVE IN OBESITY-RELATED CANCER

Given its potent anticancer and anti-inflammatory properties, vitamin D is uniquely positioned to counteract the specific oncogenic pathways activated by obesity. While it cannot reverse obesity itself, it can directly target and neutralize many of its downstream consequences.

The active form of vitamin D, calcitriol, binds to the VDR found in nearly all cells, including cancer cells, to initiate a powerful anticancer program.[24] Here is how vitamin D mounts its counteroffensive against the pro-cancer environment of obesity:

- **Countering Inflammation and Oxidative Stress:** Vitamin D directly suppresses the pro-inflammatory cytokines (IL-6, TNF-α) that are overproduced by obese adipose tissue.[25] It also bolsters the body's own antioxidant defenses, mitigating the DNA-damaging oxidative stress that drives carcinogenesis.[26]
- **Regulating the Insulin/IGF-1 Axis:** Vitamin D helps normalize the IGF-1 axis by reducing levels of the growth-promoter IGF-1 and increasing levels of its inhibitor, IGF-binding protein 3 (IGFBP-3), which prevents it from fueling cancer cell growth.[27]
- **Taming the Renin-Angiotensin System (RAS):** This is one of vitamin D's most important and direct actions. Vitamin D is a direct negative regulator of the renin gene, the enzyme that initiates the entire RAS cascade. By suppressing renin, vitamin D lowers the production of cancer-promoting angiotensin II, effectively disarming this key pathway.[28, 29]
- **Correcting Sex Hormone Signaling**: In breast cancer, vitamin D counteracts the effects of estrogen by suppressing the aromatase enzyme (reducing estrogen production) and downregulating the estrogen receptor itself, blunting its proliferative signal.[30]
- **Restoring Gut Health:** Recent groundbreaking research shows that vitamin D's anticancer effects depend partly on a healthy gut microbiome. It promotes the growth of beneficial bacteria that are important for a robust antitumor immune response, helping to reverse the gut dysbiosis associated with obesity. [31, 32]

## CLINICAL IMPLICATIONS AND STRATEGIC ACTION

The evidence leads to an undeniable conclusion: Correcting vitamin D deficiency is a critical and nonnegotiable strategy in managing the risks associated with obesity and metabolic disease. However, the sequestration and dilution effects of obesity on vitamin D mean that standard supplementation doses are simply not enough. Data from the VITAL trial stunningly revealed that while vitamin D supplementation reduced the risk of metastatic and fatal cancer by 38 percent in normal-weight individuals, no benefit was seen in participants with obesity.[33] This does not mean vitamin D is ineffective; it means the dose was too low to overcome the metabolic handicap imposed by obesity. The clinical imperative is clear. Individuals with obesity require higher doses of vitamin D to achieve the same protective serum levels as their leaner counterparts.

Research consistently shows that obese individuals need two to three times the standard dose to reach optimal serum levels.[34] For those with metabolic disease or cancer, aiming for a serum concentration of at least 50–70 ng/mL is a safe and effective target.[35] Ultimately, the most powerful strategy is a dual approach: aggressive vitamin D repletion combined with meaningful weight loss. Weight loss itself improves vitamin D status by releasing it from fat stores, creating a synergistic effect where both interventions work together to dismantle the inflammatory, pro-carcinogenic environment created by obesity.[36] Ignoring vitamin D status in an individual with obesity is to leave one of our most powerful, evidence-based tools for health restoration on the table.

# CHAPTER 14

# VITAMIN D AND THE BRAIN: QUELLING THE FIRE OF NEUROLOGICAL INFLAMMATION

The brain, long considered an immunologically privileged sanctuary, is now understood to be a site of dynamic and potent immune activity. This activity, orchestrated by a cast of specialized resident immune cells, is essential for protecting the central nervous system from pathogens and injury. However, when this immune response becomes chronic and dysregulated in the brain—a state known as neuroinflammation—it transforms from a protective force into a primary driver of neurodegeneration and disease. This chapter will explore the profound and escalating role of chronic neuroinflammation in a wide range of neurological disorders, from dementia to multiple sclerosis. We will detail the cellular and molecular mechanisms of this "fire within" and present a compelling, evidence-based argument that a widespread, modern deficiency in a critical immune-modulating hormone—vitamin D—is a key factor fueling this epidemic of brain disease.[1]

## THE RISING TIDE: A MODERN EPIDEMIC OF NEUROLOGICAL DISEASE

Since the mid-twentieth century, industrialized nations have witnessed a dramatic and alarming increase in the incidence and prevalence of a spectrum of neurological disorders. This rise has outpaced what can be explained by an aging population alone, pointing toward environmental and lifestyle factors as significant contributors.

**Alzheimer's Disease (AD) and other Dementias:** The prevalence of AD has skyrocketed. While an aging population is a factor, age-adjusted incidence rates also show an upward trend, suggesting that each successive generation faces a higher lifetime risk than the last. The global number of people living with dementia is projected to triple by 2050, highlighting a public health crisis of unprecedented scale.[2]

**Parkinson's Disease (PD):** The prevalence of PD has more than doubled globally between 1990 and 2016. It is now the fastest-growing neurological disorder in the world, a trend that cannot be solely attributed to demographic shifts.[3]

**Multiple Sclerosis (MS):** Once considered a rare disease, the global prevalence of MS has increased significantly over the past several decades, particularly in Western countries. The disease shows a distinct latitudinal gradient, with higher rates in regions farther from the equator—a classic epidemiological clue pointing toward the role of sun exposure and vitamin D.[4]

This concurrent rise across multiple, seemingly disparate conditions strongly suggests a shared underlying pathological link. A growing body of evidence identifies chronic inflammation caused by chronic vitamin D deficiency as that common, destructive thread connecting them.[5, 6]

## THE FIRE WITHIN: NEUROINFLAMMATION AS THE ENGINE OF NEURODEGENERATION

Neuroinflammation is the activation of the brain's immune system. In an acute setting, such as after a traumatic injury or infection, this response is beneficial. Microglia, the brain's resident immune cells, activate to clear debris and pathogens, then resolve, allowing for healing. However, chronic neuroinflammation is a persistent, low-grade activation of this system that inflicts continuous collateral damage on the surrounding neural tissue.[7, 8]

The mechanisms through which chronic neuroinflammation drives disease are multifaceted:

1. **Oxidative and Nitrosative Stress:** Activated immune cells, particularly microglia, release a barrage of reactive oxygen species and reactive nitrogen species. This creates a highly toxic microenvironment that damages lipids, proteins, and DNA in nearby neurons, impairing their function and triggering cell death.[9]
2. **Excitotoxicity:** Inflammatory mediators, like tumor necrosis factor-alpha (TNF-α), can cause astrocytes to release excessive amounts of the neurotransmitter glutamate. This overstimulates neurons, leading to a massive influx of calcium ions and triggering a self-destructive cascade known as excitotoxicity.[10]
3. **Protein Misfolding and Aggregation:** Neuroinflammation and the accumulation of misfolded proteins (like amyloid-beta in AD and alpha-synuclein in PD) are locked in a vicious cycle. The protein aggregates trigger an inflammatory response, and the resulting

inflammation, in turn, impairs the brain's ability to clear these toxic proteins, accelerating their accumulation.[11]

4. **Blood-Brain Barrier (BBB) Disruption**: Chronic inflammation compromises the integrity of the highly selective BBB. This allows peripheral immune cells and inflammatory molecules from the bloodstream to infiltrate the CNS, further amplifying the neuroinflammatory fire.[12]
5. **Neural Senescence:** Just as cells in the body can become senescent (a state of irreversible growth arrest), so too can brain cells. Chronic neuroinflammation is a powerful inducer of senescence in neurons and glial cells. These senescent cells cease their normal supportive functions and instead secrete a cocktail of pro-inflammatory factors known as the senescence-associated secretory phenotype (SASP), which propagates inflammation and tissue dysfunction throughout the brain, effectively accelerating brain aging.[13]

This relentless, self-perpetuating cycle of inflammation and damage is a central pathological feature of nearly all major progressive neurological diseases.

## THE CENTRAL PLAYERS: GLIAL CELLS AS DRIVERS OF NEUROINFLAMMATION

While neurons have long been the focus of neuroscience, it is the nonneuronal glial cells that are the primary orchestrators of neuroinflammation.[14] The brain contains three main types of glial cells: microglia, astrocytes, and oligodendrocytes. Microglia and astrocytes are the key drivers of the neuro-immune response.[15]

**Microglia:** Often called the brain's macrophages, microglia are the primary immune sentinels of the brain. They constantly survey their environment. In a healthy state, they exist in a resting, ready-to-act form. Upon detecting danger signals—such as pathogens, cellular debris, or misfolded proteins—they undergo a dramatic transformation. They can transform into two main functional phenotypes:

M1 (Classical Activation): This is the pro-inflammatory, "attack" mode. M1 microglia release high levels of pro-inflammatory cytokines (TNF-α, IL-1β, IL-6), reactive oxygen and nitrogen species. While necessary for fighting infection, chronic M1 activation is profoundly neurotoxic.[16]

M2 (Alternative Activation): This is the anti-inflammatory, "repair" mode. M2 microglia release anti-inflammatory cytokines (IL-10, TGF-β) and growth factors that promote tissue repair, debris clearance (phagocytosis), and the resolution of inflammation.[17]

In most neurodegenerative diseases, there is a pathological shift toward a chronic M1-dominant state.

**Astrocytes:** These star-shaped cells are the most abundant glial cells and perform a vast array of essential supportive roles for neurons. However, in response to inflammatory signals (often released by M1 microglia), they can become "reactive astrocytes." A particularly destructive subtype, known as A1 astrocytes, lose their ability to support neurons and instead acquire potent neurotoxic functions, actively killing neurons and oligodendrocytes.[18]

The dysregulated cross talk between M1 microglia and A1 astrocytes creates a powerful, self-sustaining inflammatory loop that is a cornerstone of neurodegenerative progression.

## THE VITAMIN D CONNECTION: LINKING DEFICIENCY TO DISEASE AND IMMUNITY

The epidemiological link between low sun exposure and neurological disease has a strong biological basis: vitamin D. The active form of vitamin D, calcitriol, is a potent steroid hormone that functions as a master regulator of the immune system in the brain. Importantly, the machinery needed to utilize vitamin D—both the vitamin D receptor and the enzyme that creates its active form (1α-hydroxylase)—is widely expressed throughout the brain, particularly in microglia and astrocytes.[19] This positions vitamin D to be a direct and powerful modulator of the neuro-immune functions described above.

A variety of evidence strongly links vitamin D deficiency to an increased risk and/or severity of numerous neurological conditions:

- **Multiple Sclerosis:** This is the most well-established link. Low vitamin D levels are a significant risk factor for developing MS, and among those with the disease, lower levels are associated with higher relapse rates and greater disability.[20]
- **Alzheimer's Disease:** Numerous studies have shown that vitamin D deficiency is associated with a substantially increased risk of developing AD and other dementias. Low levels correlate with poorer cognitive function and a greater burden of amyloid pathology.[21]
- **Parkinson's Disease:** A high prevalence of vitamin D deficiency is found in PD patients compared to healthy controls, and lower levels are linked to more severe motor symptoms and faster disease progression. Li et al. (2025) found that vitamin D supplementation in PD patients improved motor symptoms and shifted the immune system to a less inflammatory state.[22]

## THE MASTER REGULATOR: HOW VITAMIN D MODULATES NEURO-IMMUNITY

Vitamin D exerts its protective effects by directly targeting the cellular and molecular machinery of neuroinflammation, essentially acting as a brake on the runaway immune response.[23]

1. **Shifting Microglial Phenotype:** This is perhaps its most critical function. By binding to the VDR in microglia, vitamin D powerfully inhibits the M1 pro-inflammatory pathway while simultaneously promoting the M2 anti-inflammatory and reparative pathway. It suppresses the production of TNF-$\alpha$, IL-6, and IL-1$\beta$ and reduces the expression of inducible nitric oxide synthase (iNOS), a key source of neurotoxic RNS.[24, 25]
2. **Calming Reactive Astrocytes:** Vitamin D can suppress the activation of astrocytes, preventing them from adopting the neurotoxic A1 phenotype, thereby preserving their essential neuro-supportive functions.[26]
3. **Enhancing Debris Clearance:** Vitamin D has been shown to enhance the ability of microglia and macrophages to phagocytose (engulf and clear) amyloid-beta plaques, the hallmark pathology of Alzheimer's disease. This suggests it not only quells the inflammatory response to the plaques but also helps remove the initial trigger.[27]
4. **Direct Neuroprotection:** Beyond its immune effects, vitamin D promotes the synthesis of neurotrophic factors, such as nerve growth factor (NGF), and protects neurons directly from oxidative stress and excitotoxicity.[28]

In essence, vitamin D acts as a "rheostat" for the neuro-immune system. When levels are sufficient, it keeps the system in a state of balanced surveillance, ready to respond but biased toward resolution and repair. When levels are deficient, this rheostat is broken, leaving the system prone to hyper-activation and chronic, destructive inflammation.

## SPECIAL CASE STUDY: TRAUMATIC BRAIN INJURY, EDEMA, AND VITAMIN D

Traumatic brain injury (TBI) provides a dramatic, acute model of neuroinflammation. The initial impact triggers a massive inflammatory cascade that leads to secondary injuries, including cerebral edema (brain swelling), which is a major cause of mortality and long-term disability. This process involves glial cells and specialized water channels called aquaporins.

Aquaporins (AQPs) are a family of channel proteins that facilitate the rapid movement of water across cell membranes. Aquaporin-4 (AQP4) is the most abundant aquaporin in the brain and is located predominantly on the end-feet of astrocytes that line the blood-brain barrier and surround synapses. AQP4 is critical for maintaining water balance in the CNS. After a TBI, the inflammatory surge causes a dysregulation of AQP4. This leads to an influx of water into astrocytes, causing them to swell (cytotoxic edema), which can compress blood vessels, worsen ischemia, and increase intracranial pressure.[29]

Groundbreaking research, notably by Cekic and Stein, has highlighted that hormones with anti-inflammatory properties, like progesterone and vitamin D, can be profoundly neuroprotective after TBI. Vitamin D can mitigate post-TBI damage by reducing the initial inflammatory explosion that leads to AQP4 dysregulation. By suppressing the M1 microglial response and calming reactive astrocytes, vitamin D helps preserve the integrity of the BBB and stabilize AQP4 expression, thereby reducing the life-threatening cerebral edema that follows injury.[30] This process demonstrates how vitamin D's fundamental anti-inflammatory role translates directly into protection against acute brain injury.

## PHARMACOLOGICAL PARALLELS: MODERN DRUGS MIMICKING VITAMIN D'S EFFECTS

Many modern pharmaceuticals for neurological diseases are again, in effect, attempting to artificially replicate the specific immune-modulating functions that vitamin D performs naturally.

**Multiple Sclerosis**

Drug Class: Interferon-beta (e.g., Avonex, Betaseron)

- Pharmacological Mechanism: Modulates cytokine production, shifting the immune response to be less inflammatory.
- Parallel Vitamin D Mechanism: Shifts microglial/T cell response from pro-inflammatory to anti-inflammatory and M1 to M2 phenotype.[31]

Drug: Natalizumab (Tysabri)

- Pharmacological Mechanism: Blocks immune cells (lymphocytes) from crossing the BBB into the CNS.
- Parallel Vitamin D Mechanism: Reduces the expression of inflammatory chemokines that call immune cells to the brain and strengthens BBB integrity.[32]

Drug: Ocrelizumab (Ocrevus)

- Pharmacological Mechanism: Depletes B cells, a key immune cell type involved in attacking myelin.
- Parallel Vitamin D Mechanism: Modulates B cell function and proliferation, part of its broad immune-regulatory capacity.[33]

**Alzheimer's Disease**

Drugs: Lecanemab (Leqembi) / aducanumab (Aduhelm)

- Pharmacological Mechanism: Monoclonal antibodies that bind to and promote the clearance of amyloid-beta plaques, a process highly dependent on microglial activity.
- Parallel Vitamin D Mechanism: Directly enhances the innate ability of microglia and macrophages to clear amyloid-beta.[34]

**Parkinson's Disease**

Currently there are no drugs on the market to slow the progression or treat PD other than dopamine replacement drugs that treat the symptoms. However, there is a new focus of research in developing drugs that manipulate the immune system. Azathioprine, a commonly used drug that suppresses immune activity, has shown promise in reducing the inflammatory profile of PD.[35] You can see it, right? This wheel is being invented over and over again.

This parallel is striking. The pharmaceutical industry is spending billions to develop drugs that target specific arms of the inflammatory cascade, yet sufficient levels of the vitamin D hormone perform many of these same functions endogenously, safely, and simultaneously across multiple pathways.

## THE GRAND SYNTHESIS: A UNIFYING HYPOTHESIS FOR THE RISE IN NEUROLOGICAL DISEASE

Integrating this evidence leads to a powerful and cohesive argument:

1. **The Environmental Shift:** Since the mid-twentieth century, human behavior has radically changed. We have moved indoors, away from the sun, which is the primary source of vitamin D production. Fear of skin cancer has led to widespread sun avoidance and routine use of sunscreen, which effectively blocks vitamin D synthesis. The result is a silent, global pandemic of chronic vitamin D deficiency.
2. **The Immunological Consequence:** This chronic deficiency has left the immune systems of a large portion of the global population in a state of chronic dysregulation. Without sufficient levels of the master hormonal brake—vitamin D—the immune system is predisposed to a pro-inflammatory state attacking healthy cells.
3. **The Neurological Manifestation:** In the brain, this manifests as a lowered threshold for neuroinflammatory activation. The neuro-immune system, lacking its key regulator, overreacts to minor insults—be it aging-related cellular stress, environmental toxins, genetic predispositions, or misfolded proteins. This transforms what

should be a transient, helpful response into the chronic, smoldering fire of neuroinflammation.

4. **Disease as the Outcome:** This chronic neuroinflammation is the common soil from which a multitude of neurological diseases can grow. It accelerates brain aging (neural senescence), drives the accumulation of toxic proteins, and directly kills neurons, ultimately leading to the clinical manifestations of Alzheimer's, Parkinson's, MS, and other conditions.

The modern pharmaceuticals developed to treat these diseases are essentially reactive attempts to correct specific downstream consequences of a fundamental, upstream deficiency in vitamin D. The tragedy though is that the incidence of these neurodegenerative diseases could be greatly reduced with a population-wide adoption of a sensible sun exposure and vitamin D public health program.

Therefore, the alarming rise in neurological disease is not an unrelated collection of individual tragedies but may be, in large part, a population-wide symptom of a profound mismatch between our modern, indoor lifestyle and our ancient, sun-adapted biology.

Finally, thus far we've been discussing neuroinflammatory states caused by chronic vitamin D deficiency that can lead to neurodegenerative disease. However, neuroinflammation can also have subclinical effects, that while not indicative of neurodegeneration, can disrupt the functioning of sensitive and fragile neural networks. These subclinical effects are not obvious or dramatic but because the inflammation affects the brain, the structure that generates behavior, we must assume that pathological brain inflammation affects behavior and thought processes in recognized and unrecognized ways. This is an expansive topic that is beyond the scope of this book; however, the question must be asked: How is neuroinflammation from chronic vitamin D deficiency affecting thoughts, feelings, decision-making capability, and learning and memory capabilities? Is the vitamin D–deficient brain, with attendant neuroinflammation, functioning optimally and effectively, and rationally? A great read on the topic of neuroinflammation and decision-making capability is Michael Nehls's *The Indoctrinated Brain*.[36] Not surprisingly, his solution to the problem of neuroinflammation caused by environmental insults is . . . vitamin D.

## PREVENTION THROUGH RESTORATION

Chronic neuroinflammation is a central villain in the story of modern neurological disease. The evidence strongly suggests that chronic vitamin D deficiency is a major, modifiable risk factor that primes the brain for this destructive process. While vitamin D is not a cure for established neurodegenerative disease, its role as a fundamental requirement for a healthy and resilient neuro-immune system is undeniable.

The data implores a paradigm shift from solely focusing on expensive, late-stage pharmaceutical interventions to embracing primary prevention. Restoring physiological vitamin D sufficiency on a population-wide basis, through sensible sun exposure and/or supplementation, may be one of the most effective, accessible, and economical public health strategies available to us. By ensuring our brains have the hormonal tools they need to quell the fire of inflammation, we may be able to turn the tide against the devastating epidemic of neurological disease and safely, inexpensively, and effectively protect the brain health of generations to come.

# CHAPTER 15

# THE SHADOW OF DEFICIENCY: ALZHEIMER'S DISEASE AND THE NEUROINFLAMMATORY CRISIS

In the preceding chapter, we introduced the concept of neuroinflammation as a common thread linking various forms of dementia. We established that the brain, far from being an immunologically privileged and isolated organ, possesses a dynamic and powerful immune system. This system, when dysregulated or unbalanced, can transition from a protective force to a destructive one, driving the pathology of neurodegenerative diseases. Now, we will focus this lens on the most prevalent and feared form of dementia, Alzheimer's disease (AD), by performing a deep dive into its characteristics, potential causes, and prevention.

This chapter will show that the modern epidemic of Alzheimer's disease is inextricably linked to another, quieter epidemic: chronic, widespread vitamin D deficiency. We will explore the dramatic rise in AD incidence, delve into the mechanisms of neuroinflammation at the heart of the disease, and demonstrate how vitamin D's role as the master regulator of the neural immune system positions it as a critical, and largely overlooked, factor in the development, and potential prevention, of this devastating condition.

## THE RISING TIDE: AN UNPRECEDENTED EPIDEMIC OF ALZHEIMER'S DISEASE

For much of human history, the severe cognitive decline we now call Alzheimer's disease was considered a rare condition of "presenile dementia." However, since the mid-twentieth century, its prevalence has surged dramatically. In the 1970s, AD was still considered relatively uncommon, but by the turn of the twenty-first century, it had been recognized as a major public health crisis.[1, 2] This increase is not merely an artifact of an aging population;

while age is the single greatest risk factor, the age-specific incidence of AD has also increased, suggesting that other environmental or lifestyle factors are at play.

Today, the numbers are staggering. In the United States alone, an estimated 6.9 million people aged sixty-five and older are living with Alzheimer's dementia, a figure projected to nearly double to 13.8 million by 2060 unless medical breakthroughs are discovered to prevent, slow, or cure the disease.[3] Globally, over 55 million people live with dementia, with AD accounting for 60 to 70 percent of cases. This number is expected to rise to 78 million by 2030 and 139 million by 2050.[4]

Interestingly, there may be geographical differences in AD incidence. Studies have observed a latitude-dependent gradient, with a higher prevalence of AD in higher-latitude regions of Europe and North America compared to equatorial regions. An extensive 2025 ecological analysis of global data found a significant inverse correlation between ambient ultraviolet B (UVB) radiation—the primary stimulus for vitamin D production in the skin—and national dementia prevalence rates.[5] Remarkably, this recent study also found that ambient UVB light was more of a predictor of dementia than was age! This geographical clue provides a powerful, population-level signal that sun exposure, and by extension vitamin D status, is a significant factor in the risk of developing dementia.

## NEUROINFLAMMATION: THE SMOLDERING FIRE IN THE ALZHEIMER'S BRAIN

The classical view of AD pathology centered on two key hallmarks: extracellular plaques of amyloid-beta (Aβ) protein and intracellular neurofibrillary tangles (NFTs) of tau protein. For decades, the "amyloid cascade hypothesis" dominated research, suggesting that the accumulation of Aβ was the primary trigger for all subsequent pathology, including tau tangles and neuronal death. However, the consistent failure of Aβ-targeting drugs to halt or reverse cognitive decline has forced a paradigm shift.[6]

The new consensus, powerfully articulated in recent reviews, is that neuroinflammation is not a secondary consequence of Aβ and tau pathology but actually is the central, primary driving mechanism of the disease from its earliest stages.[7] The brain's resident immune cells—microglia and astrocytes—are at the heart of this process. In a healthy brain, microglia survey the environment, clear cellular debris (including soluble Aβ), and provide trophic support to neurons. However, in the AD brain, these cells become chronically activated and dysfunctional. They adopt a pro-inflammatory state, releasing a toxic cocktail of inflammatory cytokines like tumor necrosis factor-alpha (TNF-α), interleukin-1β (IL-1β), and interleukin-6 (IL-6).[8] This chronic inflammation damages synapses, promotes the misformation of tau, and ultimately contributes directly to neuronal death.[9, 10]

## VITAMIN D: THE MISSING CONDUCTOR OF THE NEURO-IMMUNE ORCHESTRA

As we've established, when the problem is inflammation, lack of vitamin D is a likely cause. This is where the story of vitamin D becomes critically important. Recall that the active form of vitamin D, 1,25-dihydroxyvitamin D [1,25(OH)D], is a potent secosteroid hormone that acts as a master regulator of the immune system and its machinery is fully present within the central nervous system. Both neurons and glial cells, including microglia and astrocytes, contain the vitamin D receptor (VDR) and the enzyme 1$\alpha$-hydroxylase, which converts circulating 25-hydroxyvitamin D [25(OH)D] into its active form.[11] This means the brain can both respond to and produce its own supply of active vitamin D, underscoring its vital role in neurological function.

The mechanisms by which vitamin D deficiency could fuel the neuroinflammation seen in AD are strikingly direct and overlap precisely with the known pathology of the disease:

- **Regulation of Microglia:** Vitamin D promotes the "M2" anti-inflammatory and phagocytic phenotype in microglia while suppressing the "M1" pro-inflammatory phenotype. In a state of vitamin D sufficiency, microglia are more effective at clearing A$\beta$ without triggering a damaging inflammatory response.[12, 13] In a vitamin D–deficient state, microglia become pro-inflammatory and their ability to clear A$\beta$ is impaired, leading to both increased plaque burden and inflammatory damage.
- **Control of Inflammatory Cytokines:** $1,25(OH)_2D$ directly suppresses the production of the very cytokines that are elevated in the AD brain, including TNF-$\alpha$ and IL-6, while simultaneously upregulating anti-inflammatory cytokines like IL-10.[14, 15]
- **Amyloid-Beta Clearance:** Beyond its effects on microglia, vitamin D has been shown to enhance the transport of A$\beta$ across the blood-brain barrier for removal from the brain. It also modulates the expression of genes involved in A$\beta$ production and degradation.[16]
- **Protection against Tau Pathology:** Emerging evidence suggests that the chronic inflammatory environment fostered by vitamin D deficiency can activate kinases that misform tau protein, directly contributing to the formation of neurofibrillary tangles.[17]

Therefore, a state of chronic vitamin D deficiency creates the ideal conditions for the smoldering fire of neuroinflammation to ignite and persist. It impairs the brain's ability to clear toxic proteins and pushes its immune cells toward a destructive, self-perpetuating inflammatory state. When chronic inflammation is the problem, vitamin D is the solution.

## A LIFETIME OF PROTECTION: THE DEVELOPMENTAL ORIGINS OF A HEALTHY BRAIN

Alzheimer's disease is not an event but a process that unfolds over decades. Pathological changes begin in the brain fifteen to twenty years before the first symptoms of cognitive decline appear.[18] This long preclinical phase implies that factors influencing risk must also be operative over long periods. This makes the concept of lifelong vitamin D status particularly compelling.

The epidemiological link between sunlight and dementia risk supports a "developmental origins" hypothesis for neuroprotection.[19] This idea is well-established in other neuro-inflammatory/autoimmune diseases like multiple sclerosis (MS). In MS, studies have shown that insufficient sun exposure during childhood and adolescence is a major risk factor for developing the disease later in life. Furthermore, the month of birth, which correlates with maternal vitamin D levels during pregnancy, is associated with subsequent MS risk.[20] A study on Danish MS patients found that factors related to higher vitamin D levels, such as a spring/summer birth and a rural upbringing (implying more time outdoors), were associated with a later age of disease onset, suggesting a long-lasting protective effect of sunlight and vitamin D.[21]

It is highly plausible that a similar principle applies to AD. Sufficient vitamin D exposure early in life and maintained throughout adulthood may "program" the brain's immune system for resilience, ensuring microglia remain functional and inflammation is kept in check. Conversely, a lifetime of low vitamin D status may prime the brain for the dysfunctional inflammatory responses that characterize AD, allowing pathology to accumulate silently for years until a tipping point is reached. Remember that vitamin D is the key to maintaining balance in the immune system between healthy immunity and pathological inflammation.

## THE CHALLENGE OF INTERVENTION: WHY VITAMIN D TRIALS HAVE DISAPPOINTED

Given the strong mechanistic and epidemiological evidence, numerous studies have investigated vitamin D supplementation as a potential therapy for AD. The results, however, have been mixed and often underwhelming, leading some to dismiss its role. But a closer look reveals critical flaws in the design of most of these trials.

Observational studies consistently show that low serum 25(OH)D levels are associated with an increased risk of all-cause dementia and AD.[22] A 2021 review highlighted vitamin D's potential as both a biomarker and a therapeutic agent, citing its role in Aβ clearance and neuroprotection.[23] A more recent, large-scale prospective study found that vitamin D supplementation was associated with a 40 percent lower incidence of dementia in a cohort of over 12,000 individuals. This protective effect was more pronounced in females, those without the APOE ε4 risk gene, and those with normal cognition at baseline, suggesting its primary role is in prevention rather than treatment of established disease.[24]

The failure of many randomized controlled trials (RCTs) to show a strong benefit likely stems from two fundamental problems: inadequate dosing and treating the disease far too late.

1. **The Critical Flaw of Dosing:** Most interventional trials have used low doses of vitamin D, typically 400–2,000 IU/day. These doses are often insufficient to raise serum 25(OH)D levels out of the deficient or insufficient range (<30 ng/mL), let alone to the optimal levels proposed for robust immune function. Based on extensive research, achieving serum levels of 80 to 100 ng/mL (200-250 nmol/L), which may be necessary to fully saturate the VDRs in immune and brain cells, often requires daily doses of 5,000 to 10,000 IU.[25, 26] Virtually no AD interventional trial has tested these higher doses or included a dose-response analysis to see if a greater effect is achieved at higher serum levels.
2. **The Problem of Proving Causality:** Expecting a low-dose vitamin D supplement to reverse decades of accumulated pathology in a patient with moderate AD is akin to asking a daily aspirin to reverse advanced heart disease. It is biologically implausible. The disease process is too advanced; neurons are already dead, and the inflammatory cascade is self-sustaining.

The true potential of vitamin D is not in curing AD, but in preventing the neuroinflammatory state that precedes it. Proving this requires decades-long prevention trials, which are prohibitively expensive and complex. At present, the best evidence we have that vitamin D is preventative are the geographic studies showing reduced incidence near the equator and higher in higher latitudes.[27]

## A COMPREHENSIVE MODEL: RECONNECTING THE BRAIN'S IMMUNE SYSTEM TO PREVENT ALZHEIMER'S

Let us integrate this evidence into a comprehensive model. The modern Alzheimer's crisis is exacerbated, if not substantially driven, by a dysfunctional immune system in the brain that results from chronic, population-wide vitamin D deficiency.

The pathway is as follows:

- **Chronic Deficiency:** Decades of insufficient sun exposure and dietary intake lead to a chronic state of low vitamin D (<30 ng/mL) in a large portion of the population.
- **Immune Dysregulation:** This deficiency prevents the brain's immune system from functioning optimally. Microglia lose their efficiency at clearing Aβ and shift to a pro-inflammatory state. The delicate balance of cytokines is disrupted.
- **The Vicious Cycle:** This low-grade, chronic neuroinflammation ("inflammaging") both accelerates the accumulation of Aβ and promotes the misformation of tau, leading to the formation of NFTs. These pathologies, in turn, further activate the inflammatory response, creating a vicious, self-amplifying cycle. The presence of NFTs can be seen not just as a hallmark of disease, but as a physical proxy for a long-standing state of immune dysfunction.
- **Senescence and Neuronal Death:** This toxic, inflamed environment creates "senescent zones" where stressed cells continue to release inflammatory signals, poisoning their neighbors.[28] This ultimately leads to widespread synaptic dysfunction and neuronal death, which manifests as the clinical symptoms of Alzheimer's disease.
- **Prevention:** Fortunately, this entire cascade could be largely avoided. Maintaining a sufficient vitamin D status (plausibly >50 ng/mL, and optimally 80–100 ng/mL) throughout life would keep the brain's immune system in a healthy, balanced state of readiness. It would promote efficient clearance of metabolic debris, suppress inappropriate inflammation, and protect neurons from damage.

Given the overwhelming evidence for chronic vitamin D deficiency in modern society, the dramatic increase in AD incidence, and the fundamental role of vitamin D in every aspect of neuro-immune function that is known to be dysfunctional in AD, it should not be surprising that vitamin D plays a central role. In fact, if vitamin D, the body's master immune regulator, did not play a central role in this inflammatory disease of the brain, that would be the truly shocking discovery. The optimization of vitamin D status on a population level represents one of the most promising, cost-effective, and low-risk/high-reward public health strategies available to turn the tide against the Alzheimer's disease epidemic.

## CHAPTER 16

# BUILDING THE FRAMEWORK: SUNLIGHT, VITAMIN D, AND YOUR BONES FOR LIFE

Your skeleton is not a lifeless scaffold. It is a dynamic, living organ, constantly being broken down and rebuilt in a process called remodeling. This intricate dance ensures your bones remain strong, repair microscopic damage, and serve as the body's primary reservoir for essential minerals. The undisputed conductor of this entire symphony is vitamin D, the hormone synthesized in your skin under the influence of sunlight. To view bone health as a simple matter of calcium intake is to see only one piece of a complex puzzle. The truth is that strong bones for life are not a matter of luck; they are a direct and predictable consequence of maintaining vitamin D sufficiency from birth to old age.

### A LESSON FROM THE DARK: THE INDUSTRIAL REVOLUTION AND RICKETS

History provides a stark and undeniable lesson on the importance of sunlight for human health. During the industrial revolution in the eighteenth and nineteenth centuries, a mass migration from sunlit fields to crowded, polluted cities occurred across Europe and North America. Families lived in narrow tenements, overshadowed by factories that choked the sky with thick, sun-blocking smog. Children, in particular, were deprived of sunlight, either toiling long hours in factories or playing in dark, narrow alleyways. In this sun-deprived environment, a devastating disease ran rampant: rickets. Known as "the English disease" due to its prevalence in industrial England, rickets afflicted children with a horrifying set of symptoms: Their bones failed to mineralize properly, leading to soft, pliable skeletons. This resulted in severely bowed legs, stunted growth, a deformed rib cage known as the "rachitic rosary," and chronic, debilitating pain.[1]

For decades, the cause was a mystery. It wasn't until the early twentieth century that researchers connected the dots. They observed that rickets was rare in sun-drenched regions and that it could be cured with exposure to ultraviolet (UV) light or by consuming cod-liver oil. This led to the groundbreaking discovery of a fat-soluble substance in the oil, which was named vitamin D. It was, in fact, the very same compound the body produces when skin is exposed to sunlight. Rickets was not an infectious disease but a nutritional deficiency—a disease of darkness. This historical epidemic provided the first, and perhaps most dramatic, proof of the nonnegotiable role of sunlight and vitamin D in building a healthy human skeleton.

## THE MASTER BUILDERS: HOW VITAMIN D AND CALCIUM CONSTRUCT BONE

Thinking of calcium as the "bricks" for your bones is a useful analogy, but it's incomplete. Without a foreman to direct the construction crew, those bricks would just be a useless pile. In your body, vitamin D is that master foreman. The process is elegant and efficient. When you consume calcium from your diet, it arrives in your small intestine. However, your body cannot absorb it passively. It requires a direct order, and that order comes from the active form of vitamin D, known as calcitriol. Vitamin D dramatically increases the efficiency of intestinal calcium absorption, ensuring this critical mineral gets from your gut into your bloodstream.[2] Once in the blood, vitamin D continues its work, collaborating with another hormone called parathyroid hormone (PTH). Together, they act like a thermostat, meticulously regulating blood calcium levels. If levels drop, they signal the bones to release a small amount of calcium. When vitamin D levels are adequate, they ensure that newly absorbed calcium is deposited correctly into the bone's collagen matrix, a process called mineralization. This is what gives bone its hardness and rigidity. Without sufficient vitamin D, this entire system collapses. You can consume all the calcium you want, but most of it will pass right through your body, unabsorbed and unused. Your body, desperate for calcium to maintain critical functions like muscle contraction and nerve signaling, will be forced to steal it from the only available source: your skeleton. This constant theft, day after day, year after year, is the foundation for the bone diseases that plague modern society.

## WHEN THE FRAMEWORK WEAKENS: OSTEOMALACIA, OSTEOPENIA, AND OSTEOPOROSIS

The failure to maintain adequate vitamin D status causes a spectrum of bone diseases, each representing a different stage of skeletal decay.

- **Osteomalacia:** This is the adult equivalent of rickets, literally meaning "soft bones." It occurs when there is a severe vitamin D deficiency, and the bone matrix that is laid down cannot be properly mineralized with calcium. The bones become soft, weak, and prone to aching and pain. This is a direct result of a breakdown in the fundamental bone-building process.[3]

- **Osteopenia:** This term describes low bone mass that is not yet severe enough to be classified as osteoporosis. It is a warning sign. The deep, aching bone pain often attributed to arthritis or simply "getting old" is frequently a symptom of osteopenia, signaling that the bones are suffering from a chronic lack of building materials.
- **Osteoporosis:** This is the most well-known and dangerous consequence of long-term vitamin D and calcium insufficiency. It means "porous bones." In this condition, the rate of bone resorption (breakdown) far exceeds the rate of bone formation. The internal honeycomb structure of the bone becomes thin and weak, making it catastrophically fragile and susceptible to fracture from even minor stress, like a cough or a simple fall.

Globally, osteoporosis causes more than 8.9 million fractures annually.[4] It is a silent epidemic, often undiagnosed until a debilitating fracture occurs. Epidemiological evidence strongly supports the vitamin D connection. Populations living closer to the equator with abundant, year-round sun exposure historically have demonstrated better bone density and lower fracture rates than their counterparts in northern latitudes, who endure long "vitamin D winters."[5]

It is also important to understand that modern medicine's most powerful anti-osteoporosis drugs, such as bisphosphonates, are not magic bullets. These drugs work primarily by slowing down the cells that break down bone. However, they cannot build new, strong bone out of thin air. For these medications to be effective, the body must have adequate levels of both calcium and vitamin D. Prescribing these drugs without first correcting an underlying vitamin D deficiency is like hiring a security guard to stop thieves while simultaneously failing to supply any materials to repair the building's crumbling foundation. The effort without vitamin D and calcium is fundamentally flawed and destined for failure.[6]

## A SYMPHONY OF HORMONES AND THE THREAT OF INFLAMMATION

Bone health is further governed by a synergistic relationship between vitamin D and the body's primary steroid hormones: estrogen and testosterone. These sex hormones are powerful inhibitors of bone resorption. The rapid bone loss women experience after menopause is a direct result of the sharp decline in estrogen. As we mentioned earlier, in the estrogen-depleted woman that is also vitamin D deficient, that calcium that should have been deposited into the bones instead is in the bloodstream accumulating inside inflamed arteries leading to atherosclerosis. Similarly, declining testosterone levels in men also contribute to age-related bone loss.

Vitamin D works in concert with these hormones. During our peak bone-building years in youth and young adulthood, adequate vitamin D ensures we maximize the bone-building potential that high estrogen and testosterone levels provide. Later in life, as these hormones decline, maintaining vitamin D sufficiency becomes even more critical to help slow the inevitable acceleration of bone loss.[7]

Furthermore, emerging research reveals another insidious way vitamin D deficiency damages the skeleton: by promoting chronic inflammation. Vitamin D is a potent modulator of the immune system, and its absence allows for a low-grade, systemic inflammatory state to smolder throughout the body. This inflammation releases a flood of chemical messengers called pro-inflammatory cytokines. These very same cytokines have been shown to directly stimulate osteoclasts, the cells responsible for dissolving bone.[8] Vitamin D starvation creates a vicious cycle: The deficiency causes inflammation, which in turn accelerates bone destruction.

## THE AVOIDABLE SPIRAL: RECLAIMING AGING FROM BONE DECAY

We must aggressively challenge the deeply ingrained cultural belief that frailty, bone pain, and skeletal collapse are inevitable consequences of aging. They are not. They are, in large part, the cumulative result of a lifetime of chronic, unaddressed vitamin D deficiency. The tragic and predictable downward spiral begins subtly.

1. **Accumulating Pain:** Decades of vitamin D insufficiency lead to osteopenia, causing a chronic, deep, and persistent ache in the bones and muscles. This pain is often misdiagnosed or dismissed as "normal" aches of aging.
2. **Imposed Sedentary Lifestyle:** This constant pain makes movement difficult and unpleasant. Walking, climbing stairs, and even standing become chores to be avoided. An active lifestyle gives way to a sedentary one.
3. **Muscle and Bone Atrophy:** Bones and muscles adhere to a strict "use it or lose it" principle. Without the mechanical stress of movement and weight-bearing exercise, muscle atrophy (a condition called sarcopenia) and bone decay accelerates.
4. **Misattribution to "Old Age":** This profound weakness, muscle loss, and fragility is almost universally misattributed to simply being

"old," rather than correctly identifying it as the result of a preventable cascade initiated by a nutritional deficiency.

5. **The Fall and the Fracture:** Ultimately, this combination of weak muscles, poor balance, and fragile, porous bones culminates in disaster. A simple trip or fall that a healthy person would brush off results in a broken hip, wrist, or spine.
6. **Demise:** For the vitamin D-starved elderly, a hip fracture is often a death sentence. It leads to hospitalization, surgery, immobility, a high risk of complications like pneumonia and blood clots, and a catastrophic loss of independence. Many never return home.

This entire death spiral is almost completely avoidable. These bone issues are a pathology of modern, indoor life, exacerbated by a misguided fear of the sun and not a mandatory feature of human aging. By ensuring vitamin D sufficiency through sensible, non-burning sun exposure and, where necessary, targeted supplementation throughout the entire lifespan, we can rewrite the end of our story. We can maintain strong bones, active muscles, and a pain-free, mobile life well into our later years.

# CHAPTER 17

# MORE THAN A FALL: HOW VITAMIN D FORTIFIES YOUR MUSCULAR ARMOR

In the preceding chapter, we have established the undeniable role of sunlight and vitamin D in building a strong, fracture-resilient skeleton. We have discussed how a vitamin D–replete bone is less likely to fracture. However, the story of fractures, particularly in the aging population, begins not with the snap of a bone, but with the stumble that precedes it. The overwhelming majority of fractures in the frail elderly are not spontaneous events; they are the direct result of a fall.[1] Therefore, while strengthening bones to withstand impact is critical, a far more effective strategy is to prevent the fall from happening in the first place. This shifts our focus from the skeleton to the dynamic, living armor that surrounds it: our skeletal muscle. To help prevent these falls, we must understand the mechanisms that underpin the progressive loss of muscle mass and strength, a phenomenon that robs the elderly of their stability, power, and independence. The master key to unlocking this understanding, and to reversing this decline, is vitamin D.

## SARCOPENIA: THE MISDIAGNOSED EPIDEMIC OF AGING

For decades, the gradual wasting of muscle with age was considered a simple, inevitable part of growing older. This condition, known as sarcopenia, is characterized by a progressive loss of skeletal muscle mass, strength, and function. It is the primary reason why an older person may struggle to rise from a chair, lose their balance on an uneven surface, or be unable to react quickly enough to catch themselves during a stumble. However, we must challenge the notion that sarcopenia is an unavoidable fate. Instead, we must view it as a pathological condition driven by specific, identifiable, and, most importantly, correctable factors. Foremost among these is the chronic, pervasive vitamin D deficiency that plagues aging populations worldwide. Numerous studies have established a powerful correlation: As vitamin D levels plummet, the incidence and severity of sarcopenia soar.[2] This is no coincidence. It is a direct cause-and-effect relationship rooted in the cellular biology of our muscles.

## THE LOCK AND KEY: HOW MUSCLE CELLS LISTEN TO VITAMIN D

Our bodies are intricate communication networks, and hormones are the primary messengers. For a cell to "hear" a hormonal message, it must have a specific receptor, a molecular "lock" that the hormone "key" fits into. For years, the presence of the vitamin D receptor (VDR) in muscle tissue was debated. That debate is now over. It is now definitively established that skeletal muscle cells are equipped with VDRs.[3] When activated vitamin D (calcitriol) binds to its receptor within a muscle cell, the VDR-calcitriol complex travels to the cell's nucleus. There, it binds to specific sequences on our DNA known as vitamin D response elements (VDREs). By binding to these VDREs, vitamin D acts like a genetic switch, turning on or off the genes responsible for muscle protein synthesis, growth, and contraction. The presence of this machinery is irrefutable proof that vitamin D exerts direct, genomic control over the function and health of our muscles.

## A TALE OF TWO FIBERS: THE SPRINTER AND THE MARATHON RUNNER WITHIN

To appreciate the profound impact of vitamin D on muscle, we must first understand that our muscles are not uniform. They are composed of different types of fibers, each specialized for a different task. For our purposes, we can simplify them into two main categories:

- **Type I (Slow-Twitch) Fibers:** These are our endurance fibers. They are rich in mitochondria, contract slowly, and are highly resistant to fatigue. They are essential for posture and sustained activities like walking or jogging. They are the marathon runners of our muscular system.
- **Type II (Fast-Twitch) Fibers:** These are our power and speed fibers. They contract rapidly and forcefully but fatigue quickly. They are responsible for explosive movements like jumping, lifting heavy objects, and—most critically for this discussion—making the rapid, corrective movements necessary to prevent a fall. These are the muscle fibers that determine a quick or a slower reaction time when losing our balance. They are the sprinters of our muscular system.

The tragedy of sarcopenia is that it does not affect these fibers equally. The most significant and debilitating aspect of age-related muscle loss is the selective atrophy of the type II fast-twitch fibers.[4] It is the loss of these "sprinter" fibers that critically impairs an older person's ability to react to a sudden loss of balance, turning a minor trip into a catastrophic fall.

## VITAMIN D'S MASTER PLAN FOR MAINTAINING YOUR FAST-TWITCH POWER

The connection between vitamin D and fall prevention becomes crystal clear when we examine its specific effects on muscle fiber types. Research has shown that type II muscle fibers contain a significantly higher concentration of vitamin D receptors than type I fibers.[5] This means that our fast-twitch, power-generating fibers are uniquely sensitive and responsive to vitamin D status. When vitamin D levels are optimal, it orchestrates a cascade of events specifically within these type II fibers to:

- **Direct Protein Synthesis:** By activating the VDREs, vitamin D directly stimulates the genetic machinery to build new muscle proteins, leading to an increase in the size (hypertrophy) and number of Type II fibers.
- **Enhance Calcium Handling:** A powerful muscle contraction depends on the rapid and efficient movement of calcium ions within the muscle cell. Vitamin D improves the transport and handling of calcium, leading to stronger, faster muscle contractions.[6]

Conversely, in a state of vitamin D starvation, these processes are impaired. The type II fibers, being the most dependent on the vitamin D signal, are the first and most profoundly affected. They shrink and weaken, leaving the individual vulnerable to weakness and falls. Supplementation studies have borne this out, demonstrating that raising vitamin D levels in deficient older adults leads to a measurable increase in type II fiber size and a corresponding improvement in muscle strength and a dramatic reduction in falls.[7]

## PUTTING OUT THE FIRE: VITAMIN D AS AN ANTI-INFLAMMATORY AGENT

Beyond its direct anabolic effects, vitamin D plays another important role in protecting muscle: It acts as a powerful anti-inflammatory agent. Vitamin D deficiency is associated with a state of chronic, low-grade inflammation, where the body produces an excess of inflammatory cytokines. These cytokines, particularly tumor necrosis factor-alpha (TNF-$\alpha$), are catabolic, meaning they actively promote the breakdown of muscle tissue.[8] By optimizing vitamin D levels, we suppress the production of these muscle-wasting cytokines, effectively putting out the inflammatory fire that consumes muscle mass. Vitamin

D creates a physiological environment that is permissive for muscle growth and maintenance, rather than one geared toward breakdown and decay.

## A POWERFUL ALLIANCE: VITAMIN D AND YOUR BODY'S NATURAL STEROIDS

Vitamin D does not work in a vacuum. As we have established, it is a potent steroid hormone itself, and it works synergistically with the body's other major anabolic steroids: testosterone and estrogen. Both of these hormones are well-known for their roles in building and maintaining muscle mass. What is less appreciated is that their effectiveness is intertwined with vitamin D status. Vitamin D, testosterone, and estrogen often work on similar or overlapping cellular pathways to promote muscle protein synthesis. An adequate level of vitamin D is a prerequisite for the body to respond optimally to its own natural muscle-building hormones. Think of it as a team: Testosterone and estrogen may be star players, but vitamin D is the foundational coach that ensures the entire team functions effectively to build and preserve lean muscle mass.

## MUSCLE LOSS WITH AGING IS OPTIONAL, NOT INEVITABLE

This brings us to the central, transformative idea of this chapter: Sarcopenia and age-related muscle loss are not inevitable events. They are the predictable outcomes of a modern lifestyle that combines a chronic deficit of vitamin D with a lack of physical challenge. Vitamin D governs the growth of muscle in a use-dependent plastic manner. This means the muscle's response to a stimulus is dramatically amplified by the presence of vitamin D. The key stimulus for muscle growth is resistance and weight-bearing exercise. When an elderly person engages in this type of training, they send a signal to their muscles to grow stronger. In a vitamin D–replete individual, this signal is received loud and clear. In a vitamin D–starved person, not so much.

One of the primary mechanisms, in addition to synergy with estrogen and testosterone, for this effect is vitamin D's role as a potent inhibitor of myostatin. Myostatin is a protein that acts as the body's natural "brake" on muscle growth, preventing our muscles from getting too large.[9, 10] In vitamin D–deficient states, myostatin levels are often elevated, actively suppressing muscle growth even in the face of exercise. However, when vitamin D levels are optimized, myostatin is suppressed. This effectively "releases the brake," allowing the muscle-building signals from exercise and weight training to produce a far more robust and powerful anabolic response. In essence, vitamin D unlocks the full potential of exercise to preserve and even grow new muscle fiber—primarily fast-twitch muscle fiber—in older adults. It is for this reason that we must begin to see vitamin D for what it truly is: a legal, free, natural, and essential steroid hormone that facilitates peak physical performance. Vitamin

D's role in enhancing athletic power and recovery is so significant that it will be explored in detail in a later chapter.

## TURNING BACK THE CLOCK ON MUSCLE AGING

The evidence is clear and the conclusion is inescapable. Sarcopenia is not a disease of aging; it is a disease of chronic vitamin D starvation compounded by inactivity. It is an avoidable, and for many, reversible characteristic of what we mistakenly call "normal" aging. By ensuring chronic vitamin D repletion through sensible sun exposure and supplementation, we lay the foundation for robust muscular health. When combined with the powerful stimulus of resistance exercise, this strategy becomes the definitive protocol for halting and reversing muscle loss. It is the key to maintaining the strength to stand tall, the power to catch oneself from a stumble, and the physical independence that is synonymous with a life of health and vitality.

# CHAPTER 18

# SUNSHINE FOR YOUR SMILE: HOW VITAMIN D AND SUNLIGHT AFFECT YOUR DENTAL HEALTH

Getting enough Vitamin D also helps protect your teeth. Research going back nearly a century has linked vitamin D levels to tooth decay, gum disease, and how teeth develop before birth. This chapter explains what the science says so you can make informed choices about sunlight, vitamin D, and your own dental health.

## THE GEOGRAPHY OF TOOTH DECAY: SUNLIGHT AND CAVITIES ACROSS THE UNITED STATES

One of the most fascinating bodies of evidence comes from large geographic studies showing that people who live in sunnier regions tend to have fewer cavities. This connection was first noticed in the early twentieth century and has been confirmed repeatedly since.

Using data from over 2,800 children collected in a cross-sectional survey of US adolescent males between 1933 and 1934, researchers found a striking difference between states: Children in Oklahoma had 150 cavities per 100 children, while those in Pennsylvania—a far less sunny northeastern state—had 531 cavities per 100 children. That is more than a threefold difference. A follow-up analysis of the same data found that dental cavities were inversely related to mean hours of sunlight per year. Children living in the sunny western United States (approximately 3,000 hours of sunlight per year) had roughly half as many cavities as those in the much less sunny Northeast (fewer than 2,200 hours of sunlight per year).[1]

A larger review of historical data—including dental health rankings for US servicemen from World War I (1918), Navy servicemen in 1934, and Army servicemen in 1943—found a consistent, significant inverse relationship between summertime solar UVB doses and dental health rank across states. States with higher UVB exposure consistently ranked better for dental health.[2]

Studies conducted in Oregon in the 1950s also found that dental cavities were less common in the sunnier eastern parts of that state, a pattern that held up even after accounting for other factors like water quality and diet. Researchers at the time attributed this protective effect to vitamin D's role in calcium metabolism.[3]

## WHAT CLINICAL TRIALS TELL US ABOUT VITAMIN D AND DENTAL HEALTH

Beyond geographic patterns, controlled clinical trials have also tested whether giving people vitamin D actually reduces cavities. A systematic review and meta-analysis published in the journal *Nutrition Reviews* analyzed data from 2,827 children across multiple controlled clinical trials. The results showed that supplemental ultraviolet radiation reduced cavity rates by 64 percent, vitamin D3 supplements reduced them by 49 percent, and vitamin D2 supplements reduced them by 36 percent, compared to children receiving no supplementation. The overall conclusion was that vitamin D is a "promising caries-preventive agent," though the authors noted the overall certainty of the evidence was low due to the age of many of the trials.[4]

## VITAMIN D AND CAVITIES IN CHILDREN

A systematic review and meta-analysis published in 2023 in the journal *Applied Sciences* analyzed thirteen cross-sectional studies and found that low serum Vitamin D levels increased the odds of developing dental cavities by 41 percent. This analysis also demonstrated a dose-response relationship: Every 4 ng/mL increase in vitamin D blood levels was associated with a 3 percent lower risk of cavities. This means that the higher the vitamin D level, the lower the risk of tooth decay.[5]

A 2023 systematic review and meta-analysis from *BMC Oral Health* examined 13 studies—including cross-sectional, cohort, and case-control studies—in children and found consistent evidence that lower 25(OH)D levels were associated with higher rates of dental cavities. The review noted that vitamin D insufficiency was widespread among study populations, ranging from 17.3 percent to 69.4 percent of participants depending on the region.[6]

A specific clinical study found a dramatic difference in vitamin D levels between children with severe early childhood cavities (mean: 12.19 ng/mL) versus children with no cavities (mean: 20.11 ng/mL), with a statistically significant inverse correlation between vitamin D levels and cavity severity.[7]

## VITAMIN D AND CAVITIES IN ADULTS: NHANES DATA

A large retrospective study published in 2024 used data from 18,683 participants in the US National Health and Nutrition Examination Survey (NHANES) from 2011 to 2016. The study found that the average number of decayed, missing, and filled teeth (the DMFT score) was 7.36, and that 33.2 percent of participants had untreated dental cavities. An earlier analysis from this dataset found that adults with severe vitamin D deficiency (below 25 nmol/L) were 2.48 times more likely to develop dental cavities compared to those with sufficient levels (75 nmol/L or above). Children aged 1 to 5 years in the lowest vitamin D group were 2.55 times more likely to have untreated cavities compared to children with levels at or above 75 nmol/L—a particularly important finding given that early childhood tooth decay can set the stage for lifelong dental problems.[8]

## VITAMIN D AND TOOTH DEVELOPMENT BEFORE BIRTH

Some of vitamin D's most important effects on dental health begin before a child is even born. Teeth start forming remarkably early: Primary (baby) teeth begin their development as early as six weeks into embryonic life, and the enamel and dentin layers begin mineralizing during the second trimester of pregnancy and continue after birth.[9]

Vitamin D plays a critical role in this process. The vitamin D receptor (VDR) has been found on the cells that form tooth enamel (called ameloblasts) and the cells that form dentin (called odontoblasts). This means vitamin D directly influences how these cells function.[10]

Maternal vitamin D deficiency during pregnancy can lead to enamel hypoplasia—a condition in which tooth enamel is thinner than normal, or has visible pits and grooves. The specific part of the tooth affected depends on the gestational week when deficiency occurred: Maternal deficiency at 12–16 weeks affects the tips of the front teeth; deficiency at 20–32 weeks affects the middle portion; and deficiency at 36–40 weeks affects the area near the gum line.[11]

The clinical evidence supports this: One randomized controlled trial (RCT) found that pregnant women with vitamin D levels below 15 ng/mL had a 14 percent higher risk of their children developing tooth decay in baby teeth. In contrast, high-dose vitamin D supplementation during pregnancy was associated with approximately a 50 percent reduction in the odds of enamel defects in newborns.[12]

A 2022 observational study found that children whose mothers had vitamin D insufficiency during the third trimester of pregnancy were more than three times as likely to develop cavities by age 6, compared to children of mothers with adequate vitamin D levels.[13]

## HOW DOES VITAMIN D ACTUALLY PROTECT TEETH?

Vitamin D protects teeth through several different pathways—not just by helping the body absorb calcium for strong enamel.

1. **Calcium and phosphorus absorption.** Vitamin D is essential for the intestinal absorption of calcium and phosphorus. Both minerals are needed to build and maintain hard tooth enamel and dentin. When vitamin D is low, less calcium is absorbed from food, and teeth may become weaker and more susceptible to decay.[14]
2. **Antimicrobial peptides.** Vitamin D stimulates the production of natural antibacterial proteins called antimicrobial peptides (AMPs)—particularly cathelicidin and beta-defensins. These peptides help fight the bacteria in your mouth that cause cavities. *Streptococcus mutans*, the primary bacterial species responsible for tooth decay, can be inhibited by these AMPs. Research also suggests that UVB radiation itself, by triggering Vitamin D production in the skin, promotes the production of these protective proteins.[15]
3. **Anti-inflammatory effects.** Vitamin D is a potent regulator of the immune system. It helps reduce chronic inflammation—a key driver of gum disease (periodontitis). The active form of Vitamin D, calcitriol, binds to receptors in immune cells (including macrophages and monocytes) and suppresses the production of inflammatory chemicals.[16]
4. **Saliva production and composition.** Some research suggests that Vitamin D deficiency may reduce saliva production and alter its protective chemical composition. Saliva is the mouth's first line of defense: It neutralizes acid, washes away food particles, and contains its own antimicrobial agents. Impaired saliva function can increase cavity risk.[17]

## VITAMIN D AND GUM DISEASE (PERIODONTITIS)

Gum disease—ranging from mild inflammation of the gums (gingivitis) to advanced periodontitis, which destroys the bone and tissue that hold teeth in place—is the leading cause of tooth loss in adults. Growing evidence suggests that vitamin D plays a significant protective role against gum disease as well.[18]

A systematic review published in the *Journal of Periodontal Research* in 2023 concluded that low serum vitamin D is associated with increased severity of periodontitis, and that vitamin D sufficiency—maintained through adequate sunlight exposure or supplementation—supports periodontal health. The review highlighted that experimental animal studies involving deletion of the enzyme that activates vitamin D showed significantly worse gum disease and bone loss, providing strong biological evidence for causation.[19]

A study of Canadian Forces personnel found that participants with vitamin D levels below 20 ng/mL had 63 percent higher odds of moderate to severe gum inflammation, and those below 30 ng/mL had 44 percent higher odds, compared to those with sufficient levels defined as 45 ng/mL in this study. Participants who took vitamin D supplements had significantly lower odds of gum inflammation (a 44 percent reduction).[20]

A long-term study known as the Dental Longitudinal Study found that older men who consumed less than 400 IU of vitamin D per day had more advanced alveolar bone loss (the bone that anchors teeth in the jaw) and more severe periodontal disease compared to men consuming more than 800 IU per day.[21]

Clinical research has also shown that patients who are vitamin D deficient at the time of periodontal surgery tend to have worse outcomes—less tissue reattachment and less effective pocket depth reduction—suggesting that Vitamin D status can affect the body's ability to heal gum tissue.[22]

The scientific evidence consistently shows that vitamin D—obtained primarily from sunlight, and also from food and supplements—plays an important role in dental health across the lifespan. It helps teeth form properly before birth, keeps enamel and dentin strong, fights cavity-causing bacteria through antimicrobial peptides, and reduces the gum inflammation that leads to periodontitis and tooth loss.

Geographic and epidemiological data show that populations living in sunnier regions have historically had fewer cavities, and modern clinical studies confirm an inverse relationship between vitamin D blood levels and the risk of both tooth decay and gum disease. Children and pregnant women appear to be especially vulnerable to the dental effects of vitamin D deficiency.

While vitamin D is not a magic cure for dental problems—brushing, flossing, a low-sugar diet, and regular dental visits remain essential—maintaining adequate vitamin D through sensible sun exposure, diet, or supplementation is a practical and evidence-supported step toward better oral health.

## CHAPTER 19

# THE SUN, THE CELL, AND THE SANDS OF TIME: VITAMIN D, AGING, AND THE QUEST FOR LONGEVITY

Now that we know that many of the characteristics usually associated with aging—like neurodegenerative disease and bone and muscle weakness—are in large part exacerbated, if not caused outright by chronic vitamin D deficiency, we can ask the provocative question of whether optimizing vitamin D and balancing immune system function can help us live even longer.

In the early sixteenth century, the Spanish explorer Juan Ponce de León sailed through the Caribbean, in search of a mythical fountain of youth. The legend says he sought water that could reverse the ravages of time, restore vitality, and grant eternal life. His quest, which ultimately led him to the shores of what is now Florida, is a powerful symbol of a deeply human desire to control the process of aging. For millennia, humanity has sought to slow, stop, or even reverse the ticking of our biological clock. We have searched for this power in magical waters, exotic elixirs, and elaborate rituals.

What if the secret to a healthier, longer life wasn't hidden in a remote yet undiscovered spring but was, in a sense, available to everyone, everywhere? What if a key factor in mitigating the decay of aging was not a substance to be found and drunk, but an inherent biological process to be activated by something as universal as the sun? This chapter will show that optimal levels of vitamin D, the "sunshine vitamin," are fundamentally linked to the process of healthy aging. While we presently cannot avoid aging, we can control how we age; whether it be a dreaded ache-and-pain-ridden ordeal or the fulfillment of a life well lived blessed by good health and its benefits. The idea and the mechanism driving optimal aging is straightforward: Optimal vitamin D status throughout life is a critical tool for healthy aging, primarily by reducing the cumulative effects of chronic, low-grade inflammation—a process known as inflammaging.

## THE AGING SKIN: A FADING FACTORY

One of the great ironies of aging is that the very organ responsible for producing vitamin D from sunlight—the skin—loses its ability to do so over time. As we age, our internal vitamin D factory begins to slow down, becoming progressively less efficient.

The seminal research that established this fact of life was conducted by Drs. MacLaughlin and Holick in 1985. They investigated the skin of human subjects ranging in age from eight to ninety-two years old. Their goal was to determine if the skin's capacity to produce vitamin D changed with age. They discovered that the amount of the precursor molecule, 7-dehydrocholesterol (7-DHC), which is converted into vitamin D by UVB sunlight, dramatically decreases in the epidermis as we get older. Their results were definitive and stark: The concentration of 7-DHC in the skin of a seventy-year-old was only about 25 percent of that found in the skin of a young adult.[1] This means that an older individual exposed to the exact same amount of sunlight as a younger person will produce significantly less vitamin D. This age-related decline in cutaneous synthesis creates a biological vulnerability. Just when our bodies need robust defenses against age-related diseases and optimal immune system function, our primary natural mechanism for producing a key hormonal defender falters. This biological reality makes understanding and appreciating vitamin D's role in healthy aging not just an academic exercise, but a public health imperative.

## THE FIRES WITHIN: AGING, INFLAMMATION, AND INFLAMMAGING

For decades, scientists viewed aging as a simple process of wear and tear. But recently a more nuanced picture has emerged, centered on the concept of inflammation. As such, aging is not a passive process suggested by a wear-and-tear model but instead an active process caused by chronic inflammation. Rather than tying aging to a process we can't control like the passage of time, identifying one of the mechanisms that changes as a function of time, vitamin D and inflammation, enables us to predict and control that mechanism and in turn, control aging.

As we discussed earlier, acute inflammation is a healthy, necessary response to injury or infection. It's the redness and swelling around a cut—the sign that your immune system is rushing to the site to fight invaders and repair damage. However, a different, more sinister form of inflammation has been identified as a core driver of aging. Coined "inflammaging," this term describes a chronic, low-grade, systemic inflammation that develops with age.[2] Unlike the acute inflammation of a wound, inflammaging is a quiet, persistent fire burning throughout the body. Because it is covert, subthreshold, and subclinical, it doesn't have obvious symptoms, but its long-term effects are devastating. This simmering state of low-grade, chronic inflammation contributes to nearly every major disease of aging, including heart disease, type 2 diabetes, cancer, arthritis, and neurodegenerative disorders like Alzheimer's disease.

## VITAMIN D: THE BODY'S FIRE EXTINGUISHER

This is where vitamin D plays a starring role. As we have discussed in previous chapters, vitamin D is a potent modulator of the immune system. Its active form, calcitriol, functions as a hormone that can regulate the genes involved in the inflammatory response. Vitamin D provides a guiding, finely tuned influence between protective immunity and pathological inflammation. By acting as a natural anti-inflammatory agent, adequate vitamin D can help dampen the chronic fires of inflammaging, thereby reducing the risk and progression of the many diseases associated with chronic inflammation, including aging.

## A SPECIFIC CASE: "ZOMBIE CELLS" IN THE BRAIN

One of the strangest and most compelling aspects of aging is the accumulation of "senescent" cells. These are cells that have stopped dividing but refuse to die—earning them the nickname "zombie cells." Instead of quietly being cleared away, they linger in tissues, including the brain, pumping out a cocktail of inflammatory signals that damage surrounding healthy cells, causing them to malfunction.[3] The senescent and zombie cell clusters resemble brain tumors that spread their destructive influence to more and more previously healthy brain tissue, and over time, robbing us of our faculties and stored memories. This process is a major contributor to brain aging and neurodegenerative diseases like Alzheimer's disease.

Fortunately, emerging research indicates that vitamin D can help combat this zombie cell invasion. Vitamin D receptors are found throughout the brain, and studies indicate that vitamin D can promote cellular housekeeping processes like autophagy, which helps the body clear out dysfunctional cells and debris. By supporting these clearance mechanisms and directly reducing the inflammatory output of senescent cells, vitamin D helps protect the brain from the damaging effects of inflammaging.

## MEASURING TIME: TELOMERES AS A BIOLOGICAL CLOCK

Aging is not a linear process. Just look around you, some people look and behave much older beyond their years while others are spry and active despite their advanced ages. One problem in the study of age-related biological matters is this nonlinear, somewhat subjective feature of adult aging and decline.

How can we objectively measure the rate at which someone is aging? One of the most powerful tools we have is the measurement of telomeres. Telomeres are protective caps at the ends of our chromosomes, often compared to the plastic tips on shoelaces (aglets). Every time a cell divides, these telomeres get a little shorter. Eventually, they become so short that the cell can no longer divide safely and either dies or becomes a senescent "zombie" cell. Telomere length, therefore, serves as a remarkably accurate biomarker of biological age, as opposed to chronological age. Many, many studies have shown that shorter telomeres are linked to a shorter lifespan and an increased risk of age-related diseases.

## LIFE'S BURDENS AND THE FRAYING OF OUR CHROMOSOMES

Telomere length isn't just a matter of genetics; it is profoundly affected by our lifestyle and experiences. Factors like smoking, obesity, poor diet, and lack of exercise are all known to accelerate telomere shortening. Perhaps the most groundbreaking work in this area came from Nobel laureate Dr. Elizabeth Blackburn. In a landmark 2004 study, she and her colleagues investigated the effects of chronic psychological stress on telomere length. They studied mothers who were caregivers for a chronically ill child—a situation of high, prolonged stress. The control group was mothers who had given birth to a healthy baby. Both groups certainly experienced stress caring for a baby, but the perceived psychological stress was presumed to be higher in the mothers with the chronically ill child.

The results on the biological measure of aging were stunning. The women who reported the highest levels of perceived stress had telomeres that were, on average, so much shorter than the low-stress women that it equated to at least an entire decade of additional aging.[4] This study proved that our mental and emotional state has a direct, physical impact on the very fabric of our genetic material. Stress, it turns out, literally makes us older on a cellular level.

## VITAMIN D AND THE PROTECTION OF OUR TELOMERES

If stress and poor lifestyle shorten our telomeres, can anything protect them? Again, the evidence points to vitamin D. Research has demonstrated a direct and positive relationship between vitamin D levels and telomere length. A large-scale study involving over two thousand women found that those with higher vitamin D levels had significantly longer telomeres.[5]

A more recent study found that taking just 2,000 IU of vitamin D3 daily resulted in dramatically less telomere shortening over four years compared to the placebo group. Specifically, the vitamin D group lost 140 fewer base pairs of DNA on average, which equated to nearly three fewer years of chromosomal aging compared to the placebo group.[6] Think about that: They took 2,000 IU vitamin D for four years and only aged one year. We can only imagine the magnitude of the antiaging effect if physiologically relevant quantities (5,000–10,000 IU) of vitamin D3 were used in this study.

The mechanisms for these dramatic antiaging effects are twofold. First, by reducing the chronic inflammation and oxidative stress that damage DNA, vitamin D creates a less hostile environment for our chromosomes, slowing the rate of telomere erosion. Second, vitamin D appears to influence the activity of an enzyme called telomerase. Telomerase is very similar to the "fountain of youth" for our cells; it can rebuild and lengthen telomeres. Not surprisingly, Blackburn found that psychological stress reduces telomerase activity as well. Studies have shown that vitamin D can increase the expression and activity of telomerase, actively helping to maintain and repair these critical protective chromosomal caps.[7] In essence, vitamin D not only protects telomeres from damage but may also help to rebuild them.[8]

In this model of chronic inflammation, vitamin D, and telomeres, telomerase may be the link to the healthy aging of our chromosomes while vitamin D is the key protective factor in both chronic inflammation and slower biologic chromosomal aging. The notion that vitamin D may play a role in not only protecting, but rebuilding telomeres, and its profound role in reducing chronic inflammation suggests that vitamin D is at the nexus of both the phenotypic (observable) and genomic mechanisms of aging. Vitamin D plays a central role in both observable physical signs of chronological aging that we all see and feel and its objective biologic chromosomal correlate.

## LESSONS FROM LONG-LIVED ANIMALS: A PHYLOGENETIC PERSPECTIVE ON FACTORS THAT AFFECT AGING

To find clues about longevity, it often helps to look at the champions of aging in the animal kingdom. Two creatures, in particular, offer fascinating insights: the massive bowhead whale and a tiny bird, the Leach's storm-petrel. Both animals were selected because they are such disparate opposites that any similarities between them may be noteworthy for our discussion. The bowhead whale can live for over two hundred years, making it the longest-living mammal. Despite their enormous size, adults range from 150,000 to 200,000 pounds, and vast number of cells (which should theoretically increase cancer risk), they are remarkably disease-resistant. Their genetics reveal enhanced DNA repair mechanisms and, not surprisingly, telomeres that shorten at a much slower rate than in shorter-lived mammals. In stark contrast to this behemoth is Leach's storm-petrel, a small seabird, weighing only between 1.8 to 5.3 ounces. By all metabolic rules,[9, 10] the storm-petrel should live for just a few years. Instead, it can live for over thirty-five years. It defies the standard biological rule that small animals with a fast metabolism live short lives. What could these two vastly different animals have in common?

## THE STRANGE AND TELLING CASE OF THE STORM-PETREL

The Leach's storm-petrel presents a biological puzzle that turns our understanding of aging on its head. Dr. Mark Haussmann and his team at Bucknell University made a shocking discovery: In Leach's storm-petrels, telomeres do not shorten with age. Paradoxically, they actually lengthen as the bird gets older.[11, 12] This finding is extraordinary and suggests this bird possesses a powerful, lifelong mechanism for cellular maintenance and repair.

What could explain this age-defying trait? Our compelling hypothesis (which I developed along with my daughter Laura while she was in high school) lies in its unique diet. The storm-petrel feeds far out at sea, primarily on energy-rich plankton, small fish, and crustaceans that migrate to the ocean surface at night. These organisms form the base of the marine food web and are the primary source of vitamin D in the ocean. Phytoplankton and zooplankton synthesize vitamin D from sunlight, and this vitamin becomes highly concentrated as it moves up the food chain into the fish and crustaceans the petrel eats. The storm-petrel consumes a diet that is, gram for gram, one of the most vitamin D–rich diets on the planet. This constant, high-level intake of dietary vitamin D throughout its long life could be the key factor that fuels the high telomerase activity needed to maintain and even lengthen its telomeres, allowing it to achieve a lifespan that is technically biologically "impossible" for a creature of its size and metabolic rate.

## THE MARINE DIET AND HUMAN RELEVANCE

Likewise, the long-lived bowhead whale also subsists on a diet of vitamin D–rich marine life, primarily krill and copepods. The common thread for these long-lived champions appears to be a diet supercharged with vitamin D from the ocean. To put this into perspective for humans, let's compare the vitamin D content of their foods. Marine phytoplankton, the foundation of this food web, can have vitamin D levels that are orders of magnitude higher than terrestrial food sources. A single serving of some small, oily fish or krill can contain thousands of international units (IU) of vitamin D.[13] By comparison, a cup of vitamin D–fortified milk in the United States contains only about 100 IU. The diet of these long-lived animals provides a continuous, high-dose supply of vitamin D that dwarfs what most humans consume.

## HAVE WE FOUND THE FOUNTAIN OF YOUTH?

We return to Ponce de León, searching for his mythical fountain in the sunny climes of St. Augustine, Florida. The irony is profound. He was searching for a magical source of youth while surrounded by and bathed by the very thing that would have provided him a key to healthier aging: the sun. As we age, our ability to produce our own vitamin D from the sun falters. This decline in cutaneous synthesis acts almost like programmed obsolescence—a built-in death mechanism—that leaves us vulnerable to the ravages of inflammaging. It strips us of a primary defense mechanism at the very time we need it most.

But we are not helpless. The story of aging is not yet completely written for any of us. The evidence is clear and compelling: Maintaining optimal vitamin D status is essential for combating chronic inflammation, protecting our telomeres, and promoting healthy aging. Given the decline in skin synthesis of vitamin D, relying on the sun alone is an unreliable and insufficient strategy for older adults. The modern, rational approach to healthy longevity must include ensuring optimal vitamin D levels, very likely through consistent supplementation with vitamin D3.

Ponce de León never found his fountain. But perhaps he was simply looking in the wrong place. He was looking down, at the water on the ground, when all he needed to do was look up, at the sun in the sky, and understand the power it could bestow upon us. The fountain of youth is a gift to all of us in the form of sunlight and its vitamin D which ensures that our immune systems direct their efforts against outside threats and not inward, inadvertently destroying the biological systems that support our life.

Conceptualizing aging as an active process mediated or caused by chronic inflammation may enable us to gain control of the sands of time in a meaningful way. While we may never be able to achieve immortality, we have the basic scientific understanding and simple tools to optimize and enhance our time here by working with our biological preprogramming by simply providing our bodies with what it telling us it needs for a long, healthy life: sunlight and vitamin D. Rather than striving for the unattainable goal of immortality, a more reasonable goal is the Hayflick Limit, the finite number of human cell replications until replicative senescence occurs, which appears to be around 122 years of age.[14]

Who would you rather be? A person with fewer wrinkles showered in praise by a passerby regarding how great you look in your coffin, or that passerby with a few more wrinkles?

# CHAPTER 20

# INFLUENZA AND INNATE IMMUNITY: THE ROLE OF VACCINES AND VITAMIN D

This chapter begins a series of chapters where we will apply what we've learned about sunlight, vitamin D, and health to improving our health by preventing many sicknesses and some injuries that plague the modern Western world. Most excitingly, we will also show how to use sunlight and vitamin D to optimize some measures of human performance that can make us a stronger, faster, and more resilient human and athlete.

## THE FORGOTTEN SHIELD: RECLAIMING OUR INNATE IMMUNITY IN THE AGE OF EPIDEMICS

Every year, as the days shorten and a chill enters the air, a familiar public health campaign begins. We are urged, and in some cases mandated, to line up for our annual seasonal influenza vaccine. It is presented as our primary, and often only, line of defense against the impending "flu season." This approach represents modern medicine's deep-seated faith in its ability to outsmart nature by engaging our body's sophisticated second line of defense—the adaptive immune system.

But this strategy, focused on a single invasive and expensive intervention, asks a critical question: Are we fighting the battle on the wrong front? Our relentless focus on marginally effective vaccines has led us to neglect a far more powerful, ancient, and elegant defense system. This is our innate immune system, the body's first and most important shield against pathogens. This system, powered by sunlight and regulated by vitamin D, produces its own potent antimicrobial weapons. We will show that bolstering this natural, nonspecific defense is a more prudent, less costly, and more effective public health strategy for preventing seasonal respiratory illness than a near-fanatical reliance on vaccines that often miss their mark.

## THE BODY'S FRONTLINE DEFENSE: INNATE IMMUNITY AND ITS CHEMICAL ARSENAL

Before a virus like influenza can even be identified by the specialized soldiers of your adaptive immune system (the T cells and B cells that vaccines target), it must first breach your body's external barriers. This is the domain of the innate immune system. Think of it as the castle walls, the moat, and the ever-vigilant guards who patrol them. This system is nonspecific; it doesn't need to have seen an enemy before to know it's an intruder. It attacks anything that looks like it doesn't belong there.

A key part of this defense lies in a remarkable class of molecules called antimicrobial peptides (AMPs) that we discussed earlier. These are the body's own natural antibiotics and antivirals. Two of the most important and well-studied AMPs are cathelicidin and defensins. These proteins are nature's perfect weapons. Their primary function is to physically destroy invading microbes. They are positively charged molecules, which makes them highly attracted to the negatively charged outer membranes of bacteria, fungi, and the envelopes of viruses like influenza. Once they attach, they act like molecular hole-punchers. They embed themselves into the pathogen's protective outer layer and tear it apart, causing its contents to leak out and effectively killing it before it can replicate and cause disease.[1]

Where are these potent defenders located? Exactly where you would want them: on the front lines. They line the surfaces of our skin and, most importantly for respiratory viruses, the epithelial cells of our entire respiratory tract—from our nostrils down into our lungs. This distribution creates a powerful "pathogen shield," a chemical barrier ready to neutralize threats on contact. The critical link, the one modern medicine has largely overlooked, is what turns on the production of these AMPs. The master switch is vitamin D. When immune cells and the epithelial cells lining your lungs are exposed to pathogens, they dramatically increase their expression of the vitamin D receptor (VDR). Active vitamin D then binds to this receptor, which in turn activates the genes responsible for manufacturing cathelicidin and defensins, deploying this chemical arsenal precisely when and where it is needed.[2, 3] Without sufficient vitamin D, this frontline response is limited or nonexistent.

## DECODING "FLU SEASON" AS THE SEASON OF DARKNESS

We accept the term "flu season" without question. But what if the season itself is the cause, not the flu? For the purposes of this discussion, the seasonality of influenza is a direct consequence of the seasonal availability of sunlight. The evidence for this is written across the globe. In the northern hemisphere, influenza epidemics predictably peak between December and February. This is precisely when the sun is at its lowest angle in the sky, when days are shortest, and when cold weather keeps people indoors, away from what little effective sunlight there is. In the southern hemisphere, the pattern is a mirror image. Their "flu season" arrives during their winter, from June to August, when their sun exposure is at its nadir.

The pattern is stark and simple: "Flu season" is a season of vitamin D deficiency. The sun's ultraviolet B (UVB) rays are the primary catalyst for vitamin D production in our skin. When the sun is low in the sky during winter months, the UVB rays are too weak to initiate this process, regardless of how much time you spend outside.[4] The most compelling evidence comes from looking at the tropics. In equatorial nations, where the sun is strong and high in the sky year-round, there is no predictable "flu season." Influenza cases are sporadic and do not erupt into the massive, population-wide epidemics seen in temperate climates.[5] This is not a coincidence. It is a direct reflection of populations that maintain sufficient vitamin D levels throughout the year, keeping their innate immune shields powered up. (The same set of facts exists for "cold" season. It occurs when the season is cold; starved of sunlight and vitamin D.)

## THE COVID-19 PANDEMIC: A GLOBAL VITAMIN D EXPERIMENT

The principles of seasonality and vitamin D-powered immunity were thrust from the realm of academic theory into stark reality with the arrival of the COVID-19 pandemic. The global spread of the SARS-CoV-2 virus provided the largest, most tragic, and most illuminating natural experiment in human history on the role of vitamin D in respiratory infections. The lessons were dramatic and compellingly clear for anyone willing to look.

First, the epidemiological patterns were unmistakable. From the earliest days of the pandemic, a striking geographical divide emerged. Sun-drenched countries near the equator did not experience the same devastating waves of severe illness and death that ravaged temperate nations in Europe and North America. A global analysis of 117 countries confirmed that higher ambient temperature and, importantly, higher levels of ultraviolet radiation were strongly associated with lower growth rates of COVID-19 cases.[6]

This observation was quantified in a direct comparison between tropical and nontropical countries. The differences in outcomes were not subtle; they were staggering. By mid-2020, nontropical countries reported an average of 1,775 cases and 114 deaths per million people. In sharp contrast, tropical countries reported a staggering 14 times fewer cases (125 per million) and 24 times fewer deaths (4.7 per million).[7] While factors like population age and reporting differences play a role, a disparity of this magnitude cannot be ignored. The most obvious and powerful environmental difference between these regions is the year-round availability of intense sunlight, the primary source of vitamin D.

I actually called attention to this yet-to-be-seen pattern in COVID-19 infections in April 2020 by drawing comparisons from the Spanish flu epidemic in 1918 and offered vitamin D as a remedy.[8] Using the Spanish flu pandemic as a model, the second wave of the flu was five times deadlier than the first wave. In real numbers, according to CDC figures, the peak death rate in late June 1918 was around 5 per 1000 persons. In early November 1918, it was 25 per 1000. Likewise, during COVID-19 in the United States, peak deaths occurred in January 2021, unfortunately exactly as predicted.

Second, as the pandemic progressed, research shifted from geographical observations to the biology of individual patients, and the evidence became even more compelling. The critical question was asked: Does a person's vitamin D level before they get infected determine how sick they will become? The answer was a resounding yes. A landmark study analyzed stored blood samples from over 160,000 individuals obtained before the pandemic. Researchers then tracked their outcomes after being diagnosed with COVID-19. The results were clear: Individuals who were vitamin D deficient prior to infection had a significantly higher risk of developing severe COVID-19 and dying from it.[9] This finding eliminated the possibility that the illness itself was causing low vitamin D levels; rather, the preexisting vitamin D deficiency was the predisposing factor for severe disease. This was not an isolated finding. A thorough review of the scientific literature concluded that a "vast number of studies" demonstrated this powerful association, solidifying the link between low vitamin D status and an increased risk of severe COVID-19 and mortality.[10]

Finally, the pandemic laid bare the mystery of comorbidities. Public health officials quickly identified risk factors that predisposed individuals to severe COVID-19: obesity, advanced age, darker skin pigmentation (especially in temperate climates), cardiovascular disease, diabetes, and other autoimmune-based disorders. What do all these conditions have in common? They are all strongly and independently associated with chronic, severe vitamin D deficiency. This leads to a powerful insight: Vitamin D deficiency was not just another risk factor; it was likely the unifying physiological condition that made these individuals so vulnerable. The virus was not simply preying on the old or the obese; it was preying on the vitamin D-starved, a group that happens to include many older, obese, and dark-skinned individuals living in sun-deprived regions. Their innate immune systems were running on empty, their frontline defenses crippled, leaving them exposed to the virus's most severe effects.

The COVID-19 fiasco exposed the systematic failures of the Western model of health care by revealing the effects of long-term chronic vitamin D deficiency on a population when stressed by a pandemic-scale respiratory illness. The noise inherent in the multifactorial disease syndrome with a chronic inflammation cause resolved into a clear signal when those differentially affected by adverse outcomes in COVID-19 were those same groups. That is, those with vitamin D deficiency were also the groups most harmed by COVID-19. These observations should be a national security wake-up call that a population that is vitamin D deficient is vulnerable and susceptible to attack by bad actors looking to exploit that weakness with biological weapons.

## MAKING A BAD SITUATION WORSE WITH COVID-19 VACCINE INJECTIONS

The acute phase of the COVID fiasco may be behind us, but the worst may be yet to come. A recent study of 290,727 people in Italy found a 37 percent decrease in life expectancy in those that received two doses of the COVID-19 vaccines compared to the unvaccinated.[11] This sobering glimpse into the future should motivate us to first, admit that there were problems with the COVID-19 shots and then work to fix those problems.[12] As the politicians and the powers that be posture and position, it is up to you to take action now. If you have been injected with COVID-19 shots and are chronically vitamin D deficient, it might be a good idea to start following some of the advice that you've been presented.

## THE MODERN VACCINATION STRATEGY: AN EXPENSIVE SHOT IN THE DARK AT A MOVING TARGET?

Every year, health authorities select the influenza strains they think will be most common and design a vaccine to target them. This strategy engages the adaptive immune system, creating antibodies that are highly specific to those chosen strains. The problem is, the influenza virus is a master of disguise, a moving target, constantly mutating. This makes predicting the right strains a matter of educated guesswork. The published effectiveness of the seasonal flu vaccine is often underwhelming. Depending on the year, its effectiveness in preventing any influenza illness can be surprisingly low, ranging from as low as 19 percent during the 2014–2015 season to a high of 51 percent during the 2010–2011 season.[13] On average, it often hovers in the 30–40 percent range in a "good" year.

In what can only be described as a study designed to show the effectiveness of flu vaccination blowing up in the face of Big Medicine, the Cleveland Clinic, one of the most mainstream, pro-vaccine institutions in the United States, just did a study that tracked over 53,000 of its own health-care workers during the 2024–2025 flu season. What it found was devastating to Big Medicine: Vaccinated employees caught the flu more often than the unvaccinated. Those who got the seasonal flu shot were 26.9 percent more likely to get sick with the flu during that flu season.[14] The average age of the people in this study was forty-two, so these are relatively young and healthy people. In a perfect world, it would have been interesting to measure the serum vitamin D status of the two groups.

For the purposes of our discussion, contrast this highly specific, hit-or-miss approach using vaccines with the body's innate defense capability. The antimicrobial peptides don't care if the virus is strain A or strain B , whether it is Chinese or German, or whether it's from a bird or a pig, or whether it has drifted since last season. AMPs attack a fundamental structural component—the viral envelope—making them broadly effective against a wide array of pathogens. While the vaccine is trying to pick a specific lock, AMPs simply blow the door off its hinges.

## A MORE PRUDENT PATH THAN VACCINATION ONLY: FORTIFY THE FORTRESS FIRST

This brings us to the core of our argument. A public health strategy that prioritizes invasive, expensive, and minimally effective (or apparently negatively efficacious) seasonal vaccines while ignoring the foundational role of innate immunity is misguided. A preventative strategy focused on ensuring optimal vitamin D levels, especially in our most vulnerable populations, is more prudent, less invasive, and ultimately, more effective.

Consider the frail older population, the very group most aggressively targeted for vaccination and the one that suffered the most during the COVID-19 pandemic. Frailty is often associated with weakened immune responses, making frail older people less likely to mount a strong response to a vaccine. But what if we could address both the frailty and the weak immunity with a single, simple intervention? Ample evidence shows that vitamin D deficiency is rampant in older, institutionalized populations and is a significant contributor to muscle weakness, poor balance, and frailty itself.[15] A public health initiative promoting sensible sun exposure and, where necessary, vitamin D supplementation would not only power up the elderly's innate immune system's production of cathelicidin and defensins but would also directly combat the physical decline that defines frailty. This is a double victory, promoting healthy aging and building a robust defense against infection simultaneously.

## A NEW STRATEGY FOR A NEW SEASON

The annual ritual of the flu shot is a testament to a medical system that prefers complex, expensive technological solutions over simple, inexpensive natural ones. The devastating COVID-19 pandemic provided a stark, real-world confirmation of this flawed approach. It is time for a paradigm shift. We must recognize that the first line of defense is not the needle, but the powerful innate immune system that every human is born with. A more effective, rational, and humane approach to seasonal respiratory illness would be a two-pronged strategy:

1. **Fortify the First Line of Defense for Everyone:** Launch a major public health campaign to educate the population about the critical link between sunlight, vitamin D, and innate immunity. This would involve promoting sensible, non-burning sun exposure during seasons when it is possible and advocating for routine vitamin D testing and supplementation, especially from fall through spring in temperate climates. This would be the universal, foundational strategy.
2. **Target Vaccination Strategically:** Reserve the use of vaccines for those at the absolute highest risk—such as the severely immunocompromised—who may need the additional, specific protection of the adaptive immune system. For the general population, a powered-up innate immune system should be the primary goal. By shifting our focus from a near-total reliance on the adaptive immune system to fortifying our innate shield, we can reduce the burden of respiratory viruses more effectively, at a lower cost, and in a way that promotes overall health and resilient aging. It is time to step out of the darkness and into the light.

# CHAPTER 21

# SOLAR POWER: FUELING THE ELITE ATHLETE

For millennia, the sun has been revered as a source of life and power. The greatest athletes of the ancient world, the Greek Olympians, understood this intuitively. They trained and competed in the nude, not for reasons of vanity, but to maximize their exposure to the brilliant Aegean sun. They instinctively knew what modern science is now rediscovering: The sun's rays forge stronger, faster, and more resilient bodies. This chapter will pull back the curtain on one of the best-kept secrets in sports—the profound and direct impact of sunlight and its hormonal product, vitamin D, on every aspect of athletic performance. We will explore how this "sunshine vitamin" is not merely a nutrient for bone and immune health but a potent, legal, and ethical performance-enhancing substance. We will demonstrate that many athletes, from weekend warriors to elite professionals, are performing with one hand tied behind their backs due to chronic, undiagnosed vitamin D deficiency. By understanding its mechanisms, we can unlock a new level of human potential that has been waiting, just beyond the clouds.

## LESSONS FROM HISTORY: THE SUN-SOAKED ATHLETE

The image of the Greek Olympian, a statuesque body glistening under the sun, is an iconic one. This practice provided them with a year-round vitamin D–replete status that modern, indoor-training athletes can only dream of. This historical observation is not an isolated one. In the twentieth century, both German and Russian scientists conducted extensive research on the performance-enhancing effects of ultraviolet (UV) radiation. In one stunning series of experiments, German researchers found that irradiating athletes with UV lamps improved their performance on a timed bicycle ergometer test by an average of 13 percent.[1] A second, independent group of athletes who were also irradiated—but were told the lamps were ineffective—improved by a nearly identical margin, ruling out a simple placebo effect. These findings were replicated multiple times.

The Russians, keenly interested in gaining a competitive edge, also found that UV irradiation not only improved athletic times but also lowered blood pressure and lactate levels, indicating improved cardiovascular efficiency and endurance.[2] These historical studies, largely forgotten in the modern era of sun-avoidance, are the first clues that something powerful happens when an athlete's skin meets the sun.

## THE RHYTHM OF THE SUN: SEASONALITY, LATITUDE, AND THE BIRTH OF AN ATHLETE

Peak athletic performance often follows a predictable annual pattern: It rises in the summer and falls in the winter. For years, this was attributed to training schedules and competition seasons. However, this rhythm perfectly mirrors the seasonal fluctuation of vitamin D levels in the body, which peak in late summer and hit their lowest point in late winter.[3] This is no coincidence. This effect extends beyond seasons to geography and even the month of an athlete's birth. Is there a latitudinal gradient for elite athletes? Are they born, or are they made? The evidence suggests that where and when you are born can give you a significant biological head start, largely mediated by vitamin D.

A fascinating phenomenon known as the "birth-month effect" provides compelling evidence. In his book *The Baseball Astrologer*, John Holway observed that since 1950, a baby born in the United States in August has had a 50 percent to 60 percent better chance of making the big leagues than a baby born in July.[4] An article in the magazine *Slate* reported a similar observation among US-born minor league baseball players, but also added that the birth-month pattern for Latin American minor leaguers doesn't show a birth-month peak.[5]

An interesting biological mechanism appears to be at play. Consider professional baseball, where a staggering number of players are born in August. Why? An August birth means the final trimester of fetal development—a critical period for muscle and neurological growth—occurs during May, June, and July, the months of peak sun intensity. The mother's high vitamin D levels are passed to the fetus, programming its body for superior neuromuscular function from the very beginning.[6] This suggests that early life sun exposure and vitamin D status may help "create" the raw material of an elite athlete.

What about the observation that there is no birth-month effect in Latin American players? Since the bulk of Latin American players are from the Dominican Republic, Venezuela, Cuba, and Mexico, countries near the equator where sun exposure is relatively constant throughout all twelve months, it is not surprising at all that an elite player is just as likely to be born in January as August. Because any competitive advantage of sun exposure during critical periods of prenatal development is equalized, birth month should not be a relevant factor because the entire population enjoys advantages conferred by the benefit of the sun year-round.

## THE ATHLETE'S PARADOX: FIT BUT DEFICIENT

Despite the overwhelming evidence of its importance, studies consistently show that athletes are notoriously vitamin D deficient. Their indoor training schedules, use of sunscreen, and tendency to live at higher latitudes conspire to rob them of the sun's benefits. A systematic review found that a staggering 56 percent of athletes had inadequate vitamin D levels (this means below 32 ng/mL).[7] This is the great paradox of modern sport: Athletes who meticulously manage every aspect of their diet and training are inadvertently neglecting the single most important hormonal variable for power, speed, and resilience.

## SOLAR POWER: HOW VITAMIN D BUILDS A BETTER ATHLETE

The historical and seasonal observations are compelling, but modern science has revealed the precise biological mechanisms that explain how vitamin D makes a better athlete and enhances athletic performance.

### THE MASTER SWITCH: VITAMIN D RECEPTORS IN MUSCLE

The single most important discovery in this field was finding vitamin D receptors (VDR) directly within the nucleus of human muscle cells.[8] This is the biological smoking gun regarding the mechanisms through which vitamin D affects athletic performance. The presence of VDRs in muscle means that vitamin D can directly communicate with muscle cells, switching genes on and off that control muscle growth, contraction, and repair. Vitamin D is not a passive bystander; it is an active manager of muscle function at the genetic level.

## THE ENGINE OF POWER: FAST-TWITCH MUSCLE FIBERS

Previously, we discussed the mechanisms responsible for falls in the frail elderly population. We now turn our attention to the contribution of those very same vitamin D-dependent, fast-twitch muscle fibers in elite athletic performance. Skeletal muscle is primarily composed of two fiber types: slow-twitch (Type I) for endurance and fast-twitch (Type II) for explosive power, strength, and speed. Fast-twitch fibers are what allow a sprinter to explode out of the blocks, a weightlifter to clean and jerk five hundred pounds, and a batter to react to a 100-mph fastball.

Fast-twitch muscle fibers are the engine of elite athletic performance. Importantly, research has shown that vitamin D preferentially acts on these fast-twitch (type II) fibers. Vitamin D deficiency leads to a noticeable atrophy, or shrinking, specifically of these power-generating fibers, while leaving slow-twitch fibers relatively unaffected.[9] Furthermore, fast-twitch fibers exhibit remarkable "use-dependent plasticity." This means they adapt and grow in response to training. Groundbreaking work by Gollnick and his colleagues in the 1970s demonstrated that intense training increases the enzymatic activity and can even influence the composition of these fibers, making them more powerful and efficient.[10, 11]

So, how does vitamin D fit into this plasticity? The answer lies with satellite cells, which are the stem cells of your muscles. When you train hard, you create micro-tears in your muscle fibers. Satellite cells are activated to rush in, repair the damage, and build the muscle back bigger and stronger. Vitamin D is a key activator of these satellite cells.[12] Now, connect the dots:

1. High-intensity training stimulates fast-twitch fibers.
2. This stimulation signals satellite cells to repair and build the fibers.
3. Vitamin D is required to fully activate these satellite cells.

Therefore, an athlete training in a vitamin D–deficient state is short-circuiting their own progress. Their hard work in the gym is compromised because the fundamental biological machinery for muscle repair and growth is running on empty. This is why the Greeks training under the sun and the Germans under UV lamps saw such dramatic improvements—their bodies were primed for maximal adaptation to training.

## UNLOCKING GROWTH: VITAMIN D, THE MYOSTATIN INHIBITOR

Myostatin is a protein that acts as a natural brake on muscle growth. Its job is to prevent your muscles from growing out of control. In the world of bodybuilding and strength training, finding ways to safely inhibit myostatin is a holy grail. Remarkably, vitamin D is a natural myostatin inhibitor. By binding to the VDR in muscle cells, vitamin D signaling tells the cell to produce less myostatin.[13] Releasing this "brake" allows for greater muscle protein synthesis and hypertrophy in response to training. In this sense, optimizing vitamin D levels functions similarly to a natural (legal) anabolic steroid, promoting muscle growth and strength without the dangerous side effects of banned substances.

## THE PERFORMANCE PAYOFF: MEASURABLE GAINS

The cellular mechanisms that vitamin D uses to create fast-twitch muscle fiber translate into real-world, measurable improvements in performance.

- **Reaction Time:** Basic reflexes form the foundation of reaction time. Because vitamin D improves the health and function of fast-twitch muscle fibers—the very fibers responsible for rapid contractions—it directly contributes to faster reaction times and quicker reflexes.[14]

- **Speed:** Vitamin D increases muscle protein synthesis, ATP production, muscle strength, jump height, jump velocity, jump power, and overall exercise capacity. These improvements particularly affect type II muscle fibers, which are important for explosive movements like sprinting and jumping. Studies show that vitamin D supplementation in deficient athletes improved performance metrics such as 100-meter sprint times and vertical jump height compared to placebo.[15]
- **Endurance:** While known for its effects on power, vitamin D also influences endurance. It improves cardiovascular function and mitochondrial efficiency within muscle cells, allowing them to produce energy more effectively over longer durations.[16]
- **Strength and Power:** The combined effects on fast-twitch fibers, satellite cells, and myostatin inhibition lead to documented increases in both proximal muscle strength and overall power output.

Vitamin D also affects performance by helping athletes stay healthy and in the game through:

- **Injury Prevention and Immunity:** The fastest and strongest athlete is useless if they are sitting on the sidelines. Vitamin D plays a critical role in keeping athletes healthy and in the game.
- **Bone Health and Injury Prevention:** Low vitamin D levels are a significant risk factor for stress fractures, one of the most common overuse injuries in sports. It also plays a key role in reducing inflammation, which allows for faster recovery between training sessions and after injury.[17]
- **A Fortified Immune System:** An athlete with an optimized immune system is less likely to succumb to the common colds and viruses that can derail a training session. Vitamin D is a powerful immune modulator, and maintaining sufficient levels keeps the immune system balanced and ready to fight off infections, ensuring fewer missed training days and peak performance on competition day.[18]

## THE MODERN VERDICT AND THE ETHICAL EDGE

Recent research continues to confirm what historical observation suggested. A review by Sikora-Klak et al. (2018)[19] found that athletes with low vitamin D levels (<30 ng/mL) had a significantly higher risk of stress fractures and musculoskeletal injuries. Correcting these deficiencies not only reduced injury risk but also correlated with improved markers of strength and power. This brings us to a powerful conclusion. Vitamin D is not a drug or a banned substance. It is a fundamental human hormone that our body is designed to produce in response to sunlight. Optimizing one's vitamin D status is not cheating; it is correcting a deficiency created by our modern, indoor lifestyle. It is an entirely ethical and legal performance-enhancing strategy.

The world of elite sports may be approaching a ceiling effect on human performance, where gains are measured in fractions of a second or a single kilogram. We propose that this ceiling is not the true limit of human potential, but rather a self-imposed limit of a vitamin D–deficient human potential. The amazing achievements that await the next generation of athletes may not come from a new training gadget or a designer supplement, but from stepping back into the light and embracing the solar power that fueled the very first Olympians.

## FROM WORST TO FIRST

In 2009, the Chicago Blackhawks hockey team achieved a remarkable feat: They went forty-nine years without the professional hockey championship (the Stanley Cup), a modern-day record. Just one year later in 2010, they achieved an even more remarkable feat by winning the Stanley Cup.

Did the team attribute their overnight success to better players, better coaching, or luck? No. The team attributed their newfound success to vitamin D. A 2020 review in the peer-reviewed journal *Nutrients* explicitly states, "The Chicago Blackhawks ice hockey team was supplemented with 5,000 IU/day of vitamin D3 and improved from the bottom rank in 2009 to win the Stanley Cup in 2010."[20] Another report states that "The Chicago Blackhawk team physicians began diagnosing and treating vitamin D deficiency in all Blackhawk players about 18 months ago. Apparently, most players are on 5,000 IU of vitamin D3 per day."[21]

There is a personal backstory to the above regarding how this professional team came about to experiment with vitamin D. In 2008, I was at a St. Louis Cardinals Baseball Fantasy Camp in Jupiter Florida. One of the other players and I got to talking and he commented that I looked "freakishly strong" as a fifty-year-old. I told him that I was taking high-dose vitamin D to get rid of psoriasis, and that while I've always been a good athlete, I had noticed that I had recently become a much better athlete (baseball player) than I had ever been. I was actually the MVP of that 2008 camp, so he had witnessed me in action. I told him the dosage (5,000 IU) and the frequency (every day) that I was using. I later heard that he was the conduit of information to the Blackhawks about vitamin D and athletic performance.

# CHAPTER 22

# ANOTHER DRINK FROM THE FOUNTAIN OF YOUTH: SUNLIGHT, VITAMIN D, AND MITOCHONDRIAL FUNCTION

For decades, we have praised the sun primarily for one miraculous gift: its ability to trigger the production of vitamin D in our skin. This "sunshine vitamin" is undeniably necessary for bone health, immune function, and mental well-being. But to see sunlight only through the lens of vitamin D is to miss a story that is far more profound, one that reaches into the very core of what it means to be alive and energetic. Recent, groundbreaking research is revealing that sunlight offers a second, more direct benefit that has the potential to redefine our approach to health and aging. It turns out that specific wavelengths of light from the sun can penetrate deep into our bodies and directly recharge the powerhouses of our cells.

This chapter unveils the sun's secret role as a direct source of cellular energy. We will explore how sunlight, independent of Vitamin D, communicates with our mitochondria—the tiny engines in our cells—to boost their performance, fight the decay of aging, and fill us with a sense of vitality that many of us thought was lost to time. The evidence is clear: Sunlight is a dual-action agent for health, and its ability to rejuvenate our mitochondria may just be the fountain of youth we've been seeking all along.

## MITOCHONDRIA: THE POWERHOUSES WITHIN YOU

Before we dive into the science of sunlight, we must first understand the microscopic engines that power every aspect of your existence: the mitochondria. Imagine your body is a bustling city. Every action—from the blink of an eye to the beat of your heart, from thinking a thought to healing a cut—requires energy. Mitochondria are the thousands of power plants within each of your cells, responsible for generating that energy. Their primary function is to take the food we eat (like glucose and fats) and the air we breathe (oxygen) and convert them into an energy currency called adenosine triphosphate (ATP). ATP is the fuel that powers cellular activity. When your mitochondria are working efficiently, you feel energetic, sharp, and resilient. Your body hums with vitality. However, as we age, our mitochondrial function declines. This isn't just a minor inconvenience; it is a fundamental driver of the aging process itself.

The "mitochondrial theory of aging" suggests that a slow, progressive decay in the performance of our cellular power plants underlies most of what we experience as getting older.[1] Damaged mitochondria produce less ATP, leading to that all-too-familiar feeling of fatigue and a lack of energy. Worse, inefficient mitochondria produce more "exhaust fumes" in the form of damaging free radicals, also known as reactive oxygen species (ROS). This creates a vicious cycle: Increased ROS damages the mitochondria further, which leads to even less energy and more damage. This decline is directly correlated with age-related diseases like heart disease, neurodegenerative disorders, and metabolic syndrome. In short, the subjective feeling of losing your energy as you age is not just in your head; it's in your mitochondria.

## A REVOLUTIONARY DISCOVERY: LIGHT ON YOUR BACK CAN IMPROVE YOUR SIGHT

For years, scientists believed that the biological effects of light were limited to the skin (vitamin D synthesis) and the eyes (vision and circadian rhythms). A groundbreaking study has shattered that assumption, proving that sunlight has a far deeper reach than we ever imagined. A research team led by Glen Jeffery published a landmark paper demonstrating that longer wavelengths present in sunlight—specifically red and near-infrared (NIR) light—can pass through the human body and have a systemic, rejuvenating effect on mitochondria in distant tissues.[2]

The experiment was elegant in its design and staggering in its implications. The researchers exposed participants to a panel of LED lights emitting 850nm NIR light, a wavelength abundant in natural sunlight, especially in the morning. For fifteen minutes, this light was shined on the participants' backs. Importantly, they had their heads and eyes completely shielded from the light source. The researchers needed a way to measure a change in mitochondrial performance. They chose to test vision. Why? The retina, the light-sensitive tissue at the back of the eye, has the highest concentration of mitochondria in the entire body. Its cells are incredibly energy-hungry, constantly working to process visual information. As we age, the mitochondria in our retinas decline, which is a major reason why our vision, particularly our ability to distinguish between subtle colors, fades over time. By testing for improvements in color vision, the researchers could effectively use the eye as a window into systemic mitochondrial health.

The results were astonishing. In the group where light only touched the participants' backs and their eyes were fully shielded, there was a significant improvement in color contrast sensitivity twenty-four hours later.[3] This proved that the benefits were not local, that being from the NIR light shining on the eyes. The light penetrated the torso, was absorbed by mitochondria in the tissues of the back, and somehow, this triggered a signal that improved mitochondrial function all the way in the retinas. This research provides the first concrete evidence in humans that NIR light from the sun has a systemic, whole-body effect, directly boosting the performance of our cellular engines.

## THE MECHANISM: HOW LIGHT RECHARGES OUR CELLULAR BATTERIES

How can light possibly interact with our mitochondria? The answer lies in the intricate machinery of the electron transport chain—the assembly line inside our mitochondria where ATP is produced. A specific enzyme in this assembly line, called cytochrome C oxidase (also known as complex IV), acts as a photoreceptor, meaning it is designed to absorb certain wavelengths of light. Research has shown that near-infrared light, in the 650nm to 900nm range, is perfectly absorbed by this enzyme.[4] When a cell is under stress, a molecule called nitric oxide can build up and effectively "clog" cytochrome C oxidase, slowing down the entire energy production assembly line. This is like a traffic jam on the energy highway. When NIR light strikes cytochrome C oxidase, it provides the energy to "kick off" the nitric oxide, breaking up the traffic jam and allowing oxygen to bind more efficiently. This simple action has two profound effects:

1. **Increased ATP Production:** With the assembly line unclogged, the electron transport chain runs faster and more efficiently, generating significantly more ATP. This translates directly to more cellular energy.
2. **Reduced Oxidative Stress:** A more efficient energy production process creates fewer damaging ROS "exhaust fumes." This helps break the vicious cycle of mitochondrial damage and protects the cell from premature aging.

In a study on cardiac arrest, researchers demonstrated that applying NIR light to the brain reduced injury by improving mitochondrial function and lowering oxidative stress, showcasing the powerful protective and restorative capabilities of this light therapy.[5] Sunlight, therefore, contains the exact wavelengths needed to penetrate our tissues and perform this microscopic tune-up on our cellular engines, boosting energy and reducing damage.

## THE VITAMIN D CONNECTION: A SECOND PATHWAY TO MITOCHONDRIAL HEALTH

While the discovery of NIR's direct effect is revolutionary, we cannot forget sunlight's other gift: Vitamin D. It turns out that Vitamin D is also intimately involved in maintaining mitochondrial health, creating a powerful synergy.

The Vitamin D Receptor (VDR), the protein that allows Vitamin D to exert its effects, has been found not only in the nucleus of our cells but also directly inside our mitochondria.[6] When Vitamin D binds to these mitochondrial receptors, it orchestrates a symphony of beneficial effects. Research shows that adequate Vitamin D levels promote mitochondrial biogenesis (the creation of new, healthy mitochondria), enhance their ability to produce energy, and help protect them from oxidative damage.[7] In essence, sunlight provides a two-pronged attack to support our mitochondria:

1. **Direct Stimulation:** Red and near-infrared light directly penetrates tissues to energize Cytochrome C Oxidase, immediately boosting ATP production and reducing oxidative stress.
2. **Indirect Regulation:** UVB light triggers Vitamin D production, which then acts as a long-term regulator, ensuring our cells have a healthy and robust population of high-performing mitochondria.

This dual mechanism underscores just how critical a relationship our species has evolved to have with the sun. Vitamin D receptor activation directly influences how cells manage and replace mitochondria (mitophagy and mitochondrial turnover), which are vital for energy production and cellular repair, particularly in older tissues. For athletes, this could mean faster muscle recovery and reduced inflammation. For older adults, it suggests potential protection against age-related neurodegenerative conditions.

We are, in a very real sense, solar-powered beings.

## SUNLIGHT: A FREE AND POWERFUL ANTIAGING THERAPY

If declining mitochondrial function is a primary driver of aging, then any intervention that can safely and effectively restore it holds the key to a longer, healthier life. The evidence we've explored strongly suggests that sunlight is one such intervention—and it's free, safe in appropriate doses, and available to everyone. By strategically exposing ourselves to sunlight, we can leverage both the direct NIR pathway and the indirect Vitamin D pathway to combat aging at its cellular source. Morning sunlight is particularly rich in the red and near-infrared wavelengths that energize cytochrome C oxidase. A daily practice of morning sun exposure can serve as a powerful therapy to:

- Increase baseline energy levels.
- Reduce systemic inflammation and oxidative stress.
- Improve cellular repair and regeneration.
- Support the function of energy-demanding organs like the brain, heart, and eyes.

This is not a complicated or expensive biohack. It is a return to an ancestral practice that our bodies are exquisitely designed for. Manipulating mitochondrial health is one of the most promising frontiers in antiaging medicine, and sunlight offers a natural, holistic way to do it.

## THREATS TO YOUR MITOCHONDRIA AND HOW TO FIGHT THEM

While sunlight is a powerful ally, our modern lifestyle is filled with threats to our mitochondrial health. To get the most out of the sun's benefits, we must also be mindful of what damages our cellular power plants. Key threats include:

- **Diet:** A diet high in processed foods, refined sugars, and industrial seed oils bombards mitochondria with excessive fuel that they cannot process cleanly, leading to a massive increase in damaging free radicals.
- **Environmental Toxins:** Pollutants, pesticides, heavy metals, and chemicals found in plastics can directly poison the mitochondrial electron transport chain, crippling energy production.
- **Sedentary Lifestyle:** Physical activity, particularly exercise that challenges your muscles and cardiovascular system, is a primary signal for the body to create more mitochondria. A lack of movement allows the mitochondrial population to shrink and weaken.
- **Chronic Stress and Poor Sleep:** Both psychological stress and a lack of restorative sleep disrupt hormonal balance and increase inflammation, which places a heavy burden on mitochondria and accelerates their decline. Protecting your mitochondria involves both adding positives, like sunlight and exercise, and removing negatives, like processed foods and toxins.

## THE SUN IS A MULTIFACETED FOUNTAIN OF YOUTH

We stand at the cusp of a new understanding of sunlight and human health. The story is no longer just about vitamin D. It is about a direct, energetic transfer between the sun and the deepest parts of our cells. Sunlight is a powerful, dual-action antiaging agent. Its UVB rays provide the raw material for vitamin D, which builds a strong and resilient mitochondrial network over time. Simultaneously, its red and near-infrared rays penetrate deep within us to provide an immediate energy boost, cleaning and recharging our existing mitochondria on a daily basis.

This rejuvenating effect of near-infrared light, delivered free of charge by the morning sun, is nothing short of a biological fountain of youth. It offers a simple, profound, and deeply human way to combat the primary driver of aging—the decline of our energy. By embracing the sun, we are not just warding off disease; we are actively turning back the clock on a cellular level, recharging our bodies with the very energy that powers life itself.

## CHAPTER 23

# CONCUSSION, NEUROINFLAMMATION, AND THE PROTECTIVE SHIELD OF VITAMIN D

In the world of sports, from the peewee football field to the professional arena, the specter of concussion looms larger than ever. Once dismissed as merely "getting your bell rung," a concussion is now understood to be a traumatic brain injury (TBI) with a complex and potentially devastating aftermath. While helmets and rule changes aim to reduce the initial impact, a critical question has been largely overlooked: What if the severity of a concussion and its long-term consequences are not just about the force of the blow, but about the biochemical state of the brain before the injury ever occurs?

This chapter will explore the dramatic rise in concussion diagnoses and make the case that this modern epidemic is profoundly exacerbated by a silent, widespread deficiency in a critical neuro-steroid hormone: vitamin D. We will detail how an impact to the head triggers a cascade of events—an energy crisis, rampant inflammation, and cellular dysfunction—and how a brain lacking sufficient vitamin D is dangerously unprepared to manage and resolve this trauma. Ultimately, we will show that concussion should be reframed not just as a biomechanical injury, but as an aberrant immune and inflammatory response to trauma, a response that can be normalized and controlled by maintaining optimal vitamin D status.

### THE RISING TIDE: AN EPIDEMIC OF CONCUSSION AND DEFICIENCY

The incidence of diagnosed concussions has skyrocketed since the mid-twentieth century. While some of this increase is due to better awareness and reporting, the sheer numbers across a wide variety of activities are staggering. In the United States, emergency room visits for sports-related head injuries in young people have more than doubled in the last decade for which data is available. It's not just high-contact sports like American football. A 2013 analysis revealed that cycling was the leading cause of sports-related head injuries in emergency rooms, followed by football, baseball, and basketball.[1] Soccer, particularly for female athletes, also shows alarming concussion rates, rivaling those of male football players.[2]

The long-term consequences are also coming into sharper focus, with research showing that the risk of being diagnosed with chronic traumatic encephalopathy (CTE), a degenerative brain disease, increases by 30 percent for each year of playing American football and by 15 percent for each year of ice hockey play.[3]

This dramatic rise in concussion incidence has occurred in parallel with the growing recognition of widespread vitamin D deficiency. This is not a coincidence. Vitamin D, once thought to be important only for bone health, is now understood to be a potent steroid hormone that regulates the immune system, inflammation, and cellular health throughout the body, including the brain.

Since vitamin D is indeed neuroprotective, one would expect to find a high prevalence of deficiency among populations at high risk for concussion, such as athletes. The data confirm this hypothesis in dramatic fashion. A landmark 2015 study on players in the National Football League (NFL) found that a staggering 86 percent had either insufficient or deficient levels of vitamin D.[4] Another study presented to the American Academy of Orthopaedic Surgeons found that NFL players with vitamin D deficiency were significantly more likely to suffer muscle injuries, highlighting a systemic vulnerability.[5] This is not an isolated finding; low vitamin D status is common across collegiate and professional sports, leaving the very individuals most susceptible to head trauma biochemically unprepared for the insult.

## NEUROINFLAMMATION: THE FIRE WITHIN

To understand how vitamin D deficiency amplifies the damage resulting from a concussion, we must first understand the modern model of TBI. It is a multistage process that begins with a physical force and rapidly descends into a biochemical and metabolic crisis.

**Phase I:** The Initial Biomechanical Insult: The Axonal Stretch
The injury is not primarily about the brain bruising against the skull. The most significant damage comes from rotational and acceleration/deceleration forces that cause a shearing and stretching strain on the brain's delicate wiring. This strain physically stretches axons, the long fibers that connect neurons, triggering the entire pathological cascade.[6]

**Phase II:** The Neurometabolic Cascade: The "Energy Crisis"

The stretching of neuronal membranes forces ion channels to open, leading to a massive, chaotic influx of calcium ($Ca^{2}+$) into the cells. This "electrical storm" forces the neuron's energy pumps to work frantically to restore balance, consuming enormous amounts of ATP (the cell's energy currency).[7] Simultaneously, blood flow to the brain is often reduced after the impact. This creates a severe "energy crisis": skyrocketing energy demand coupled with a plummeting energy supply. This mismatch is responsible for the classic concussion symptoms of brain fog, fatigue, and slowed thinking.

**Phase III:** Microstructural Damage and Inflammation: The Lingering Aftermath

The energy crisis and calcium overload damage mitochondria (the cell's power plants) and trigger a devastating inflammatory response. The brain's resident immune cells—microglia and astrocytes —are activated. In a healthy response, they clean up debris and promote healing. However, in an uncontrolled state, they release a flood of pro-inflammatory chemicals that cause secondary damage, impair neuronal function, and can lead to the breakdown of the blood-brain barrier (BBB).[8] This allows more inflammatory agents to pour in from the bloodstream, fanning the flames of neuroinflammation.[9] This chronic inflammatory state is now believed to be the driving force behind long-term damage, including the tau protein dysfunction seen in CTE.[10]

## THE VITAMIN D DEFICIENCY DISADVANTAGE: ADDING INSULT TO INJURY BY FUELING THE FIRE

A brain operating with insufficient vitamin D is at a profound disadvantage at every stage of this TBI cascade. Vitamin D is not merely a vitamin; it is a hormone that the brain relies on for protection and immune regulation. Neurons and glial cells are rich with vitamin D receptors (VDR) and the enzymes needed to convert circulating vitamin D into its active hormonal form, 1,25-dihydroxyvitamin D.[11] When vitamin D levels are low, the brain's defenses are down.

**During the Energy Crisis:** Active vitamin D is critical for regulating calcium channels and supporting mitochondrial function.[12] In a vitamin D–deficient state, the neuron is already less capable of managing calcium influx and producing the ATP needed to survive the energy crisis. The initial metabolic damage is therefore deeper and more prolonged.

**During the Inflammatory Response:** This is where vitamin D's role is most critical. Vitamin D is a master regulator of the brain's immune system. It acts on microglia and astrocytes to suppress the production of pro-inflammatory cytokines (like TNF-$\alpha$ and IL-6) and promote the release of anti-inflammatory signals.[13] In a vitamin D–deficient brain, this regulation is lost. Upon activation by trauma, glial cells become hyper-inflammatory, spewing out destructive chemicals that damage healthy, neighboring neurons and degrade the blood-brain barrier. Concussion in a vitamin D–deficient athlete is, therefore, an aberrant and exaggerated immune response to trauma.

## AQUAPORINS: A KEY MECHANISM OF VITAMIN D'S PROTECTION

A critical and often overlooked component of post-concussion damage is cerebral edema, or brain swelling. Much of this swelling is controlled by tiny water channels on the surface of glial cells, particularly astrocytes, called aquaporins. The most abundant of these is Aquaporin-4 (AQP4).

After a TBI, AQP4 channels become dysfunctional. This disrupts the brain's delicate water balance, leading to cytotoxic edema—water rushing into damaged cells, causing them to swell and burst. This swelling increases intracranial pressure and is a major cause of secondary brain injury after a TBI.

Here again, vitamin D plays a direct, protective role. Research by Dr. Donald Stein and colleagues at Emory University, pioneers in TBI research, has highlighted that vitamin D helps regulate the expression and proper function of AQP4.[14] By ensuring these water channels work correctly, vitamin D can help mitigate the dangerous brain swelling that follows an injury. A brain with sufficient vitamin D is better equipped to manage water balance and resist the damaging effects of edema, while a deficient brain is more susceptible to this life-threatening complication. The proper function of aquaporins, regulated by vitamin D, can be seen as a proxy for the overall health of the brain's immune and support systems.

## MITIGATION AND SYNERGY: THE POWER OF PROACTIVE SUPPLEMENTATION

If vitamin D deficiency exacerbates concussion, can supplementation mitigate it? The evidence, though still emerging, is encouraging and compelling. One striking case study involved a high school football team in New York. After the team experienced fifteen concussions in just two seasons, the team's coaches, working with medical professionals, implemented a program to test and optimize the players' vitamin D levels. Over the next two seasons, with the team maintaining sufficient blood levels of vitamin D, they suffered only one mild concussion.[15] While anecdotal, this real-world result aligns perfectly with the known biological mechanisms.

Furthermore, vitamin D's protective effects can be amplified when combined with other neuroprotective agents. Dr. Stein's research group has extensively studied the hormone progesterone, which has been shown to be highly effective in reducing brain damage after TBI. Their preclinical work has revealed a powerful synergy: Pretreating with vitamin D to ensure sufficient levels before an injury occurs significantly potentiates the protective effects of post-injury progesterone treatment.[16] They conclude that the combination of the steroid progesterone and vitamin D is a "novel and compelling approach to TBI treatment" and that deficiency can "significantly affect recovery after CNS injury."[17]

Another interesting finding of the Stein experiments was a complex relationship between the timing of the injury and the application of the vitamin D intervention. They found that vitamin D only enhanced the protective effects of the progesterone if the brain was in a state of chronic vitamin D repletion before the TBI. That means that waiting until the TBI occurs and administering vitamin D after the fact to treat the TBI is not effective. There must be a state of chronic vitamin D sufficiency in place before the TBI for the progesterone to have maximal therapeutic effect.[18]

This synergy between vitamin D and progesterone, both steroid hormones, is key. It demonstrates that the brain's baseline health, established by adequate vitamin D status, is a prerequisite for optimal healing and response to another therapy (progesterone). You cannot expect a therapy to work effectively on a system that is already compromised by a fundamental vitamin D deficiency. This interesting finding raises many issues regarding the effects of other drugs and treatments on a vitamin D starved population, and calls into question whether vitamin D status is an unaccounted-for and profound uncontrolled variable in human pharmaceutical research.

## A NEW PARADIGM: FROM REACTION TO PREVENTION OF CONCUSSION

The evidence paints a clear and coherent picture. The modern concussion crisis is not just a story of bigger, faster athletes and harder hits. It is a story of a collision between the unavoidable trauma of sport and the avoidable vulnerability of chronic vitamin D deficiency.

Let us integrate this into a final, comprehensive model:

A blow to the head causes axonal stretching, triggering a massive energy crisis and calcium overload. In a vitamin D–replete brain, the immune system responds with controlled efficiency. Glial cells are activated but the response is modulated and balanced by the calming presence of hormonal vitamin D. Glial cells clean up debris, release anti-inflammatory factors, support neuronal survival, and help maintain the integrity of the blood-brain barrier and aquaporin function, thus limiting edema. The healing process is orderly and efficient.

In a vitamin D–deficient brain, the same blow triggers a catastrophic, unregulated cascade. The initial energy crisis is more severe due to preexisting deficits in calcium regulation and mitochondrial support. The subsequent immune response is aberrant and hyper-inflammatory. Glial cells, lacking hormonal vitamin D's modulating and balancing signal, unleash a firestorm of destructive chemicals. The blood-brain barrier breaks down, aquaporin function is disrupted (leading to severe edema), and the inflammatory fire rages unchecked for days or weeks, causing widespread secondary damage. This chronic neuroinflammation not only worsens the acute symptoms but also likely paves the road for long-term neurodegenerative diseases like CTE.

Concussions will always be a risk in sport. The trauma is, to some degree, unavoidable. The brain's response to that trauma, however, is not. We can choose to send our athletes onto the field with a brain that is biochemically prepared to heal, or one that is primed to self-destruct. In essence, there are two ways to deal with concussions: either don't engage in sports that risk head injury, or accept that risk and do all that is possible to mitigate the effects of those blows. Realization that concussion is a symptom of a dysfunctional immune response caused by chronic vitamin D deficiency and that maintaining an optimal vitamin D status is a rational, safe, inexpensive and scientifically valid policy is a giant step forward in this mitigation effort.

## A CALL TO ACTION: A PROACTIVE VITAMIN D PLAN FOR ATHLETE BRAIN HEALTH

Given the overwhelming evidence of its importance for neurological health and the high prevalence of deficiency, optimizing vitamin D status should become a standard of care for every athlete, at every level. A simple, proactive plan includes:

1. **Baseline Testing:** Every athlete should have their serum 25(OH) D level tested at the beginning of the preseason to establish their baseline.
2. **Define Optimal Levels:** The goal should not be to simply avoid deficiency (<20 ng/mL) or even insufficiency (<30 ng/mL). For optimal neuro-immune function and athletic performance, levels should be targeted in the range of 80–100 ng/mL.
3. **Personalized Supplementation:** Based on baseline levels, a personalized supplementation plan using vitamin $D_3$ should be implemented. This often requires doses between 5,000 and 8,000 IU/day, but should be guided by a health care professional.
4. **Year-Round Maintenance and Retesting:** Vitamin D levels can fall during the winter months. Supplementation should be maintained year-round, with levels retested annually to ensure the target range is being maintained.

This simple, safe, and inexpensive strategy represents one of the most powerful tools available to us to protect the brains of our athletes. It is time to move beyond a reactive approach to concussion and embrace a proactive strategy of building a more resilient brain from the inside out to prevent concussions or at least lessen their severity. The physiological shield that vitamin D offers may be the single most important piece of protective equipment an athlete can have.

# CHAPTER 24

# SHINING SUNLIGHT ON EQUITY: HOW VITAMIN D CAN BRIDGE RACIAL HEALTH DISPARITIES

It's a stark reality: Significant health gaps exist between racial groups in the United States, with chronic diseases disproportionately affecting minority populations. While many point to social and economic factors, a powerful biological explanation—one that's often overlooked, especially in relation to skin pigmentation—lies in something as fundamental as sunlight and a vital nutrient: vitamin D.

## THE ALARMING REALITY OF HEALTH DISPARITIES

Let's look at the numbers: African Americans experience dramatically higher rates of chronic conditions. Hypertension is 25 percent higher, diabetes 49 percent higher, and obesity 59 percent higher compared to white individuals.[1] The Centers for Disease Control and Prevention (CDC) reported that nearly 44 percent of African American men and 48 percent of African American women live with some form of cardiovascular disease. Autoimmune diseases also show a higher incidence among African Americans.[2, 3]

For years, the focus has been on socioeconomic conditions as the primary drivers of these disparities. While these factors undoubtedly play a role, a groundbreaking finding reveals a deeper layer to the problem: Even affluent African Americans, with access to superior resources, still experience worse health outcomes than their white counterparts of similar socioeconomic status.[4] This insight begs the question: Are we systematically ignoring the biological influence of dark skin?

## THE EVOLUTIONARY DANCE OF SKIN COLOR AND SUNLIGHT

Why do we have different skin colors? It's an adaptive marvel, directly tied to our evolutionary journey and the sun's powerful rays. Skin color is essentially a finely tuned regulator of ultraviolet (UV) radiation penetration.[5] The process of tanning, where skin darkens after sun exposure, is a temporary, on-the-fly mutation to protect our DNA. Dark skin, rich in melanin, offers a significant selective advantage in regions with intense sunlight, like those near the equator. Melanin is a highly efficient absorber of UV-B photons, acting as a natural sunscreen to prevent or reduce DNA damage.[6] But as ancestors migrated away from the sunlight-drenched equator, skin evolved. Melanin content decreased, indicating that sunlight provided another important benefit. That benefit is vitamin D.

## DARK SKIN'S DOUBLE-EDGED SWORD: PROTECTION AND DEFICIENCY

While dark skin excels at protecting against sun damage—skin cancer is 70 times less likely in dark skin compared to white skin[7]—this protective mechanism comes with a significant trade-off. Dark skin dramatically diminishes the body's ability to produce essential vitamin D. Here's how it works: UV-B light that isn't absorbed by melanin triggers vitamin D synthesis in the skin. Considering that nearly every one of the estimated 37 trillion cells in the human body has a receptor for vitamin D, its widespread influence is undeniable.[8, 9] However, dark skin is remarkably inefficient at producing this vital nutrient. Studies have shown that white skin exposed to UV-B light can experience a fifty-fold increase in vitamin D levels within hours, while dark skin may show no increase at all under the same conditions. To achieve even a thirty-fold increase, dark skin requires five to ten times more UV-B exposure.[10]

This biological reality translates directly into widespread vitamin D deficiency among African Americans compared to white Americans. A National Health and Nutrition Examination Survey (NHANES) found average vitamin D levels of 14 ng/ml for African Americans, significantly lower than the 24 ng/ml for white individuals (which is also drastically low as well)—a 42 percent difference. Even more concerning, the percentage of African Americans with severe vitamin D deficiency (below 10 ng/ml) skyrocketed from 9 percent in 1988 to 29 percent in 2006, a staggering 222 percent increase.[11] The reappearance of rickets, a disease once largely eradicated by vitamin D fortification in milk, is a tragic indicator of the severity of the deficiency among African American infants and children.[12]

## THE "FISH OUT OF WATER" EFFECT: WHEN ANCESTRY MEETS ENVIRONMENT

Imagine people whose ancestors thrived in year-round sunshine now living in environments with limited sun exposure. This "fish out of water" scenario highlights the profound health consequences of chronic vitamin D deficiency for dark-skinned individuals in sun-poor regions.

Comparing African immigrants to the United States with multigenerational African Americans provides a compelling illustration. Recent black African immigrants show significantly lower rates of risk factors for heart attacks, strokes, hypertension, and other cardiovascular diseases compared to multigenerational African Americans.[13] This difference strongly suggests that environmental factors, particularly sunlight exposure, play a critical role.

As we've learned, a common thread linking many of these cardiovascular conditions is chronic inflammation, often fueled by long-term vitamin D deficiency.[14] This idea is further supported by the observed low incidence of autoimmune diseases among Black populations in equatorial Africa.[15] Furthermore, African Americans consistently exhibit higher levels of serum inflammatory markers compared to white individuals.[16] Importantly, low-grade systemic inflammation is a key player in the development and progression of cardiovascular disease and hypertension.[17, 18]

## VITAMIN D: A MASTER REGULATOR OF HEALTH

Chronic vitamin D deficiency and its resulting inflammatory state are linked to increased risks of autoimmune diseases, various cardiovascular conditions, epithelial cancers (breast, prostate, lung, and colon), and many other debilitating health issues.[19, 20] While socioeconomic status, health-care access, lifestyle, and cultural factors undoubtedly contribute partly to health disparities,[21] vitamin D deficiency—exacerbated in dark-skinned people living in sun-poor environments—offers a powerful and plausible biological explanation for the observed health outcomes. African Americans demonstrate a significantly higher prevalence of vitamin D insufficiency and suffer worse outcomes for cardiovascular disease, certain cancers, diabetes mellitus, and renal disease, all conditions linked to low vitamin D levels.

Given vitamin D's profound impact on overall health and the documented deficiencies among African Americans, addressing vitamin D status immediately is not just practical; it's critical. Vitamin D is inexpensive, safe, and easily accessible—a simple solution to a serious problem. While complex social and economic factors deserve attention, we cannot afford to wait when a readily available remedy is at hand. As filmmaker Tyler Perry recently urged, increasing vitamin D intake among the African American population can strengthen the immune system and reduce the incidence of autoimmune disease, a message resonating especially during public health crises.[22]

## UNPACKING THE VITAMIN D CONNECTION: THREE CRITICAL EXAMPLES

The health disparities compared to whites observed in the African American community offer profound insights into the underestimated role of vitamin D in various health conditions. Let's examine three wildly different examples: infant mortality, cardiovascular disease, and COVID-19.

### Infant Mortality

African American mothers face significantly higher risks during pregnancy. They are 2.3 times more likely than white mothers to experience intrauterine fetal death.[23] They are also 1.5 to 2.5 times more likely to deliver preterm or very preterm infants, and more likely to have term low-birth-weight infants.[24] Preeclampsia, a serious pregnancy complication, is also more prevalent and severe among African American women.[25, 26, 27]

Maternal vitamin D deficiency may contribute to the increased inflammatory response characteristic of preeclampsia.[28, 29] The link between vitamin D, immune function, and dark skin as a risk factor for exacerbated vitamin D deficiencies in adverse birth outcomes is becoming increasingly clear.[30]

### Cardiovascular Disease (CVD)

NHANES data consistently demonstrate a high prevalence of CVDs—including coronary heart disease, heart failure, stroke, and peripheral artery disease—among all groups with vitamin D deficiency. This risk is further amplified in the African American population with vitamin D deficiency.[31] Vitamin D's protective effects against CVD stem from its role in maintaining healthy vascular endothelial tissue (the inner lining of blood vessels) by promoting nitric oxide availability. Nitric oxide is essential for healthy endothelial function[32] through its ability to suppress inflammation-induced vascular dysfunction.[33] A compelling study on the effects of vitamin D on blood pressure in African Americans found that daily vitamin D supplementation (1,000 IU, 2,000 IU, or 4,000 IU) for three months significantly reduced mean arterial pressure in a dose-dependent manner compared to a placebo group.[34] Again, the connection between vitamin D, immune function, and dark skin acting as a risk factor for vitamin D deficiencies affecting CVD is evident.

### COVID-19

The COVID-19 pandemic has disproportionately affected African American communities. An analysis by the *Washington Post* revealed that counties with African American majorities had three times the rate of COVID-19 cases and six times the death rate compared to predominantly white communities.[35] A study published in *JAMA* in April 2020 described the clinical outcomes of 5,700 hospitalized COVID-19 patients in the New York area: 94 percent had at least one chronic health problem, and 88 percent had two or more. The most prevalent conditions were hypertension (57 percent), obesity (42 percent), and diabetes (34 percent).[36] Given the documented chronic vitamin D deficiency among African Americans, vitamin D's role as a risk factor for these comorbidities, and its critical function in immune system regulation, enhancing vitamin D status in the African American community is clearly warranted. A recent paper even suggested that vitamin D is "very important in preventing the cytokine storm and subsequent acute respiratory distress syndrome that is commonly the cause of mortality" in COVID-19, noting lower population mortality rates in countries closer to the equator with higher vitamin D production.[37]

## A CLEAR PATH FORWARD

The bad news is undeniable: Significant health disparities persist within the African American community, many appearing to be directly linked to chronic vitamin D deficiency exacerbated by dark skin. The good news, however, offers a clear path forward: Vitamin D supplements are an effective, safe, inexpensive, and readily available remedy. As Tyler Perry and many health experts urge, embracing vitamin D supplementation carries minimal risk and offers tremendous, potentially lifesaving benefits particularly for dark-skinned people in the West.

## WHAT YOU CAN DO

Consult your doctor. Get your 25(OH)D blood levels tested. Optimal levels typically fall between 60–100 ng/ml. If you are deficient and year-round sun exposure is a challenge, supplement with vitamin D3, the most bioavailable form. If you have dark skin, it's highly probable you need to supplement. Start building and maintaining healthy vitamin D levels now.

# CHAPTER 25

# IS SUNSCREEN THE NEW MARGARINE?

For decades, we were given a simple, authoritative command by doctors, health organizations, and the media: Fat is the enemy.[1] For example, the saturated fat found in butter was demonized as a direct path to heart disease. The solution, we were told, was margarine—a triumph of food science, a heart-healthy alternative that would save us from ourselves.[2] Millions of people made the switch, confident they were making the healthier choice. We now know this advice was not just wrong; it was catastrophically harmful. The industrial process used to create margarine produced trans fats, toxic substances that we now understand are far more dangerous than the natural butter they replaced, actively contributing to cardiovascular disease, inflammation, and a host of other health problems. The well-intentioned advice contributed to a public health disaster of obesity, chronic inflammation, and cardiovascular disease.

In 2019, writer Rowan Jacobson posed a provocative question that perfectly frames our modern relationship with the sun: "Is Sunscreen the New Margarine?"[3] The parallels are striking and deeply unsettling. For the past fifty years, we have been given another simple, authoritative command: The sun is the enemy. We have been told to avoid it at all costs, to seek shade, and to slather ourselves—and our children—in chemical sunscreens from head to toe. The advice, intended to protect us from skin cancer, has created a different and arguably more widespread health crisis: a global pandemic of vitamin D deficiency and a daily exposure to potentially toxic chemicals in those sunscreens that are absorbed directly into our bloodstreams. Just as we replaced natural butter with a synthetic, harmful substitute, we have blocked the life-giving rays of the sun—our primary source of essential vitamin D—and replaced them with a chemical shield whose long-term safety is far from guaranteed, known, or understood. This chapter will explore the mounting evidence that this advice has also been profoundly misguided, examining the paradoxical nature of melanoma, the risks of the chemicals in sunscreen, and the devastating environmental cost caused by our neurotic fear of the sun.

## THE MELANOMA PARADOX: A CANCER THAT PREFERS THE DARK

The public health message is simple and unwavering: Sun exposure causes malignant melanoma, the deadliest form of skin cancer. If this were the complete story, we would expect to find melanoma primarily on the areas of the body that receive the most cumulative sun exposure—the face, the neck, the forearms, and the hands. But this is not what the data shows. In a baffling paradox, melanoma often occurs in places rarely, if ever, exposed to the sun. It is found on the soles of the feet, the palms of the hands, between the toes, under the fingernails, on the buttocks, in the armpits, and even in internal areas like the anal fissure.[4] This simple observation fundamentally challenges the narrative that solar UV radiation is the sole cause of this deadly cancer. While severe, blistering sunburns, especially in childhood, are a known risk factor, the relationship between chronic, sensible sun exposure and melanoma is far more complex, nuanced and uncertain. This suggests that something else is at play. If the sun is not the only factor, what is? A growing body of research points to an internal, protective mechanism that is crippled by a modern, sun-avoidant indoor lifestyle: vitamin D.

## THE VITAMIN D DEFENSE: YOUR BODY'S BUILT-IN MELANOMA FIGHTER

While public health campaigns have focused exclusively on the sun as a carcinogen, they have ignored its role as the primary source of vitamin D, a potent hormone that regulates thousands of functions in the human body, including the suppression of cancer. The evidence linking vitamin D deficiency to worse melanoma outcomes is now overwhelming. A 2022 retrospective study published in *Melanoma Research* found that melanoma patients who were vitamin D deficient had significantly worse overall survival rates than those with sufficient levels.[5] This wasn't a minor effect; the deficiency was a powerful predictor of a poorer prognosis. Similarly, research published in *Oncotarget* on patients with metastatic melanoma—cancer that has already spread—found a clear association between vitamin D deficiency and a worse prognosis.[6]

The connection is so strong that researchers are now actively investigating the role of vitamin D status as a critical biomarker in melanoma. A comprehensive review in the *European Journal of Cancer Prevention* concluded that sufficient vitamin D levels are associated with less-aggressive tumors and improved survival rates for melanoma patients.[7] The vitamin D hormone appears to work by promoting cell differentiation and apoptosis (programmed cell death) and inhibiting cell proliferation and angiogenesis (the formation of new blood vessels that feed tumors). In simple terms, vitamin D produced from sun exposure or diet helps your immune system identify and destroy cancerous cells before they can become life-threatening tumors. By avoiding the sun and living in a state of chronic vitamin D deficiency, we may be inadvertently disabling one of our body's most essential, built-in cancer defense systems.

The danger of sun avoidance extends far beyond melanoma. A landmark study of nearly thirty thousand Swedish women over twenty years produced a truly shocking finding. The researchers concluded that avoidance of sun exposure was a risk factor for all-cause mortality of a similar magnitude to smoking.[8] Let that sink in: Actively avoiding the sun was as dangerous a cancer risk factor as was being a smoker. The nonsmokers who avoided the sun had a life expectancy similar to smokers in the highest sun exposure group, indicating that sun avoidance negated the health benefits of not smoking. The evidence is clear: The risk of avoiding the sun and the resulting vitamin D deficiency is a far greater threat to our overall health than sensible, non-burning sun exposure itself.

## A FALSE SENSE OF SECURITY: THE DANGERS IN THE BOTTLE

Sunscreens provide a false sense of security. People who apply them tend to stay in the sun for much longer periods than they otherwise would, believing they are completely protected. This can lead to overexposure and the kind of burning that is a known risk factor for skin cancer.

But the danger is not just behavioral; it is also chemical. The US Food and Drug Administration (FDA) regulates sunscreens not as cosmetics, but as over-the-counter drugs. This is because their active ingredients are designed to be absorbed into the body to do their work. For decades, the industry operated on the assumption that absorption of those drugs was minimal. That assumption has been proven false. In a series of studies, the FDA confirmed that common chemical sunscreen ingredients are absorbed systemically into the bloodstream after just a single use.[9] Chemicals in popular sunscreens like oxybenzone, octinoxate, octocrylene, and avobenzone were found in blood plasma at levels far exceeding the FDA's threshold for safety testing. More alarmingly, these chemicals lingered in the body for days or even weeks. You are not just putting a protective layer of sunscreen on your skin; you are absorbing a cocktail of synthetic, potentially harmful drugs through your skin.

Once these drugs are absorbed, what are these drugs doing inside our bodies? A review in *Toxicology Reports* highlighted the neurotoxic effects of many of these active ingredients.[10] The review detailed how common sunscreen chemicals like octyl methoxycinnamate, benzophenone-3 and -4, 4-methylbenzylidene camphor, 3-benzylidene camphor, and octocrylene can interfere with normal nervous system function. Most disturbingly, several of these fat-soluble chemicals have been shown to cross the blood-brain barrier, a highly selective membrane that is supposed to protect the brain from toxins. The long-term consequences of this continuous, low-dose exposure to neurotoxic chemicals, especially for the developing brains of children, are simply unknown.

Many of these same chemicals are also known endocrine disruptors, meaning they can mimic or interfere with the body's natural hormones, potentially impacting reproductive health, thyroid function, and brain development. In response to this crisis of relatively no information on the long-term toxicity of these ubiquitous substances, a study by Hiller et al. said "high in-vivo loads call for a critical toxicological assessment of the UV filters and their metabolites."[11]

In sum, once absorbed, these active sunscreen chemicals disrupt normal nervous system activities at molecular and cellular levels, cross protective brain barriers, alter neurotransmitter and hormone signaling, and may induce structural neuronal damage. Their known endocrine disrupting properties add further concern about reproductive and developmental risks from chronic exposure

Let's return to our comparison. We have spent over fifty years proving the undeniable dangers of smoking. We are only now, after decades of widespread, daily use, beginning to investigate the systemic, long-term risks of the synthetic and dangerous drugs in sunscreen. Is it responsible to continue slathering our bodies in these chemicals while the safety data is so alarming and incomplete?

## SUNSCREEN CHEMICALS: ACCUMULATING TO UNHEALTHY LEVELS IN YOUR BODY WITH EACH USE

FDA-funded studies revealed that certain sunscreen ingredients can accumulate in the body at unsafe levels.[12, 13] These studies investigated avobenzone, oxybenzone, octocrylene, homosalate, octisalate, and octinoxate. The findings indicated that some of these chemicals accumulate to levels exceeding what is considered safe. And that the chemicals remained above accepted levels even seven days after a single application.[14]

One study found detectable levels of benzophenone-3 (oxybenzone) in 96.8 percent of sunscreen samples.[15] Oxybenzone is particularly concerning because, in addition to being toxic, it also enhances the skin's permeability, increasing the absorption of other chemicals, including potentially toxic herbicides, pesticides, and insect repellents. Another study demonstrated that oxybenzone significantly increased the absorption of the herbicide 2,4-D, a serious concern for agricultural workers and farmers.[16] Oxybenzone, along with at least eight other sunscreen ingredients, has been found in alarming levels in breast milk, amniotic fluid, urine, and blood.[17]

A subsequent FDA-funded study expanded its investigation into the time-course of sunscreen ingredients.[18] Participants applied 2 mg per square centimeter over 75 percent of their body at two-hour intervals at baseline and on days 2, 3, and 4. Over the following 21 days, blood samples were collected, revealing a mean maximum plasma concentration for oxybenzone of 258.1 nanograms per milliliter (ng/mL) when applied as a lotion and 180.1 ng/mL when applied as an aerosol spray.[19] These concentrations were over 500 times higher than the presumed safety threshold of 0.5 ng/mL after just a few days of use.[20]

A variety of additional studies on the toxicity of oxybenzone found that it:

- **Acts as a phototoxicant:** Its adverse effects and ability to generate harmful free radicals are amplified upon light exposure, which is precisely when sunscreen is used.[21]
- **Is neurotoxic:** It is harmful to brain cells.[22]
- **Exhibits significant reproductive and fertility effects:** It can "significantly lower" testosterone levels in adolescent boys,[23] alter hormone levels in men,[24] reduce sperm count,[25] and decrease male fertility by affecting calcium signaling in sperm, partly by mimicking progesterone.[26] It is also linked to endometriosis in women[27] and can lead to lower male birth weight and decreased gestational age.[28]

Despite their own funded research highlighting the dangers of systemic absorption of sunscreen chemicals, the FDA continues to advocate for sunscreen use. The justification for this recommendation, as noted by doctors in an accompanying editorial[29] and discussed by the American Academy of Dermatology, is a purported "lack of evidence" that the chemicals in sunscreens are dangerous.[30] This stance is baffling, given the mounting research demonstrating oxybenzone's multisystem harmful effects.

## THE HIDDEN DANGERS OF NANOPARTICLES IN SUNSCREEN

Given the endocrine-disrupting and neurotoxic effects of oxybenzone, its high absorbability, and the availability of demonstrably safer mineral-based sunscreens (those containing non-nanometer-sized zinc oxide and titanium dioxide), the continued use of oxybenzone-containing sunscreen for sun protection is illogical. However, unfortunately the latest advancements in sunscreen technology also present their own set of dangers. While titanium dioxide and zinc oxide are recognized as safe sunscreen ingredients, this safety does not extend to their nanosized versions. Most nanoparticles measure less than 100 nanometers. Sunscreens formulated with nanoparticles typically contain titanium dioxide or zinc oxide, and many are aerosol spray products.

Animal research indicates that inhaling nanoparticles allows them to reach areas of the lungs that are difficult for the body to clear. This can enable them to enter the bloodstream. Once in the lungs or after penetrating the skin, nanoparticles have the potential to inflict widespread damage to cells, organs, the immune system, the nervous system, the heart, and the brain.[31, 32] Some scientists suspect that the toxic effects of nanoparticles in the body are directly related to their minute size, which can trigger an adverse immune response.[33] Inhaling high doses of titanium dioxide is classified as a possible human carcinogen by the International Agency for Research on Cancer.[34] Inhaling zinc oxide can lead to metal fume fever, a condition occurring within hours afterward, characterized by symptoms such as chest pain, cough, nausea, reduced lung volume, and leukocytosis.[35]

## AN OCEAN OF TROUBLE: SUNSCREEN'S ENVIRONMENTAL TOLL

The toxicity of these sunscreen chemicals is not limited to the human body. When we swim in the ocean or shower after a day at the beach, these toxic chemicals wash off our skin and into the environment, with devastating consequences for marine ecosystems. Coral reefs, the vibrant rainforests of the sea, are particularly vulnerable.[36] According to the Smithsonian Institution, chemicals like oxybenzone and octinoxate are profoundly toxic to coral.[37] They can induce coral bleaching even at low concentrations, damage coral DNA, cause deformities in young coral, and disrupt their reproduction. It only takes a tiny amount—equivalent to a single drop of water in six and a half Olympic-sized swimming pools—to cause damage. Each year, an estimated 14,000 tons of sunscreen wash into coral reef areas, contributing to their rapid, worldwide decline.[38]

The toxic effects are not limited to corals. The Australian government has found that sunscreen chemicals can also harm other marine organisms, including algae (the base of the marine food web), sea urchins, fish, and marine mammals.[39] They can accumulate in the tissues of these animals and cause reproductive and developmental problems. In response to this overwhelming evidence, some regions, like Hawaii and Palau, have banned the sale of sunscreens containing oxybenzone and other harmful chemicals to protect their precious marine ecosystems.[40]

We are not just poisoning ourselves; we are poisoning the planet in our misguided quest to hide from the sun.

## SMARTER ALTERNATIVES TO A CHEMICAL SHIELD

The solution is not to embrace sunburns. The solution is to develop a new, healthier relationship with the sun. Instead of relying on a chemical shield, we can adopt a set of simple, time-tested strategies:

1. **Seek Shade During Peak Hours:** The sun is strongest between 10 a.m. and 4 p.m. Enjoy the sun in the morning and late afternoon, and use a tree or umbrella for cover during peak intensity.

2. **Cover Up:** Lightweight, long-sleeved shirts, pants, and wide-brimmed hats provide excellent, nonchemical protection.
3. **Build a Base Tan Slowly:** A tan is the body's natural, protective response to UV radiation. Allow your skin to adapt gradually to the sun in the spring, starting with just ten to fifteen minutes of exposure and slowly increasing the duration. Never burn.
4. **Choose Mineral Sunscreens:** If you must use sunscreen for extended periods of intense exposure (e.g., a long day at the beach or on the water), choose sunscreens that use minerals like zinc oxide and titanium dioxide as their active ingredients. These create a physical barrier that sits on top of the skin rather than being absorbed into it. Do not use nanoformulations as mentioned above.
5. **Consider Natural Oils:** For mild protection during nonpeak hours, some natural oils like coconut oil can offer a very low SPF (around 4 to 8).

Finally, there are also natural substances that function as indirect "sunscreens," discussed in chapter 30.

## THE FINAL VERDICT: A PUBLIC HEALTH CATASTROPHE

We return to the central question: Is sunscreen the new margarine? The evidence strongly indicates the answer is yes. A vast majority of the population uses it to protect against a manufactured and overstated threat, while in reality it is that protection, in the form of toxic sunscreen chemicals, that is itself the threat. Furthermore, the misguided, dogmatic advice for complete sun avoidance over the past fifty years, issued without any compensatory plan to replace the lost vitamin D, may well be one of the most destructive acts in the history of modern medicine. By treating the sun as a poison, our connection to the primary source of a hormone critical for preventing cancer, autoimmune diseases, infectious diseases, and mental health disorders has been severed. Western populations have been driven indoors and a pandemic of vitamin D deficiency has resulted. Furthermore, we have been instructed that to venture outside, we must coat ourselves in systemically absorbed drugs with known toxic properties. Western civilizations are now reaping the results of this destructive advice in the form of skyrocketing rates of chronic disease, premature aging, and preventable death. Just like with margarine, the "cure" appears to have become far worse than the perceived disease. It is time to reject the fear, step out of the poisonous chemical shadow, and intelligently, respectfully, and gratefully step back into the sun.

# CHAPTER 26

# THE SUNSHINE CONNECTION: VITAMIN D, NEURODEVELOPMENT, AND THE PUZZLE OF AUTISM

In this chapter, we will apply some of what we've learned about the sun, vitamin D, and health by delving into the intriguing and increasingly compelling link between vitamin D, neurodevelopment, and the rising incidence of autism spectrum disorder (ASD). We will explore how geographical location and even birth month might offer critical clues, examine the intricate role of vitamin D in brain development, pinpoint specific brain regions potentially affected, and consider the tantalizing possibility of reversing some aspects of autism through vitamin D optimization.

## THE SHIFTING LANDSCAPE OF AUTISM

The past few decades have witnessed a striking increase in the reported incidence of autism in the United States. Since the 1950s, diagnostic criteria and awareness have evolved, but the numbers suggest a genuine rise in prevalence. For instance, the Centers for Disease Control and Prevention (CDC) reported that in 2000, approximately one in 150 children were identified with ASD, a figure that has steadily climbed to one in 36 by 2020.[1] Compare these figures to the incidence of autism in the 1960s, the pre-sunscare and sunscreen era, one in 2000. An apples-to-apples comparison of incidence across these time periods is staggering: 1960s, .05 percent; 2000, .286 percent and 2020, 2.78 percent, a tenfold increase since 2000 and a 55.6x greater incidence of autism over the past 60 years.

These numbers don't indicate a typical trend or gradual genetic process at play, they indicate a, relatively speaking, overnight ubiquitous, catastrophic environmental insult. That ubiquitous catastrophic environmental insult may be chronic vitamin D deficiency during critical periods of neurodevelopment, compounded by the neurotoxic effects of the drugs in sunscreens that are absorbed through the skin, enter the bloodstream, and cross through the placenta and blood-brain barrier.

One of the most compelling observations regarding autism's incidence is its potential geographic and latitudinal gradient. Evidence suggests a higher incidence of autism in sun-starved temperate latitudes compared to equatorial regions.[2] This pattern raises an important question: Are populations living further from the equator, and thus receiving less intense sunlight exposure and subsequently having lower vitamin D levels, experiencing a disproportionate burden of autism? This observation hints at a possible environmental connection that warrants closer examination.

Further supporting a link to environmental factors, specifically those tied to seasonal changes, is the phenomenon of birth-month effects in autism. Research indicates that the month a child is born can influence their risk of developing ASD. A study by Lee et al found a significant association between birth seasonality and the risk of ASD.[3] While the specific months with higher risk can vary depending on the hemisphere and methodology, the consistent finding of birth-month effects points toward prenatal environmental exposures that fluctuate throughout the year. Given that vitamin D levels in pregnant mothers often exhibit seasonal variations, with lower levels typically seen during winter months, this observation further strengthens the hypothesis that maternal vitamin D status during critical periods of fetal brain development may be a contributing factor to autism risk.[4]

## SUNLIGHT, VITAMIN D, AND THE AUTISM ENIGMA

The intriguing geographic and seasonal patterns in autism incidence lead us to consider a prominent environmental factor: sunlight and its pivotal role in vitamin D production. In the search for causes of prenatal developmental disorders, we tend to look for an agent that is differentially present in one group that is causing the issue. For example, the introduction of thalidomide to treat morning sickness resulted in horrendous birth defects. Once thalidomide was identified as the cause, it was eliminated, as were the birth defects. One logical obstacle regarding the role of vitamin D in autism is the fact that its *absence* may be a potential cause. It is difficult for us to see what is not there. Therefore, when the status quo is population-wide vitamin D deficiency, a maternal environment deficient in vitamin D becomes the norm, making the identification of the absence of vitamin D as a causative factor in a multifaceted disease like autism all the more difficult. In other words, vitamin D deficiency as a cause of autism is hidden in plain sight, we look right past it examining every other possible agent because we've assumed vitamin D has no role.

The idea that vitamin D deficiency might contribute to autism is gaining traction, supported by several compelling lines of observational evidence. A particularly insightful observation comes from a relocated group of Somalis, as highlighted in *Scientific American*.[5] The article discusses the significantly higher rates of autism observed in Somali children living in cooler, less sunny climates, such as Minnesota, compared to those living in Somalia.

Another group of fifteen thousand relocated Somalis in Stockholm, Sweden, had no word for the newfound scourge of autism affecting their community, so they call it the "Swedish Disease." Somalis, often characterized by darker skin pigmentation, require more sun exposure to produce adequate vitamin D. When living in regions with less intense sunlight compared to Somalia, like Minnesota or Sweden, they are at an increased risk of vitamin D deficiency. This stark contrast in autism prevalence between the two groups (resident vs. relocated Somalis), with the same genetic background but differential sun exposure, strongly suggests an environmental factor at play, with vitamin D deficiency being a prime candidate.

A paper by Grant and Soles provides comprehensive epidemiological evidence supporting the role of maternal vitamin D deficiency as a risk factor for infantile autism.[6] Their analysis suggests that populations with lower sunlight exposure, and consequently lower vitamin D levels, tend to have higher rates of autism. This ecological study, while not establishing causation, powerfully illustrates a consistent correlation across different populations and geographic regions, reinforcing the potential significance of vitamin D.

A systematic review and meta-analysis by Wang et al. further solidified the association between vitamin D status and ASD.[7] By synthesizing data from numerous studies, they concluded that lower vitamin D levels are associated with an increased risk of ASD. Serum vitamin D levels are indeed lower in autistic children compared to age-matched controls.[8] This robust analysis provides stronger evidence for the connection, moving beyond individual observations to a more generalized understanding of the relationship between vitamin D deficiency and autism spectrum disorder.

Integrating and synthesizing this epidemiological and incidence data reveals a clear and consistent pattern: Geographic location, with its inherent variations in sunlight exposure and subsequent vitamin D production, appears to play a significant role in the incidence of autism. The higher prevalence in sun-deprived regions, the birth-month effects, and the observations in specific vulnerable populations like the Somali cohort all point toward a compelling link between vitamin D status and autism risk.

## VITAMIN D'S INFLUENCE ON NEURODEVELOPMENT

Given the strong epidemiological link between geographic incidence and autism, with vitamin D emerging as a key factor, it becomes essential to examine the direct role of vitamin D in neurodevelopment and the potential pathological mechanisms related to autism. Vitamin D's influence extends profoundly into the intricate processes of brain development and function. Importantly, vitamin D receptors (VDRs) and the enzyme 1-alpha-hydroxylase, responsible for converting inactive vitamin D to its active form, are widely distributed throughout the brain. Buell and Dawson-Hughes highlighted the widespread presence of VDRs in various brain regions, including the cortex, hippocampus, and cerebellum.[9] Eyles et al. further detailed this distribution in human brain tissue, confirming that key areas involved in cognitive and behavioral processes are equipped to respond to vitamin D.[10] This extensive presence indicates that vitamin D is not merely a passive bystander but an active participant in brain physiology and function.

The timing of vitamin D's influence is also critical. Studies, such as the one by Voltas et al., investigated the impact of maternal vitamin D status during pregnancy on child neurocognitive functioning. Insufficient maternal 25(OH)D throughout pregnancy was linked to poorer visual-motor precision in children. Inadequate 25(OH)D levels in the third trimester were associated with poorer executive functioning, specifically lower working memory scores and deficits in metacognition and inhibition.[11]

These prenatal stages are periods of intense brain development, where nutrient availability can have lasting consequences. Inadequate maternal vitamin D during these critical windows may disrupt the normal trajectory of brain development, potentially contributing to neurodevelopmental disorders.

Darryl Eyles provided an insightful overview of vitamin D's role in brain and behavior, emphasizing its multifaceted functions. Vitamin D is known to be involved in neuronal differentiation, proliferation, and survival, as well as neurotransmitter synthesis and brain detoxification.[12] These processes are fundamental to the establishment of healthy neural circuits. When vitamin D is deficient, these important developmental steps can be compromised, leading to subtle yet significant alterations in brain architecture and function.

Further supporting the importance of vitamin D, Ye et al. explored the synaptic and circuit functions of vitamin D in neurodevelopmental disorders. They highlight how vitamin D influences synaptic plasticity—the ability of synapses to strengthen or weaken over time—a process vital for learning and memory.[13]

Dysregulation of synaptic function is a hallmark of several neurodevelopmental conditions, including autism. In fact, some have characterized the neural correlates of autism as "the disease of the synapses."[14] Vitamin D's ability to modulate these intricate synaptic processes suggests that its deficiency could contribute to the synaptic dysfunction observed in ASD. In essence, vitamin D acts as a neurosteroid, influencing a broad spectrum of cellular and molecular events essential for a healthy developing brain. Its widespread presence in brain regions critical for cognition and behavior, coupled with its role in neuronal growth, neurotransmission, and synaptic plasticity, firmly establishes vitamin D as a key player in neurodevelopment. Disruptions in its availability during critical prenatal and early postnatal periods can have profound implications for brain health, potentially contributing to the neuroanatomical and corresponding behavioral pathology observed in autism.

## THE CEREBELLAR VERMIS—A KEY ANATOMICAL INTERSECTION

One persistent obstacle in the study of brain mechanisms of autism is the simple issue of knowing where to look. Fortunately, within the complex landscape of the brain, a particular region, the midline cerebellar vermis, has emerged as a compelling anatomical location differentially affected in autism. This area is drawing significant attention for several reasons: Anatomical studies consistently show reduced cerebellar vermis volume in individuals with autism, cerebellar Purkinje cells—critical neurons within this region—are known to possess vitamin D receptors, the cerebellum undergoes extensive development both prenatally and postnatally, and, intriguingly, animals with midline cerebellar damage exhibit behavioral deficits strikingly similar to those observed in autistic humans.[15, 16]

The pioneering work of Eric Courchesne has been instrumental in illuminating the role of the vermis in autism. His MRI study published in *Neurology* revealed unusual brain growth patterns in early life in children with autistic disorder, specifically highlighting abnormalities in cerebellar development .[17] This seminal research underscored that the cerebellum, and particularly the vermis, is not merely a motor control center but plays a critical role in higher cognitive, emotional and social functions[18, 19] including learning and memory[20, 21] areas significantly impacted in autism.

A consensus paper by Fatemi et al. further solidified the pathological role of the cerebellum in autism.[22] This comprehensive review, drawing on the expertise of numerous researchers, established that cerebellar abnormalities are a consistent finding in autism, with particular emphasis on the vermis. The paper details the evidence for reduced cerebellar volume, alterations in neuronal cell counts, and other structural deviations within this region in individuals with ASD.

Importantly, these brain changes in autism appear to be distinct from those seen in other developmentally delayed brains. Webb et al. demonstrated that cerebellar vermal volumes in children with autism spectrum disorder were uniquely associated with specific behavioral correlates of autism, distinguishing these findings from other forms of developmental delay.[23] This specificity further emphasizes the unique involvement of the cerebellar vermis in the pathophysiology of autism.

Focusing on the cellular level, Purkinje cells, which are the sole output neurons of the cerebellar vermal cortex, are of particular interest. Sudarov discussed the critical role of these cells in autism spectrum disorders.[24] If, as Sudarov says, autism is a "disease of the synapses" then the cerebellar Purkinje cell, which is among the largest neurons in the brain (receiving around 200,000 synapses per cell), is the place to look. For comparison, typical cerebral cortical pyramidal neurons receive about 10,000 to 30,000 synapses, highlighting the unique complexity and connectivity of Purkinje cells in generating and affecting complex behaviors. Studies have consistently reported a reduction in Purkinje cell numbers in the cerebellar vermis of individuals with autism.

Importantly for our discussion, Purkinje cells are known to express vitamin D receptors, indicating they are directly influenced by vitamin D levels.[25] This connection provides a likely cellular mechanism by which vitamin D deficiency could impact cerebellar development and function. Furthermore, activation of the maternal immune system—a factor sometimes linked to altered vitamin D status—can significantly alter cerebellar development, including effects on Purkinje cells, in offspring.[26]

Beyond structural and cellular changes, the functional implications of vermal abnormalities are profound. Pierce and Courchesne provided evidence for a cerebellar role in reduced exploration and stereotyped behavior in autism.[27] These behavioral characteristics, central to the autism diagnosis, are remarkably similar to deficits observed in animal models with damage to the midline cerebellum.[28] This parallel between animal models and human autism strengthens the argument for the cerebellum, and specifically the vermis, as a critical nexus for the behavioral manifestations of ASD.

In conclusion, the midline cerebellar vermis stands out as a highly significant anatomical location in the study of autism. Its consistent structural and cellular abnormalities in autistic individuals, the presence of vitamin D receptors on its Purkinje cells, its protracted postnatal developmental timeline, and its established link to key autistic behaviors all point to this region as a prime candidate for neurodevelopmental changes influenced by vitamin D, changes that appear intrinsically related to autism.

## THE STRANGE CASE OF WILLIAMS SYNDROME—A VERMAL MIRROR OF OPPOSITES

To truly appreciate the significance of the cerebellar vermis in autism, it is instructive to consider its potential role in another condition called Williams syndrome. Behaviorally, autism is characterized by a constellation of symptoms including significant social withdrawal, difficulties with social communication, repetitive behaviors, and specific learning challenges. Individuals with autism often prefer solitary activities and may struggle with reciprocal social interactions. In stark contrast, Williams syndrome is defined by a remarkably different social behavioral profile. Individuals with Williams syndrome are typically overly friendly, highly outgoing, and often exhibit an excessive drive for social engagement, displaying a pronounced lack of social inhibition. This makes them almost the diametric behavioral opposite of individuals with autism in terms of their social behavior.

Intriguingly, this behavioral dichotomy is mirrored by distinct and opposing neuroanatomical representations within the cerebellar vermis. As discussed, autism is characterized by neuroanatomical pathology in the midline cerebellar vermis, frequently observed as atrophy, reduced cell counts, and even an absence of specific cell types like Purkinje cells. This structural reduction aligns with the idea of a compromised or underdeveloped vermal region. Conversely, and quite amazingly, Williams syndrome is characterized by a hypertrophic, or enlarged, midline cerebellar vermis. Jones et al. documented these cerebellar abnormalities in infants and toddlers with Williams syndrome, specifically highlighting the increased size of the vermis.[29] This fascinating comparison offers a compelling argument for the vermis as the central anatomical hub for the behavioral and neuroanatomical distinctions between these two neurodevelopmental conditions.

The argument is clear: These two distinct and behaviorally opposite syndromes—autism with its social withdrawal and repetitive behaviors, and Williams syndrome with its hyper-sociability—have remarkably opposite neuroanatomical representations in the vermis. Autism is associated with a smaller, potentially underactive and dysfunctional vermis, while Williams syndrome is linked to a larger, potentially overactive, yet still dysfunctional vermis. This striking inverse relationship strongly suggests that the cerebellar vermis plays a pivotal role in modulating social behavior and repetitive actions, and that its developmental trajectory, potentially influenced by pre- and postnatal factors like vitamin D, is critical in shaping the distinct behavioral phenotypes of these two conditions.

## CAN AUTISM BE REVERSED? THE PROMISE OF VITAMIN D AND CEREBELLAR PLASTICITY

The evidence linking vitamin D deficiency to autism, coupled with the critical role of the highly plastic cerebellar vermis in the disorder's neuroanatomy and behavior, raises a profound and hopeful question: Can autism be reversed? It is estimated that between 3 percent and 25 percent of autistic kids will lose their diagnosis in a process known as spontaneous remission.[30, 31] The very existence of instances of spontaneous recovery from autism suggests that a permanent cure or significant amelioration is indeed possible, challenging the notion of autism as an immutable lifelong condition.[32, 33]

This optimism is fueled by the growing understanding of vitamin D's multifaceted restorative and healing role in brain function. A 2015 study found that vitamin D supplementation improved autistic symptoms.[34] A more recent study published in *BMC Psychiatry* in March 2025 by Tian et al. investigated the effects of vitamin D on brain function in preschool children with ASD. The findings revealed that lower serum levels of 25-hydroxyvitamin D were significantly associated with multiple brain functional abnormalities. Importantly, children with lower vitamin D levels exhibited more severe autism symptoms.[35] This research indicates a potential causal link between vitamin D deficiency and the severity of ASD, suggesting that optimizing vitamin D levels could positively impact brain function.

Further reinforcing the potential for intervention, a double-blind randomized clinical trial published in *BMC Pediatrics* in August 2025 by Javadfar et al. focused on the effects of vitamin D supplementation on inflammatory status and behavioral symptoms in children with ASD. The results were encouraging: After fifteen weeks of supplementation, there was a significant increase in serum 25(OH) levels, alongside a notable decrease in inflammatory markers. Importantly, the behavioral symptoms in the group receiving vitamin D showed significant improvement.[36] This study provides direct clinical evidence that vitamin D supplementation may have a beneficial effect on some aspects of autism, particularly by mitigating inflammation, which is often implicated in ASD.

Beyond broad behavioral improvements, vitamin D's influence extends to specific neurological functions relevant to autism. For instance, Burne et al. demonstrated that combined prenatal and chronic postnatal vitamin D deficiency in rats impaired a simple sensorimotor behavior: prepulse inhibition of acoustic startle.[37] Another paper found that damage to the cerebellar vermis blocked acoustic startle habituation, a form of sensorimotor learning, in rats.[38] Prepulse inhibition of startle is where a weak stimulus (the prepulse) reduces the reaction to a stronger stimulus (the pulse) that follows closely afterward. This serves as a measure of the brain's ability to filter out unnecessary information. Prepulse inhibition (PPI) is a neurological measure of sensorimotor gating, a process often found to be deficient in individuals with autism. This animal model provides a mechanistic link, showing that vitamin D deficiency can directly impact neural circuits responsible for critical sensory processing, a core deficit in ASD.

In conclusion, the cumulative evidence paints a compellingly hopeful picture. We have seen that vitamin D deficiency is epidemiologically linked to the incidence of autism, with geographic and seasonal patterns strongly suggesting its involvement. This observation is supported by the growing understanding of vitamin D's multifaceted restorative and healing role in brain function.

Regarding which part of the brain could be affected, the cerebellar vermis, a highly plastic brain region involved in social behavior and repetitive actions, is anatomically affected in autism and harbors vitamin D receptors. Furthermore, this part of the cerebellum is anatomically and physiologically linked to many brain regions involved in a variety of complex behaviors.[39, 40]

This convergence of evidence, coupled with direct intervention studies showing improvements in autism symptoms with vitamin D supplementation, suggests a powerful opportunity. Given the cerebellar vermis's remarkable postnatal plasticity and its profound impact on core autistic behaviors, and vitamin D's known role in neurodevelopment and anti-inflammatory processes, the prospect of reversing or significantly ameliorating autism through vitamin D therapy and/or sensible sun exposure is not merely a hope but a tangible possibility. We will explore these ideas more thoroughly in the next chapter.

Optimizing vitamin D levels during critical developmental windows, both prenatally and postnatally, could serve as a powerful and accessible intervention, potentially reshaping the neurodevelopmental trajectory and offering a path toward improved outcomes for individuals with autism. While more research is undoubtedly needed, the available data strongly advocates for a proactive approach to ensure adequate vitamin D status, viewing it not just as a supplement, but as a critical pre- and postnatal neurodevelopmental nutrient with the potential to profoundly impact the landscape of autism.

# CHAPTER 27

# CRITICAL PERIODS, NEUROTOXINS, AND VITAMIN D DEFICIENCY: A POTENTIAL CAUSE AND TREATMENT OF AUTISM

## THE SILENT TRIPLE THREAT: MATERNAL VITAMIN D DEFICIENCY, SUNSCREEN CHEMICALS, AND FETAL NEURODEVELOPMENT

The miracle of life unfolding within the womb is a delicate dance, meticulously choreographed by nature. Every nutrient, every chemical, every environmental exposure plays a role in shaping the developing human. For too long, the importance of vitamin D in this intricate process has been underestimated, especially concerning fetal neurodevelopment. Simultaneously, our modern lifestyle, characterized by the widespread use of sunscreen, has introduced new players into this complex equation—chemicals that, while protecting our skin, may subtly yet profoundly impact the developing brain. This chapter will explore the alarming relationship between chronic maternal vitamin D deficiency and fetal neurodevelopment, further complicated by the pervasive presence of neurotoxic sunscreen chemicals, and consider their potentially devastating synergistic effects on the developing brain.

## SUNSCREEN CHEMICALS: AN UNSEEN JOURNEY

The very sunscreens we've been conditioned to apply with the best intentions to shield ourselves from UV rays contain chemicals that are not merely confined to the skin's surface. As discussed, many common sunscreen drugs readily penetrate the skin, enter the systemic circulation, and, disturbingly, can cross the placental barrier, reaching a vulnerable fetus.[1] This means that when a pregnant woman applies sunscreen, the chemicals aren't just protecting her; they are embarking on an unseen journey into her unborn child's developing nervous system. While it may seem that the baby is conceptually protected because the sunscreens are applied to the mother's skin, nothing could be further from the truth. These sunscreen drugs enter the bloodstream no less differently than if they were injected by a syringe directly into the mother's circulation and then into the vulnerable baby's developing brain.

One pivotal study, highlighted in *Environmental Health Perspectives*, specifically examined the systemic absorption of active ingredients in sunscreens.[2] Again, read your sunscreen container: These chemicals are listed as drugs because they enter the bloodstream. The findings were stark: After a single application, all fourteen active ingredients studied were detected in the plasma at concentrations exceeding the FDA's threshold for waiving further safety studies. More concerning, some of these chemicals, such as oxybenzone, octocrylene, avobenzone, and octinoxate, were found to persist in the bloodstream for several days, even after cessation of use. The implications of these circulating chemicals for fetal exposure are profound, as they can readily traverse the placenta and cross the delicate blood-brain barrier of the developing fetus.[3, 4] This establishes a direct pathway for these compounds to influence critical stages of neurodevelopment.

## TERATOGENIC NEUROTOXICITY: A MULTI-PRONGED ASSAULT

The mechanisms by which various drugs such as sunscreens can disrupt the intricate process of neurodevelopment are multifaceted and often insidious and subtle. Teratogenic neurotoxicity (poisoning the baby's brain) can occur through several pathways, including the induction of hyperinflammatory states, the generation of oxidative stress, and the disruption of endocrine and neuroendocrine systems by the sunscreen chemicals, all of which can disrupt brain development, especially so during critical periods of development.

**Hyperinflammatory States and Oxidative Stress:** Inflammation, while a necessary immune response, can become detrimental when chronic, dysregulated, and/or misdirected. Certain chemical exposures, including those from sunscreen drugs, can trigger persistent inflammatory responses in the developing brain, potentially damaging to the formation of delicate neural structures.[5] Similarly, oxidative stress, an imbalance between the production of reactive oxygen species and the body's ability to detoxify them, can also lead to cellular damage and death. The developing brain, with its high metabolic rate, is particularly vulnerable to oxidative stress. Both hyperinflammation and oxidative stress are known to impair neuronal growth, differentiation, and synaptic plasticity—all critical components of healthy brain formation.[6]

**Endocrine and Neuroendocrine Disruption:** The endocrine system, a network of glands that produce and release hormones, plays a paramount role in orchestrating brain development. Hormones like thyroid hormones and sex steroids are important for neuronal migration, synapse formation, and myelination. Endocrine-disrupting chemicals (EDCs) are exogenous agents that interfere with any aspect of hormone action, from synthesis and secretion to transport, binding, and elimination. Many sunscreen chemicals are recognized EDCs, capable of mimicking or blocking natural hormones, thereby throwing the delicate hormonal balance of the developing fetus into disarray.[7] This disruption can have profound and lasting effects on brain architecture and function, including those that are seen in autism.

## VITAMIN D: THE BRAIN'S SILENT GUARDIAN

Now, imagine these neurotoxic mechanisms attacking a brain already weakened and compromised by chronic vitamin D deficiency. Remember, the baby can only get its vitamin D from the mother, so if the mother is deficient, so is the baby. Vitamin D is a powerful neurosteroid with widespread receptors throughout the brain, including areas critical for cognition, mood, and social behavior. It plays a critical role in neuronal proliferation, differentiation, migration, and synaptic plasticity. It also exhibits anti-inflammatory and antioxidant properties, helping to protect the brain from damage.[8] Therefore, a vitamin D–deficient brain is a vulnerable brain. When vitamin D is insufficient, these neuroprotective mechanisms are weakened, making the developing brain exceptionally susceptible to the damaging effects of neurotoxins.

Research indicates that vitamin D deficiency during critical periods of fetal brain development can indeed be devastating. While brain development is a continuous process, certain windows of vulnerability exist. These are known as critical periods. The second and third trimesters of pregnancy, characterized by rapid neuronal growth and synapse formation, are particularly sensitive to vitamin D availability.[9] Insufficient vitamin D during these periods can lead to altered brain structure, impaired cognitive function, and increased risk for neurodevelopmental disorders. Not surprisingly, studies have linked maternal vitamin D deficiency during pregnancy to an increased risk of autism spectrum disorder (ASD) and schizophrenia in offspring.[10, 11]

## SYNERGY AND VULNERABILITY: A PERFECT STORM TO DISRUPT THE DEVELOPING BRAIN

The concept of synergy is critical when considering the impact of multiple environmental insults. Synergy describes a phenomenon where the combined effect of two or more agents is greater than the sum of their individual effects. In the context of teratogenic neurotoxicity, this means that while individual exposures to sunscreen chemicals or even moderate vitamin D deficiency might have subthreshold, or undetectable effects, their interaction or co-occurrence can create a "perfect storm" of neurodevelopmental disruption, especially if they occur during critical periods of development.

The idea here is that chronic maternal vitamin D deficiency doesn't just act in isolation; it creates a profound vulnerability to neurotoxic insult in the developing brain. In this vitamin D–starved environment the developing brain becomes hypersusceptible to the neurotoxic effects of agents like sunscreen chemicals. Imagine a delicate house of cards in which each card represents a critical neurodevelopmental process. Vitamin D deficiency weakens the foundational cards, making the entire structure unstable. When neurotoxic sunscreen chemicals are introduced, they might simply nudge a few cards, but in this preexisting state of vulnerability, the entire structure can collapse. The mechanisms previously discussed—hyperinflammation, oxidative stress, and endocrine disruption—are all exacerbated in a vitamin D–deficient state, creating a devastating cycle of damage.

## ENDOCRINE DISRUPTION AND THE AUTISM SEX DISPARITY

The endocrine-disrupting effects of sunscreen chemicals on the developing brain warrant particular attention, especially when considering the puzzling sex disparity observed in autism. Autism spectrum disorder is diagnosed approximately four times more frequently in boys than in girls.[12] This dramatic sex difference has long been a subject of intense scientific inquiry. Endocrine-disrupting agents can have subtle, yet profound, "organizational effects" on the developing brain. These effects refer to the permanent changes in brain structure and function that occur during critical periods of development due to altered hormone exposure. For example, exposure to certain endocrine disruptors during specific critical periods of development can permanently alter the brain's sensitivity to sex hormones, influencing later behaviors and neurological function.

Several sunscreen chemicals, such as oxybenzone and octinoxate, have been shown to possess estrogenic and antiandrogenic properties.[13] This means they can mimic or block the actions of natural sex hormones such as estrogen and testosterone. It should come as no surprise that endocrine-disrupting chemicals, like those in sunscreens, impair vitamin D synthesis and availability, essentially making a bad situation worse with respect to maternal vitamin D availability and stores.[14] And, again, it should not be surprising that studies show that vitamin D protects the developing brain from toxic insults from endocrine disrupting chemicals as well.[15]

Given the critical role of sex hormones in shaping sexually dimorphic brain structures and functions during development, the introduction of exogenous endocrine disruptors at critical junctures could significantly alter these organizational processes. Could the endocrine-disrupting effects of sunscreen chemicals, particularly their antiandrogenic potential, contribute to the observed sex difference in autism incidence by differentially and subtly altering male brain development? This is a compelling hypothesis that warrants further investigation, suggesting a plausible mechanism for how environmental factors could contribute to complex neurodevelopmental disorders with a strong sex bias like that seen in autism.

## OXIDATIVE STRESS: A COMMON THREAD

Beyond endocrine disruption, neurotoxic sunscreens are also implicated as a source of oxidative stress, a phenomenon we've already identified as a key mechanism of cellular damage and malformation in the developing brain. The very act of detoxifying these chemicals can generate reactive oxygen species, further burdening an already vulnerable developing neuroanatomical system. It's important to recognize that sunscreen chemicals are not the sole environmental culprits. Exposure to maternal infection, heavy metals like mercury and lead, and various pesticides are also well-established sources of oxidative stress and have been independently implicated in ASD. For instance, a study by Sajdel-Sulkowska and colleagues highlighted increased oxidative stress markers in the cerebellum of individuals with autism, suggesting a link between oxidative damage and the disorder's neuropathology.[16] This emphasizes a critical point: The developing brain is constantly assailed by a myriad of environmental factors, many of which converge on the common pathway of oxidative stress. The vitamin D–starved brain, including the fetal brain, is at a severe disadvantage and hyper-vulnerable when dealing with oxidative stress as we have detailed previously.

## THE CUMULATIVE BURDEN DISRUPTING NEURODEVELOPMENT LABELED AS AUTISM

This brings us to an important understanding: The etiology of complex neurodevelopmental disorders like autism is rarely attributable to a single factor. Instead, it is likely the result of an intricate interplay of genetic predispositions and environmental exposures, creating a "cumulative burden." Imagine a scenario where chronic maternal vitamin D deficiency weakens the baby's brain's resilience, sunscreen chemicals introduce subtle neurotoxic insults, and other ubiquitous environmental toxins like pesticides, herbicides, and even adjuvant metals like aluminum and mercury found in some vaccines contribute their own subthreshold neurotoxic effects. Individually, each of these factors might not be sufficient to trigger a full-blown neurodevelopmental disorder. However, when combined, their additive or synergistic effects can be devastating. Each seemingly minor insult chips away at the developing brain's capacity, pushing it closer to a threshold of dysfunction. What might be a harmless exposure for a mature brain operating optimally or a developing brain operating in an optimal vitamin D environment can become profoundly damaging when combined with multiple other stressors. This concept challenges us to look beyond single-cause explanations and embrace a more holistic, multifactorial view of environmental influences on neurodevelopment, like chronic vitamin D deficiency and sunscreen toxins (one absent, one added), that may be involved in autism, including the most obvious ones like vitamin D and sunscreen chemicals!

## AUTISM: A DISEASE OF THE SYNAPSES

To truly appreciate the profound impact of these environmental insults, we must delve into the very fabric of brain function: the synapse. Autism is increasingly understood as a "disease of the synapses"—the microscopic junctions where neurons communicate. The Purkinje cell, a magnificent neuron in the cerebellum, exemplifies this complexity, boasting an astounding 200,000 synapses.[17] The cerebellum itself is a powerhouse processor of sensory and motor information, and its dysfunction is strongly implicated in the complex sensorimotor challenges characteristic of autism. While autism spectrum disorder is currently diagnosed based on behavioral criteria—deficits in social reciprocity, communication challenges, repetitive behaviors, and insistence on sameness—a deeper understanding of the disease, and ultimately its treatment and cure, lies in unraveling the effects of these environmental insults on the intricate synaptic microanatomy of neurons like the Purkinje cell. Subtle alterations in synaptic structure, function, and connectivity, driven by factors like vitamin D deficiency and neurotoxic exposures, can profoundly impact information processing and lead to the diverse range of symptoms observed in ASD.

Consider the facts of presented in the previous chapter regarding the visible differences in the midline cerebellar regions of autistic children compared to non-affected children. Their cerebellar vermal regions were visibly smaller with fewer Purkinje cells. If each Purkinje cell receives 200,000 synaptic connections, each Purkinje cell lost is potentially devastating to the information processing capability of the cerebellum and linked regions. However, one amazing characteristic feature of the brain is redundancy and associated recovery of function. Whether it be an injury, stroke, or degeneration, there are remarkable instances of recovery of function from those neural insults. Recovery of function is also seen in autism in the form of spontaneous recovery as mentioned earlier. We also covered a study where vitamin D supplementation lessened autistic symptoms. A double-blind randomized clinical trial published in *BMC Pediatrics* in August 2025 by Javadfar et al. focused on the effects of vitamin D supplementation on inflammatory status and behavioral symptoms in children with ASD. The results were encouraging: After fifteen weeks of supplementation, there was a significant increase in serum 25(OH) levels, alongside a notable decrease in inflammatory markers. Importantly, the behavioral symptoms in the group receiving vitamin D showed significant improvement. This study provides direct clinical evidence that vitamin D supplementation may have a beneficial effect on some aspects of autism.[18]

Just one instance of spontaneous recovery or promising restorative vitamin D interventional studies provide hope to all those afflicted that it can happen to them too, if only we understood the mechanisms. As mentioned earlier, one issue that plagues brain research is identification of the structures involved in the behavior of interest. That is, we don't know where to look. Fortunately, with autism, it looks like the midline cerebellar vermis is an important place to examine.

In yet another stroke of luck, the cerebellum happens to be a brain structure that has extensive postnatal development capability. Think about how babies crawl then walk. This is the cerebellum in action. Now think about all the higher-order complex behaviors that we showed the cerebellar vermis was involved in, such as emotion, learning, and memory.[19] Now think about how those higher-order complex behaviors develop over time. It looks like the cerebellum plays a big role there as well. Now, factor in that the cerebellum continues to develop and mature to at least age five.[20, 21] Purkinje cells show remarkable regenerative capacity in other species, and there do appear to be critical period effects as well, consistent with the notion that the window for effect in humans may be open for at least five years.[22, 23] We may be on to something exciting regarding reversing the neuroanatomical damage and corresponding behavioral correlates of autism.

Does this mean that kids with autism can be helped? Maybe. Will exposing autistic kids to sunlight and optimizing their serum vitamin D levels help with their symptoms or possibly reverse the condition? Some research has encouraging results with vitamin D supplementation, and it certainly will not hurt to try.

Hopefully, what we've covered here provides a testable explanation for the exponential growth in the incidence of autism since the 1970s. That is, chronic vitamin D starvation creates a precondition in the developing brain for differential vulnerabilities to environmental neurotoxic insults. One of those insults is ubiquitous, overlooked and hidden in plain sight: sunscreens with neurotoxic effects. The vitamin D–starved brain does not have the capabilities to effectively deal with these neurotoxins due to disrupted inflammatory and oxidative stress mechanisms. In contrast, a vitamin D–replete mother imparts the tools for her baby's brain to effectively deal with some neurotoxic insults like sunscreen and other toxins. Her baby can be exposed to the same toxic insult, but, because her baby's developing brain can mitigate the insult because vitamin D status is adequate, that baby wards off the threat and develops normally.

The insidious and subtle mechanisms of this transient neurotoxic developmental process are hidden in plain sight. First, most women, including pregnant women, are vitamin D deficient, creating the precondition and laying the foundation for exacerbated and dysfunctional inflammatory responses for themselves, and most importantly, in their baby's developing brain, to environmental insults. A recent study found only 1.36 percent of pregnant women to have sufficient serum vitamin D levels.[24] Second, application of sunscreens, in addition to avoiding the sun, contributes to the vitamin D deficiency noted above. But sunscreens are also one of those environmental insults, in the form of neurotoxins, mentioned above. Whether the law of unintended consequences, perverse effect or *Verschlimmbesserung* (an attempted improvement makes things worse) best describes this situation is unclear, but what *is* clear is that combining a preexisting chronic vitamin D deficiency with known neurotoxic sunscreens is a likely recipe for disaster in the vulnerable developing brain.

## A PATH FORWARD: SIMPLE SOLUTIONS TO COMPLEX PROBLEMS

In conclusion, while the precise mechanisms underlying autism are complex and multifaceted, we can no longer ignore the compelling evidence suggesting a significant role for chronic maternal vitamin D deficiency and ubiquitous environmental neurotoxins, including those found in common sunscreens. While individually these factors may be subthreshold teratogenic agents, when combined their effects can create a devastating synergistic outcome, contributing to the neuroanatomical pathology characteristic of autism. What we can no longer ignore is the palette for pathology presented to environmental toxins by chronically vitamin D starved brains upon which they paint their destructive murals. The vitamin D–deficient developing brain that becomes autistic is one such mural.

Whether these exact mechanisms are borne out as precisely accurate in every detail by future research is, in many ways, irrelevant to the urgent task at hand today. We possess actionable knowledge that can profoundly impact the health of present and future generations. The proposed solution, in its essence, is surprisingly simple, despite the complexity of the problem:

1. **Ensure adequate vitamin D:** Prioritize optimal vitamin D levels for both mother and fetus throughout pregnancy and early childhood. This often requires supplementation, as dietary intake and sun exposure alone are frequently insufficient. Optimal vitamin D status should be a lifestyle choice that will positively affect every component of your physical and mental well-being. Popping vitamin D supplements or going out in the sun for a brief period will not correct a lifetime of deficiency overnight. Furthermore, there are yet to be understood processes operating with phasic vs. chronic vitamin D use.[25]

2. **Avoid neurotoxic chemicals:** Exercise vigilance in minimizing exposure to toxic chemicals, particularly those found in sunscreens and other personal care products. If you must use sunscreen after obtaining sensible sun exposure, opt for mineral-based sunscreens (zinc oxide and titanium dioxide) which are generally considered safer and are not absorbed systemically. Furthermore, be mindful of other environmental toxins such as pesticides, herbicides, and the adjuvant metals like aluminum and mercury that may be found in some vaccines, and strive to reduce exposure where possible.

Lastly, for those now struggling with ASD, given the tremendous neuroplastic capability of the brain and the cerebellum in particular, it is by no means a wasted effort to eliminate neurotoxins and optimize sun exposure and the vitamin D status of yourself or your child through supplementation (in consultation with your medical professional, of course). The wonders of the brain, the extended window of development in the cerebellum, and the miracle that is vitamin D appear to be offering a second chance.

By embracing these simple measures, we can empower ourselves to protect the delicate developing brain from known threats, fostering a healthier neurodevelopmental trajectory for our children. This proactive approach offers a beacon of hope in the ongoing quest to understand and mitigate the rising incidence of autism.

## CHAPTER 28

# THE PROMISE OF A SUNNY DAY: SUNLIGHT AND VITAMIN D FOR A BETTER NIGHT'S SLEEP

A truly healthy waking life is built upon a foundation of restorative sleep. It is only fitting, then, that vitamin D is intricately involved in the complex processes of sleep. Far from being a mere bystander, vitamin D acts as a silent conductor, orchestrating a complex symphony of molecular and neuroendocrine pathways that are essential for a sustained, restful night of restorative sleep.

Vitamin D has a profound influence on the quality and stability of your sleep. A comprehensive 2025 review in *Frontiers in Nutrition* consolidated extensive evidence, painting a clear picture of vitamin D's deep involvement in sleep regulation.[1] As we've seen previously, the key to understanding vitamin D's role lies in the widespread presence of the vitamin D receptor throughout the brain, particularly in areas critical for sleep modulation, such as the hypothalamus, prefrontal cortex, and brainstem.[2] This extensive distribution underscores vitamin D's foundational role in maintaining brain health, extending naturally to its involvement in sleep.

When vitamin D activates these brain receptors, a cascade of beneficial effects unfolds, directly supporting the mechanisms of healthy sleep:

- **Neurotransmitter Balance:** Vitamin D is a major modulator of key neurotransmitters directly impacting sleep. It influences the delicate balance of serotonin, dopamine, and GABAergic signaling—all essential for both initiating and maintaining sleep.[3] Serotonin, for instance, is a precursor to melatonin, the hormone that signals your body it's time to sleep. This modulation by vitamin D is vital for achieving the calm and readiness required for sleep.

- **Circadian Gene Expression:** Your internal clock, or circadian rhythm, governs your sleep-wake cycles and is fundamental to a predictable waking life. Sunlight and vitamin D plays a direct role in synchronizing this rhythm by interacting with core circadian genes like Clock, Bmal1, and Per2 through the vitamin D receptor.[4] This ensures your body's natural sleep patterns remain aligned with the twenty-four-hour day, promoting consistent energy levels and cognitive function during waking hours.
- **Melatonin Synthesis:** While not directly producing melatonin, vitamin D indirectly enhances its synthesis. It achieves this by regulating tryptophan hydroxylase, the enzyme responsible for converting tryptophan into serotonin, which then becomes the building block for melatonin.[5] By supporting melatonin production, vitamin D facilitates the natural progression into sleep.
- **Neuroimmune and Glial Regulation:** Chronic inflammation not only disrupts waking behavior, it also severely disrupts sleep. Optimal vitamin D levels are shown to suppress proinflammatory cytokines such as IL-6 and TNF-α, which are often associated with sleep fragmentation.[6] Furthermore, vitamin D helps maintain the delicate balance of microglial cells, the immune cells of the brain, thereby reducing neuroinflammation that can interfere with sleep quality.[7] This anti-inflammatory role is necessary for maintaining a healthy brain environment conducive to restorative sleep and sharp cognition during the day.

## CLINICAL EVIDENCE: THE LINK BETWEEN VITAMIN D AND RESTFUL NIGHTS

The molecular insights above are consistent with a wealth of clinical observations and controlled trials. Many studies have shown a clear correlation between vitamin D deficiency (defined as less than 20 ng/mL) and poorer sleep outcomes.[8] Individuals with insufficient vitamin D often experience reduced sleep efficiency, longer times to fall asleep (increased latency), and shorter overall sleep duration. This is particularly noticeable in middle-aged and elderly populations.[9] A frequent finding is that low vitamin D levels are frequently observed in patients with various sleep disorders, prompting calls for further investigation into supplementation as a potential therapeutic avenue.[10] These clinical findings reinforce the idea that robust vitamin D status is a cornerstone for a well-rested and productive waking life.[11]

The good news is that vitamin D supplementation can make a significant difference. Controlled trials have demonstrated that supplementing with vitamin D (at doses of 4,000 IU/day or more) leads to measurable improvements in sleep latency, overall sleep quality, and even mood.[12] These benefits are especially pronounced in vulnerable groups such as the elderly, pregnant women, and shift workers, who often face unique sleep challenges.[13] Another study found that vitamin D supplementation significantly improved sleep quality in individuals with a variety of sleep disorders.[14]

Furthermore, combining vitamin D with other beneficial supplements like melatonin or magnesium has shown synergistic improvements in both sleep onset and the depth of sleep.[15] Clinical data also reinforces the broader impact, showing that improvements in vitamin D levels often parallel a reduction in depressive symptoms and better alignment of circadian rhythms, underscoring its multifaceted neuroendocrine role.[16] This idea is consistent with a study that found vitamin D supplementation to be effective in improving sleep quality in individuals with primary sleep disorders and depression.[17] These improvements in sleep and mood are directly conducive to a more engaged, energetic and satisfying waking life.

## SUNLIGHT: THE ORIGINAL SOURCE AND CIRCADIAN MAESTRO

While vitamin D's internal mechanisms are potent, its initial synthesis is intrinsically linked to sunlight exposure, which itself plays a significant and direct role in sleep regulation. Sunlight exposure, particularly in the morning, acts as a powerful external cue for our body's internal clock (circadian pacemaker) via specialized retinal light sensors.[18] Sunlight striking these receptors signals wakefulness to the brain, suppressing melatonin production and raising cortisol levels to promote alertness, effectively synchronizing our internal rhythm to the external environment.[19]

As daylight fades in the evening, the absence of sunlight triggers melatonin synthesis, promoting natural sleepiness. This inverse relationship between sunlight and melatonin production means more sunlight and higher vitamin D levels in summer can contribute to suppressed melatonin during the day, while reduced sun exposure in winter often leads to lower vitamin D and increased melatonin sensitivity.[20] This finely tuned balance, orchestrated by both direct light cues and vitamin D's influence on melatonin, is essential for healthy sleep-wake cycles.[21]

## STABILITY IN SLUMBER: VITAMIN D AND SLEEP CONSISTENCY

Beyond just quality, vitamin D plays a critical role in the stability of sleep—a key factor for a consistent and productive daytime routine. A study on healthy adults revealed a significant finding: Lower circulating vitamin D levels were directly linked to greater variability in both sleep duration and timing.[22] This suggests that vitamin D acts as an important buffer for circadian resilience. Participants with 25(OH)D levels (above 30 ng/mL) maintained more consistent sleep timing, even when faced with environmental changes or behavioral shifts, highlighting vitamin D's role in promoting a more predictable and stable sleep schedule.[23] This consistency in sleep directly translates to greater stability and effectiveness during waking hours.

## AGE-SPECIFIC INSIGHTS AND PEDIATRIC FINDINGS

Vitamin D affects sleep spans across all age groups, emphasizing its lifelong importance on a healthy waking existence. Emerging pediatric research indicates that higher vitamin D levels are associated with fewer sleep disturbances and improved overall sleep efficiency in children.[24] For children, good sleep is paramount for development, learning, and daytime behavior.

In older adults, the higher the serum vitamin D level the lower the reported sleep difficulties. Those with 35 ng/mL or greater serum vitamin D slept longer, fell asleep faster and had fewer disruptive sleep disorders like sleep talking, sleep walking or frequent awakenings.[25] Another study found that lower 25(OH)D concentrations were associated with shorter sleep duration, with subjects whose vitamin D concentrations were below 20 ng/mL having double the risk of total sleep time less than five hours compared with those subjects whose vitamin D concentrations were above 40 ng/mL.[26] Higher serum levels of vitamin D were also found to be associated with falling asleep faster and fewer nighttime awakenings.[27]

## DREAMS OR NIGHTMARES

In addition to being related to diminished sleep quality, vitamin D deficiency increases the likelihood of unpleasant dreams, including troubling nightmares. A comprehensive study of 382 individuals with chronic musculoskeletal pain found that those with vitamin D deficiency had significantly higher rates of bad dreams and nightmares compared with those with normal vitamin D levels. The authors proposed that vitamin D may improve dream quality indirectly by reducing psychological distress and promoting healthier calcium and melatonin homeostasis in the brain.[28]

Returning to the notion of melatonin regulation in the brain, it is important to remember that vitamin D receptors are widely distributed in brain regions involved in sleep and emotion, including the hypothalamus and brainstem nuclei. These regions are also intimately involved in REM (rapid eye movement dreaming) sleep and emotional behavior. Low vitamin D impairs melatonin production, disrupting circadian rhythms and REM sleep quality. Vitamin D supports serotonin and melatonin synthesis, which modulate dreaming and emotional tone during REM cycles. Because REM sleep is when most dreaming occurs, disturbances affecting this phase of sleep may cause more fragmented, intense, or negatively toned dreams.[29] It is important to appreciate that some hallucinogenic drugs like LSD manipulate serotonin usage in the brain, which may provide insight into how imbalance in the serotonin-melatonin system could lead to altered dream states.[30]

## THE ROLE OF VITAMIN D IN SLOW-WAVE RESTORATIVE SLEEP

Sleep is far more than a period of passive rest or dreaming; it is an active, indispensable state of systemic restoration. During the deep, non–rapid eye movement (NREM) stages of sleep, the brain's glymphatic system actively clears metabolic by-products and neurotoxins, such as beta-amyloid, which are linked to neurodegenerative disease.[31] During slow-wave sleep, the body's metabolic rate decreases, enabling the replenishment of cellular energy stores and the neutralization of damaging reactive oxygen species through enhanced antioxidant production.[32] This period of biological maintenance also involves the pruning of excess synapses to consolidate learning and memory, the regulation of essential neurotransmitters and hormones, and the repair of mitochondrial damage, which collectively ensure cellular health, neural plasticity, and physiological equilibrium in the brain.[33]

The effectiveness of these restorative functions is determined by neuroendocrine factors, with vitamin D being the key modulator of sleep architecture and quality. The vitamin D receptor is expressed in key brain regions that govern sleep-wake cycles, including the suprachiasmatic nucleus of the hypothalamus, which functions as the body's master circadian pacemaker.[34] By regulating the transcription of enzymes essential for melatonin synthesis, vitamin D directly supports the hormonal patterns required for achieving deep, restorative sleep.[35] This biochemical influence ensures that the body's internal clock remains synchronized, promoting consistent and high-quality sleep. Furthermore, vitamin D exerts powerful anti-inflammatory effects within the central nervous system, controlling the expression of inflammatory cytokines and reducing oxidative stress that will also disrupt sleep and impair neural function.[36]

This neuroprotective role is validated by clinical evidence linking vitamin D deficiency to poor sleep quality, increased sleep variability, and specific sleep disorders. Conversely, targeted supplementation has demonstrated marked improvements in sleep parameters, especially in individuals whose sleep is compromised by chronic pain or depression.[37] Therefore, vitamin D is not merely associated with sleep; it is functionally integrated into the very mechanisms of neurochemical balance, circadian regulation, and cellular repair that enable sleep to be truly restorative.[38]

## SUNLIGHT AND VITAMIN D ARE ESSENTIAL FOR A HEALTHY BRAIN AND SLEEP

This latest research firmly establishes vitamin D as a powerful, multifunctional hormone essential for regulating sleep. It seamlessly integrates neural, endocrine, and immune networks to ensure restorative rest and sleep. Optimized vitamin D3 supplementation and sunlight exposure—especially in deficient or circadian-stressed populations—is now understood to significantly enhance sleep quality, stability, and emotional restoration through its systemic and intricate neurochemical actions. These effects are not isolated; they are fundamental to supporting a vibrant and healthy waking life.

Understanding and optimizing your vitamin D status is not just about strong bones or even just good sleep; it's a foundational step toward achieving consistently high-quality, stable, and truly restorative sleep that directly underpins a healthy and thriving waking life. It's time to recognize vitamin D as the silent conductor of your sleep symphony, ensuring every note is played in harmony for your overall well-being.

# CHAPTER 29

# SUNSHINE, SEROTONIN, AND SANITY: VITAMIN D'S ROLE IN COGNITIVE AFFECTIVE STATES

The sun is a potent modulator of our mood, a silent conductor of our emotional symphony. While its physical benefits are widely acknowledged, the profound impact of sunlight and its ensuing vitamin D production on our affective states, particularly depression, is often underestimated. Research strongly suggests that vitamin D deficiency is linked to an increased risk of depression, anxiety, ADHD, and suicide, with supplementation showing promising benefits.[1] This chapter will illuminate the intricate connections between sunlight, vitamin D, and mental well-being, delving into both familiar and lesser-known relationships.

## THE WINTER BLUES AND BEYOND: VITAMIN D AND SEASONAL AFFECTIVE DISORDER

Perhaps the most recognized link between sunlight, vitamin D, and mood is seasonal affective disorder (SAD). This condition, often dubbed "the winter blues," is characterized by recurrent episodes of depression that typically begin in the fall or winter and remit in the spring.[2] The prevailing theory suggests that reduced exposure to sunlight during shorter, darker days disrupts the body's circadian rhythm, leading to imbalances in neurotransmitters like serotonin and melatonin. Vitamin D, synthesized in the skin upon exposure to UVB radiation from sunlight, plays a critical role in this complex interplay. It acts as a neurosteroid, influencing brain function and mood regulation.[3] Lower vitamin D levels are observed in individuals with SAD, and studies have shown that vitamin D supplementation can improve depressive symptoms, particularly when combined with light therapy.[4] Early studies showed improved mood in healthy individuals and those with SAD during winter months with vitamin

D supplementation.[5, 6] The exact mechanism is still under investigation, but it's believed that vitamin D may enhance serotonin synthesis and modulate inflammatory pathways in the brain, both of which are implicated in depression.

## BEYOND SAD: VITAMIN D'S BROADER INFLUENCE ON DEPRESSION

While SAD highlights a clear seasonal pattern, the impact of vitamin D on nonseasonal depression is equally compelling. Numerous studies have established a significant association between low vitamin D levels and an increased risk of depression in the general population.[7] An analysis of observational studies found that individuals with vitamin D deficiency had a substantially higher risk of depression compared to those with sufficient levels.[8] Further research extended these findings to other forms of depression, with larger studies demonstrating benefits of vitamin D in overweight individuals with depression and when used as an adjunctive treatment alongside standard medication.[9, 10]

Vitamin D can also reduce the symptoms of depression. People who took 1,000 IU of vitamin D3 per day experienced a slight reduction in symptoms, whereas those that took 8,000 IU per day experienced a dramatic improvement.[11] The mechanisms underpinning this broader association are multifaceted. Vitamin D receptors are found throughout the brain, including areas involved in mood regulation such as the hippocampus, cerebellum, and hypothalamus.[12] Through these receptors, vitamin D influences the production and activity of various neurotransmitters, including serotonin, dopamine, and norepinephrine, all of which are critical for maintaining a stable mood.[13]

Furthermore, vitamin D possesses anti-inflammatory properties. Chronic low-grade inflammation is increasingly recognized as a contributing factor to depression, and vitamin D's ability to modulate immune responses may offer a protective effect.[14]

Despite some methodological limitations in earlier research, research consistently shows that low vitamin D levels correlate with depression, and supplementation significantly improves depressive symptoms.[15, 16]

## THE POSTPARTUM PERIOD: VITAMIN D AND THE "BABY BLUES"

The period following childbirth is a time of immense physiological and emotional upheaval for new mothers. While "baby blues"—mild mood disturbances, anxiety, and sadness—are common and often resolve quickly, a significant number of women experience a more severe and persistent form of depression known as postpartum depression (PPD). This serious condition can profoundly impact a mother's well-being and her ability to care for her infant.

Emerging research suggests that vitamin D may play an important, yet often overlooked, role in PPD. During pregnancy, a woman's vitamin D requirements increase, and deficiencies are common due to various factors, including reduced sun exposure, dietary inadequacies, and the demands of fetal development.[17] Low vitamin D levels at the end of pregnancy or in the postpartum period have been consistently associated with an increased risk of PPD.[18] One study found the incidence of PPD increased by 330 percent in mothers with less than 20 ng/mL 25(OH)D vs. those over 20 ng/mL.[19]

The mechanisms are likely similar to those in general depression, involving vitamin D's influence on neurotransmitter synthesis, inflammatory pathways, and brain plasticity. The dramatic hormonal shifts during and after pregnancy, combined with potential vitamin D insufficiency, could create a vulnerable state for mood dysregulation.[20] Ensuring adequate vitamin D levels throughout pregnancy and into the postpartum period may therefore offer a valuable, easily implementable strategy to mitigate the risk and severity of PPD.

## POST-TRAUMATIC STRESS DISORDER

Research has also identified a link between vitamin D and PTSD. Studies have found lower vitamin D levels in individuals with PTSD.[21] Interestingly, researchers also noted that specific genetic variations in vitamin D–binding protein were correlated with lower vitamin D status in these patients.[22] This suggests a complex interplay between genetics and vitamin D status in the context of PTSD.[23]

## SUICIDE

Alarmingly, vitamin D deficiency is identified as a common risk factor for suicide. Studies have found a correlation between low vitamin D levels and increased suicide risk. For instance, a 2013 study found that active military service members with the lowest vitamin D levels had a higher risk of suicide.[24] Another study on depressed patients who attempted suicide revealed lower vitamin D levels and higher inflammation compared to those who did not attempt suicide.[25]

A 2023 study confirmed the association between low vitamin D and suicidal behaviors.[26] Most notably, a retrospective study of over 300,000 veterans demonstrated that vitamin D supplementation nearly halved the risk of suicide, with an even more significant reduction (64 percent) in individuals with darker skin or existing vitamin D deficiency.[27]

Given the ease of testing and treatment, addressing vitamin D deficiency is a simple yet potentially lifesaving strategy in suicide prevention.[28]

## ANXIETY

Vitamin D shows potential in alleviating anxiety symptoms. A small study involving patients with generalized anxiety disorder (GAD) and vitamin D deficiency found that those receiving vitamin D alongside standard treatment experienced a nearly one-third reduction in anxiety levels, unlike the control group.[29] Similar improvements in anxiety were observed in women with prediabetes and low vitamin D, with even greater reductions when combined with fish oil, suggesting a neuroinflammation basis.[30] Adolescents with premenstrual syndrome and severe vitamin D deficiency also saw a significant 61 percent reduction in anxiety scores with supplementation.[31]

## ATTENTION DEFICIT HYPERACTIVITY DISORDER

Vitamin D is necessary for healthy brain development in children. A systematic review noted positive effects of vitamin D supplementation on various aspects of children's mental health.[32] Supplementation is recommended for deficient pregnant mothers, as it may protect against the development of ADHD and autism in their offspring.[33] Meta-analyses have confirmed that children with ADHD have significantly lower vitamin D levels.[34] Furthermore, when used as an adjunctive therapy, vitamin D supplementation has been shown to decrease ADHD symptoms and improve vitamin D status without serious adverse effects.[35] In particular, a study using high-dose vitamin D (7143 IU/day) for eight weeks raised baseline serum vitamin D from 16 ng/mL to almost 50 ng/mL and dramatically improved behavioral and cognitive measures indicative of ADHD and overall mental health of children with ADHD.[36]

## COGNITIVE FUNCTION AND MOOD: AN INTERTWINED RELATIONSHIP

The intricate connection between our cognitive abilities and our emotional states is undeniable. When our minds aren't functioning optimally—when we struggle to focus, remember, or process information—it can significantly impact our mood. This is where vitamin D's role in cognitive function becomes particularly relevant to affective well-being. Studies have consistently demonstrated a link between lower vitamin D levels and impaired cognitive performance across various domains. Specifically, research indicates that vitamin D insufficiency can negatively affect executive function, which encompasses critical skills like planning, problem-solving, decision-making, and working memory.[37, 38] When these executive functions are compromised, daily tasks become more challenging, leading to frustration, reduced productivity, and a diminished sense of accomplishment. Imagine constantly struggling to organize your thoughts or finding it difficult to focus on a task at hand; such experiences can quickly erode self-esteem and contribute to feelings of hopelessness or anxiety.

Vitamin D has also been implicated in memory function and information-processing speed. Lower levels of the vitamin have been associated with poorer verbal fluency and visual memory.[39] A sluggish mind, slower reaction times, and difficulty recalling information can make social interactions awkward, make learning new things daunting, and generally reduce one's engagement with the world. This sense of cognitive decline, even subtle, can foster feelings of inadequacy and social withdrawal, acting as a direct pathway to depressive symptoms.[40]

The mechanisms behind vitamin D's influence on cognition are diverse. Vitamin D receptors are widely expressed in brain regions importantly involved in complex cognitive processes, such as the hippocampus, cortex, and cerebellum.[41] Through these receptors, vitamin D directly participates in neurogenesis (the birth of new brain cells), synaptic plasticity (the brain's ability to adapt and change), and the protection of neurons from damage.[42] It also modulates calcium homeostasis, a vital process for neuronal signaling, and reduces oxidative stress and inflammation, both of which can impair cognitive function.[43]

By ensuring these fundamental brain processes are supported, adequate vitamin D levels contribute to sharper thinking, better memory, and quicker processing. When our cognitive faculties are robust, we are better equipped to handle life's challenges, learn new skills, maintain social connections, and experience a greater sense of control and accomplishment, all of which indirectly but powerfully contribute to a more positive and stable affective state.

## THE GUT-BRAIN AXIS: A SURPRISING CONNECTION

An emerging area of research explores the intricate relationship between vitamin D, the gut microbiome, and mental health. The "gut-brain axis" refers to the bidirectional communication system between the gastrointestinal tract and the central nervous system. A healthy gut microbiome, the community of microorganisms residing in our intestines, produces a variety of compounds that can influence brain function and mood.[44] Intriguingly, vitamin D has been shown to influence the composition and diversity of the gut microbiome.[45] Deficiencies in vitamin D can lead to dysbiosis—an imbalance in gut bacteria—which in turn may contribute to inflammatory processes and altered neurotransmitter production, potentially exacerbating depressive symptoms. While this field is still in its early stages, it presents a fascinating avenue for understanding the holistic impact of vitamin D on mental well-being.

## SUNLIGHT, VITAMIN D, AND SCHIZOPHRENIA: AN EARLY LIFE LINK

The connection between vitamin D and mental health extends even to severe psychiatric conditions like schizophrenia, though the relationship here is more complex and often rooted in early life development. Research suggests that vitamin D deficiency during critical periods of brain development, particularly during gestation and early childhood, may increase the risk of developing schizophrenia later in life. One prominent theory, known as the "prenatal vitamin D deficiency hypothesis of schizophrenia," posits that insufficient maternal vitamin D during pregnancy can disrupt normal fetal brain development.[46]

Vitamin D is known to be critical for neurodevelopmental processes, including neuronal proliferation, differentiation, and migration, as well as the formation of synaptic connections.[47] Disruptions in these processes due to vitamin D insufficiency could lay the groundwork for neurological vulnerabilities that manifest as schizophrenia in adulthood.

Epidemiological studies have observed higher rates of schizophrenia in individuals born in winter or spring, in higher latitudes, and in urban environments—all factors associated with reduced sunlight exposure and lower vitamin D levels.[48] The authors also refer to animal studies demonstrating that vitamin D deficiency during gestation can lead to brain abnormalities and behavioral deficits relevant to schizophrenia. While these are associations and not direct causation, they strengthen the hypothesis. Furthermore, studies have shown that individuals with schizophrenia often have lower circulating vitamin D levels compared to healthy controls.[49] While vitamin D supplementation in adulthood may not reverse established schizophrenia, maintaining optimal vitamin D levels throughout pregnancy and early life could be a preventative strategy.

## PRACTICAL APPLICATIONS AND MOVING FORWARD

The evidence strongly suggests that maintaining adequate vitamin D levels is an important component of a comprehensive approach to mental health. While sunlight exposure remains the primary natural source, geographical location, skin type, and lifestyle factors can significantly impact an individual's ability to synthesize sufficient vitamin D. In fact, the connections between lack of sunlight, vitamin D, and schizophrenia suggest a cost of the insane behavior of denying our reality as solar-based beings by shunning the sun is, ironically, a break from reality in the form of depression and schizophrenic insanity. For many, supplementation becomes a necessary strategy, particularly during darker months or in cases of confirmed deficiency. A prominent psychiatrist adds that his "clinical experience often highlights the importance of testing vitamin D levels in patients struggling with any mental health diagnosis, as supplementation can help reduce symptoms and improve overall well-being."[50]

Armed with the knowledge of vitamin D's profound influence on our brains and our moods, we can confidently embrace strategies that ensure optimal levels, paving the way for brighter days, both literally and figuratively.

# CHAPTER 30

# ILLUMINATING THE MIND: SUNLIGHT, VITAMIN D, AND COGNITIVE PROWESS

Beyond their profound impacts on mood, sunlight and vitamin D stand as formidable forces in shaping our cognitive function. The notion that a simple sunbath or a daily supplement could sharpen our minds, enhance our focus, and bolster our memory might seem almost too good to be true. Yet, a growing body of scientific evidence asserts this very truth. This chapter will delve into the compelling research demonstrating how vitamin D deficiency disrupts cognitive performance; explore the intricate dance between sunlight, vitamin D, and circadian rhythms; and illuminate the profound effects of vitamin D and sunlight on arousal, attention, learning, and memory.

## THE COGNITIVE FALLOUT: WHEN VITAMIN D LEVELS DIP

The evidence is clear: When our vitamin D levels are insufficient, our cognitive abilities often suffer. This isn't just about feeling a bit "off"; it translates to measurable disruptions in how effectively our brains process information and execute complex tasks. Research consistently links vitamin D deficiency to impaired performance across several critical cognitive domains. One of the most frequently observed impacts is on executive function. This umbrella term covers high-level mental processes like planning, problem-solving, decision-making, and working memory—the ability to hold and manipulate information in your mind. Individuals with lower vitamin D blood levels often demonstrate poorer scores on tests assessing these vital skills.[1, 2] Imagine trying to manage a busy schedule, learn a new skill, or make complex financial decisions when your brain struggles with these fundamental operations. The implications for daily life, productivity, and overall well-being are substantial.

Furthermore, vitamin D deficiency has been associated with reduced information-processing speed. This refers to how quickly an individual can take in new information, think about it, and respond.[3] A sluggish processing speed can make conversations challenging, slow down learning, and lead to feelings of being overwhelmed. Memory function also takes a hit; studies have reported connections between low vitamin D and deficits in verbal fluency and visual memory, affecting our ability to recall words, recognize faces, or remember important events.[4] These cognitive impairments, while not always manifesting as a diagnosed disorder, can significantly diminish quality of life and contribute to frustration and reduced self-efficacy.[5]

Again, we return to the foundational message that neuroanatomy dictates the underlying mechanisms involved in these widespread cognitive disruptions. That message is the presence of vitamin D receptors throughout brain regions vital for complex cognitive processes, including the hippocampus (critical for memory), the prefrontal cortex (executive function), and the cerebellum (learning, memory, motor control and cognition).[6] Through these receptors, vitamin D influences neurogenesis (the creation of new brain cells), synaptic plasticity (the brain's ability to adapt and form new connections), and the protection of neurons from damage.[7] It also plays a role in calcium homeostasis, which is essential for neuronal signaling, and acts as an anti-inflammatory agent, reducing oxidative stress—factors that, when out of balance, can significantly impair cognitive function.[8] Receptors for vitamin D on and within brain cells is proof that vitamin D or its metabolites have an important role in the function of that cell.

## THE RHYTHMIC PULSE OF COGNITION: SUNLIGHT, VITAMIN D, AND CIRCADIAN RHYTHMS

Our cognitive performance is not a static state; it fluctuates throughout the day, heavily influenced by our internal "body clock" or circadian rhythm. This twenty-four-hour cycle regulates our rest-active or sleep-wake patterns, hormone release, and even our core body temperature. Sunlight is the primary synchronizer of this internal clock, and vitamin D plays a role in its regulation. Exposure to bright light, especially in the morning, signals to the brain that it's daytime, suppressing melatonin production (the sleep hormone) and promoting alertness.[9] Disruptions to this natural rhythm, often caused by insufficient daylight exposure, can lead to a cascade of cognitive problems. When our circadian rhythms are out of sync, we experience fragmented sleep, which directly impairs attention, arousal, and alertness. A poorly rested brain struggles to maintain focus, leading to errors, decreased productivity, and a general feeling of mental fogginess.[10]

While sunlight directly impacts circadian rhythms, vitamin D's involvement is also significant. Vitamin D receptors are present in the suprachiasmatic nucleus (SCN), the brain's master clock.[11] Research suggests that vitamin D may influence the expression of circadian clock genes, helping to maintain their rhythmicity.[12] When vitamin D levels are low, this regulatory influence might be compromised, further exacerbating circadian disruptions. Deficits in attention, arousal, and alertness that manifest due to misaligned circadian rhythms—whether from lack of natural light or potentially insufficient vitamin D—can masquerade as fundamental cognitive impairments. Individuals might struggle with concentration, exhibit slower reaction times, and find it difficult to stay engaged in tasks, all of which are symptoms often attributed to "poor cognition" but are, in essence, a result of a dysregulated internal clock.

## SHARPENING THE MIND: EFFECTS ON AROUSAL, ATTENTION, LEARNING, AND MEMORY

Delving deeper, sunlight and vitamin D exert specific, beneficial effects on key cognitive faculties:

**Arousal and Attention:** Direct exposure to natural light has an immediate impact on arousal and attention. Bright light, particularly blue-enriched light found in natural daylight, stimulates pathways in the brain that promote wakefulness and vigilance.[13] This isn't just about feeling awake; it's about being mentally prepared to receive and process information. Vitamin D further supports this by its widespread influence on neurotransmitter systems. For instance, it affects dopamine and norepinephrine pathways, which are critical for regulating attention and executive control.[14] Sufficient vitamin D ensures these systems operate efficiently, allowing for sustained focus and quick shifts in attention when needed.

**Learning and Memory:** The brain areas most important for learning and memory, such as the hippocampus and cerebellum, are rich in vitamin D receptors. This is no coincidence. Vitamin D plays a vital role in neurogenesis, the process of generating new neurons, particularly in the hippocampus, which is essential for forming new memories.[15] It also enhances synaptic plasticity, strengthening the connections between neurons—the very foundation of learning and memory consolidation.[16] Furthermore, vitamin D's anti-inflammatory and antioxidant properties protect brain cells from damage, creating an optimal environment for these complex processes to thrive. When these protective and supportive mechanisms are compromised by vitamin D deficiency, the ability to acquire new knowledge and recall existing information becomes significantly hampered.

## VITAMIN D EFFECTS ON COGNITION NOT RELATED TO INFLAMMATION

Vitamin D deficiency causes neuroinflammation which can disrupt normal brain function. Is there evidence that vitamin D directly affects brain function separate from preventing disruptive neuroinflammation? Yes, several studies show a primary and direct effect of vitamin D on cognition beyond its role in preventing neuroinflammation. Why is this important? Because it shows that vitamin D, in addition to removing inflammation as an obstacle to normal function, is also directly involved in regulating the brain mechanisms involved in a given cognitive function. This suggests the opportunity to enhance brain function and cognition by optimizing vitamin D in the brain. Vitamin D receptors are present in key brain areas involved in cognition such as the hippocampus, cerebral cortex, cerebellum, and limbic system, suggesting a direct genomic effect on neuronal function.[17]

Experimental studies in animals show vitamin D promotes neurite outgrowth, synaptic function, and gene expression linked to learning and memory.[18] This suggests that vitamin D has positive and perhaps enhancement effects on cognition and associated behaviors.

In rodent models, sufficient vitamin D improved hippocampal-dependent memory and enhanced synaptic transmission. This study found that high-dose vitamin D (10,000 IU/kg) enhanced learning, memory and performance in middle aged rats and that the effects were likely related to enhanced synaptic efficiency in the hippocampus, a part of the brain involved in the maze-learning behavior studied. This study, and others like it in middle-aged subjects, indicates that vitamin D plays an important role in the optimal functioning of brain regions–in normal brains– involved in complex cognitive behaviors and, as such, suggests that optimal vitamin D status is necessary for optimal cognitive performance.[19]

Observational studies in humans link higher dietary vitamin D intake and serum vitamin D levels to better cognitive performance, executive function, and reduced risk of cognitive decline and dementia.[20] Some evidence also suggests vitamin D may influence cognition via effects on calcium regulation, neurotransmitter synthesis, and neurotrophin production in the brain.[21]

While research is in the early stages, the body of molecular, animal, and human research supports a direct role of vitamin D in maintaining and enhancing cognition independently of neuroinflammation.[22]

The accumulated research leaves no room for doubt: Sunlight exposure and adequate vitamin D levels are not merely beneficial for cognitive function; they are foundational to its proper function. While much of the research effort is focused on neurodegenerative disease states that result from chronic vitamin D deficiency like Alzheimer's disease, there is an entire domain of untapped knowledge waiting to be exploited in understanding the roles of vitamin D in complex cognitive processes like emotion, learning and memory in the normal human brain. From the basic alertness needed to navigate our day to the complex processes of learning and memory, our brains perform at their peak when bathed in sufficient sunshine and fueled by essential vitamin D. Prioritizing both is a confident step toward a sharper, more agile mind.

# CHAPTER 31

# THE "-IB" AND "-AB" DRUG REVOLUTION: SYMPTOM MANAGEMENT IN A VITAMIN D-DEFICIENT WORLD

The Western world is grappling with an undeniable crisis: a surge in autoimmune diseases that has mirrored our retreat from the sun and its vital vitamin D. Health and Human Services Secretary Kennedy recently stated that 76.4 percent of Americans have a chronic disease; below we discuss most of these diseases.[1] Since the 1970s, the incidence of autoimmune diseases has risen significantly, with some conditions nearly doubling in prevalence.[2, 3] In response, a new generation of pharmaceuticals, often identifiable by their "-ib" (kinase inhibitors) and "-ab" (monoclonal antibodies) suffixes, has emerged. These drugs are triumphs of scientific ingenuity, offering much-needed relief from the debilitating symptoms of autoimmune disorders, where the body's own immune system mistakenly attacks healthy tissues. However, a critical question demands our attention: Are these sophisticated medications primarily manipulating biological pathways that are inherently and profoundly influenced by vitamin D?

In an era defined by insufficient sunlight exposure and widespread vitamin D deficiency, it is highly probable that these powerful drugs are treating the symptoms of a fundamental imbalance, rather than addressing the root cause. Autoimmune diseases are characterized by an overactive or misdirected immune response. Our immune system, a complex biological marvel, is designed to differentiate between "self" and "nonself," defending us against pathogens while leaving our own cells untouched. When this delicate balance is disrupted—as by chronic vitamin D deficiency—chronic inflammation and tissue damage ensue. The "-ib" and "-ab" drugs aim to restore order by targeting specific components of this intricate immune system.

## TARGETED THERAPIES AND THEIR AUTOIMMUNE TARGETS: A DUAL PERSPECTIVE

Let's examine common autoimmune conditions and the modern pharmaceuticals used to treat them, juxtaposing their mechanisms of action with the established roles of vitamin D.

### Rheumatoid Arthritis (RA)

Rheumatoid arthritis is a chronic inflammatory disorder predominantly affecting the joints, leading to pain, swelling, stiffness, and potentially severe joint damage.

Common "-ib" and "-ab" Drugs for RA:

- **Adalimumab (Humira), Etanercept (Enbrel), Infliximab (Remicade)**: These are TNF-alpha inhibitors ("-ab"). Tumor necrosis factor-alpha (TNF-α) is a key pro-inflammatory cytokine driving the inflammatory cascade in RA. These drugs bind to TNF-α, preventing its interaction with receptors, thereby reducing inflammation and joint destruction.[4]
- **Tofacitinib (Xeljanz), Baricitinib (Olumiant):** These are JAK inhibitors ("-ib"). Janus Kinase (JAK) enzymes are important for signaling pathways that orchestrate inflammation and immune responses. By inhibiting these enzymes, JAK inhibitors reduce the production of various inflammatory cytokines, including interleukins.[5]
- **Vitamin D's Role:** Vitamin D is a potent immunomodulator that directly influences TNF-α production. Research demonstrates that vitamin D can suppress TNF-α synthesis and activity, effectively dampening inflammatory responses.[6] Furthermore, vitamin D receptors are present on various immune cells, and calcitriol, the active form of vitamin D, regulates the expression of genes involved in inflammation and immune cell differentiation, including those influenced by JAK-STAT signaling pathways.[7, 8]

### Psoriasis and Psoriatic Arthritis

Psoriasis is a chronic autoimmune skin condition marked by red, scaly patches. Psoriatic arthritis, a related condition, causes joint inflammation and pain.

Common "-ib" and "-ab" Drugs for Psoriasis:

- **Ustekinumab (Stelara), Secukinumab (Cosentyx), Ixekizumab (Taltz):** These are IL-12/23 or IL-17 inhibitors ("-ab"). Interleukin-12 (IL-12), IL-23, and IL-17 are pivotal cytokines in the inflammatory pathways driving psoriasis. By blocking these specific interleukins, these drugs reduce the proliferation of inflammatory cells and the excessive production of skin cells.[9]

- **Apremilast (Otezla):** This is a PDE4 inhibitor, a targeted immune modulator that increases intracellular cyclic AMP (cAMP), regulating the production of pro-inflammatory and anti-inflammatory mediators.[10]
- **Vitamin D's Role:** Vitamin D is indispensable for skin health and immune regulation. It can inhibit the proliferation of keratinocytes (skin cells) and reduce inflammation in psoriatic lesions.[11] Vitamin D also influences the balance of T-helper cell subsets, including Th17 cells, a primary source of IL-17. Adequate vitamin D levels can promote a more balanced immune response, potentially mitigating the excessive IL-17-driven inflammation observed in psoriasis.[12]

**Inflammatory Bowel Disease (IBD)**—Crohn's Disease and Ulcerative Colitis

IBD involves chronic inflammation of the digestive tract, leading to symptoms such as abdominal pain, diarrhea, bloating, constipation and weight loss.

Common "-ib" and "-ab" Drugs for IBD:

- **Vedolizumab (Entyvio):** This is an integrin receptor antagonist ("-ab"), preventing certain immune cells from migrating into the gut, thereby reducing gut inflammation.[13]
- **Ustekinumab (Stelara):** As noted for psoriasis, this IL-12/23 inhibitor is also effective in IBD, targeting inflammatory pathways contributing to gut inflammation.[14]
- **Tofacitinib (Xeljanz):** This JAK inhibitor is used for ulcerative colitis, working to reduce the broad inflammatory response.[15]
- **Vitamin D's Role:** The gut is a major site of immune activity, and vitamin D is essential for maintaining gut barrier integrity and regulating intestinal immune responses. Vitamin D deficiency is highly prevalent in IBD patients and is associated with more severe disease and increased relapse rates.[16] Vitamin D modulates the expression of cytokines like IL-12 and IL-23 and supports the function of regulatory T cells, which are necessary for maintaining immune tolerance in the gut.[17]

**Multiple Sclerosis (MS)**

Multiple sclerosis is a chronic, often progressive autoimmune disease of the central nervous system, where the immune system attacks the myelin sheath protecting nerve fibers.

Common "-ab" Drugs for MS:

- **Natalizumab (Tysabri):** This is an integrin receptor antagonist ("-ab"), preventing immune cells from crossing the blood-brain barrier and attacking the central nervous system.[18]
- **Ocrelizumab (Ocrevus):** This is an anti-CD20 monoclonal antibody ("-ab") that targets and depletes B cells, which play a role in the pathogenesis of MS.[19]
- **Vitamin D's Role:** The link between vitamin D and MS is one of the most extensively researched in autoimmune diseases. The geographic prevalence of MS strongly correlates with latitude, indicating a significant role for sunlight exposure, which drives vitamin D synthesis. Vitamin D modulates various immune cells, including T cells and B cells, influencing their differentiation and function to promote an anti-inflammatory and neuroprotective environment.[20] It also influences the integrity of the blood-brain barrier.

## CHRONIC VITAMIN D STARVATION: THE UNADDRESSED ROOT CAUSE OF AUTOIMMUNE DISEASE

The striking overlap between the mechanisms of action of these advanced pharmaceuticals and the known functions of vitamin D is not a mere coincidence. It shows that in a state of chronic vitamin D starvation, which afflicts a vast segment of the global population, these autoimmune disease states result from the systemic immune disruption caused by insufficient vitamin D. Our modern lifestyles often keep us indoors, shielded from the very sunlight our bodies require to produce this essential hormone. Sunscreen use also blocks vitamin D synthesis. Dietary sources are limited, and fortification efforts are often insufficient to overcome widespread deficiency. The consequence is a silent epidemic of suboptimal vitamin D levels, subtly eroding the fine-tuned balance of our immune systems.

Imagine a highly complex machine, designed to operate optimally within specific environmental parameters. If one critical input is consistently missing or below optimal levels, the machine will eventually malfunction. Our immune system is that machine, and vitamin D is a critical input. When this input is deficient, the delicate checks and balances within the immune system can falter, leading to an exaggerated inflammatory response and a breakdown in immune tolerance—precisely the conditions that characterize autoimmune diseases.

## VITAMIN D: THE FOUNDATION FOR IMMUNE RESILIENCE

It should be clear that with adequate vitamin D, these autoimmune diseases would be less prevalent. Maintaining optimal vitamin D levels provides the immune system with the fundamental support it needs to regulate inflammation, differentiate immune cells correctly, and maintain self-tolerance. It is akin to providing the "machine" with the fuel it was designed to run on, allowing it to perform its protective functions without overreacting or misfiring. This is not to say that vitamin D is a magic bullet or a cure-all. Autoimmune diseases are complex, with multifactorial causes, including genetic predispositions and environmental triggers. However, vitamin D's pervasive influence on immune function shows it is an important, yet often overlooked, foundational factor in disease prevention and management.

## BIOLOGICS: TREATING THE BRANCHES, IGNORING THE ROOTS?

Consider the immense success of modern biologic pharmaceuticals like Humira, Enbrel, Stelara, and Xeljanz. These drugs represent a leap forward in treating debilitating autoimmune conditions, offering relief and improved quality of life to millions. However, their very efficacy, often by meticulously blocking inflammatory cytokines or specific immune cell pathways, underscores a critical point: These modern biologic pharmaceuticals are essentially treating a symptom that is likely a result of chronic vitamin D deficiency causing immune system disruption leading to autoimmune symptoms and disease.

When an individual's immune system is chronically deprived of vitamin D, it struggles to maintain its normal regulatory functions. Inflammatory pathways become overactive, and the ability to distinguish "self" from "nonself" is compromised. The result is the emergence of autoimmune symptoms and ultimately, full-blown disease. The biologics then step in, not to correct the underlying vitamin D deficiency, but to suppress the downstream inflammatory consequences. They are, in essence, cutting off the branches of a diseased tree, while the roots—the chronic vitamin D starvation—remain unaddressed.

## CONDITION CREEP: A DEEPER VITAMIN D CONNECTION

Have you noticed that some biologics are becoming quite the jack of all trades with respect to one drug being found to be effective in treating more than one autoimmune condition? The remarkable expansion of diseases treated by biologic drugs like guselkumab (Tremfya) exemplifies a phenomenon that may be termed "condition creep" within the pharmaceutical landscape.

Initially approved solely for the treatment of moderate to severe plaque psoriasis, guselkumab, a monoclonal antibody that targets the p19 subunit of interleukin-23 (IL-23), has demonstrated efficacy in other autoimmune conditions.[21] This has led to its subsequent approval for psoriatic arthritis and the inflammatory bowel diseases Crohn's disease and ulcerative colitis. This expansion underscores a broader understanding of the interconnectedness of inflammatory pathways in various autoimmune disorders.

This "condition creep" phenomenon is not unique to guselkumab. Many other "-ib" (kinase inhibitor) and "-ab" (antibody) drugs have followed similar trajectories. For instance, adalimumab (Humira), one of the earliest and most widely used anti-TNF-alpha biologics, was initially approved for rheumatoid arthritis. Its utility soon broadened to encompass a wide array of autoimmune and inflammatory conditions, including psoriasis, psoriatic arthritis, ankylosing spondylitis, Crohn's disease, ulcerative colitis, and hidradenitis suppurativa.[22] Similarly, tofacitinib (Xeljanz), a Janus kinase (JAK) inhibitor, started with use for rheumatoid arthritis and has since gained approval for psoriatic arthritis, ulcerative colitis, and ankylosing spondylitis.[23] Recall that my wife and I experienced this phenomenon similar to condition creep when we discovered that high-dose vitamin D eradicated both my psoriasis and her ulcerative colitis. These examples highlight a growing trend in which drugs designed to target specific inflammatory mediators or cellular pathways demonstrate a broader therapeutic reach due to shared underlying pathological mechanisms across different autoimmune diseases.

This observed "condition creep" is not merely coincidental; it points to a deeper, more fundamental connection, particularly when considering the ubiquitous role of vitamin D in immune regulation. Vitamin D is a critical immunomodulator with profound effects on both innate and adaptive immunity. It influences the differentiation of immune cells, the production of cytokines, and the overall balance of immune responses.[24] Specifically, vitamin D has been shown to suppress inflammatory pathways, including those involving IL-23, the very target of drugs like guselkumab. In individuals with vitamin D deficiency, which is highly prevalent in populations suffering from autoimmune diseases, the immune system can become dysregulated, leading to chronic inflammation and the manifestation of various autoimmune conditions.[25]

Therefore, it is entirely unsurprising that in a vitamin D–deficient individual with multiple autoimmune diseases, drugs like guselkumab would be found to affect other autoimmune diseases as well. These biologic drugs, by manipulating a specific component of the inflammatory cascade, are essentially intervening in a system that vitamin D holistically regulates. The success of the biologics in diverse conditions merely reinforces the critical, overarching role of vitamin D in maintaining immune balance and underscores the potential for a foundational vitamin D repletion strategy to augment or even reduce the need for such targeted drug therapies by making the diseases less likely to occur. Essentially, these drugs treat the symptoms of the diseases that adequate vitamin D would likely prevent from ever occurring. Again, this is the concept proven out in my personal experience when my wife and I resolved our psoriasis and UC, respectively, simply by using adequate amounts of vitamin D.

## THE DOUBLE-EDGED SWORD: WHY BIOLOGIC DRUGS CAN CAUSE SIDE EFFECTS AND VITAMIN D RARELY DOES

Biologic drugs, with their highly targeted mechanisms, have revolutionized the treatment of many diseases, from aggressive cancers to debilitating autoimmune conditions. Yet, this precision comes at a cost for some patients: a range of undesirable side effects. We will now delve into the underlying mechanisms that contribute to these adverse reactions, particularly contrasting them with the generally side-effect-free physiological regulation and immune system balance offered by vitamin D. We will explore the idea that the selective, "piecemeal" manipulation of the immune system by biologics creates an imbalance that manifests as side effects, in stark contrast to the holistic, synergistic balanced control exerted by side-effect-free vitamin D.

## THE TARGETED APPROACH: HOW BIOLOGICS WORK AND WHY IT CAN LEAD TO TROUBLE

Recall that biologic drugs, such as those ending in "-ib" (tyrosine kinase inhibitors) and "-ab" (monoclonal antibodies), are designed to interfere with very specific molecular pathways or targets within the body. Tyrosine kinase inhibitors (TKIs) block the activity of enzymes called tyrosine kinases, which play critical roles in cell growth, division, and signaling. Monoclonal antibodies (mAbs) are engineered proteins that can bind to specific targets on cells or circulating proteins, either blocking their activity or flagging them for destruction. While this targeted approach is intended to maximize efficacy against a disease, it often overlooks the intricate interconnectedness of biologically complex immune systems. Imagine trying to fix a sophisticated machine by only adjusting one specific gear. While that gear might be directly involved in the problem, its movement influences many other gears, and an isolated adjustment could throw the entire machine out of whack. This analogy helps explain why targeting a single component of a highly complex and interconnected system like the immune system can lead to unforeseen consequences. In the case of "-ib" and "-ab" drugs, we're referring to adverse side effects.

## SIDE EFFECTS OF "-IB" DRUGS (TYROSINE KINASE INHIBITORS): A CASCADE OF UNINTENDED CONSEQUENCES

Tyrosine kinases are not just involved in disease-specific pathways; they are ubiquitous and essential for a wide range of normal cellular functions. When TKIs block these enzymes, they can inadvertently disrupt these vital processes, leading to a spectrum of side effects:

- **Gastrointestinal Issues (Nausea, Vomiting, Diarrhea, Abdominal Pain):** Tyrosine kinase pathways are involved in the normal functioning and regeneration of cells lining the digestive tract. Disrupting these pathways can impair gut integrity and motility, leading to common gastrointestinal complaints.[26]

- **Skin Reactions (Rashes, Dry Skin, Itching):** Skin cells also rely on various tyrosine kinase pathways for their growth, differentiation, and repair. Inhibition can lead to altered skin barrier function, inflammation, and abnormal cell turnover, manifesting as rashes, dryness, or itching.[27]
- **Fatigue:** The mechanisms behind cancer-related fatigue are complex, but disrupting energy metabolism and cellular signaling through TKI inhibition can contribute to profound tiredness.[28]
- **Liver Function Changes (Elevated Liver Enzymes):** The liver is a central organ for metabolism and detoxification. Tyrosine kinase inhibition can interfere with hepatic cell function or cause direct cellular stress, leading to elevated liver enzymes—a sign of potential liver damage.[29]
- **Cardiovascular Effects (Hypertension, Heart-Related Issues):** Tyrosine kinase pathways are critical for the healthy function of blood vessels and heart muscle cells. Disrupting these can lead to changes in blood pressure regulation and direct cardiac toxicity.[30]
- **Blood Disorders (Anemia, Thrombocytopenia, Neutropenia):** Hematopoiesis, the process of blood cell formation, relies on finely tuned signaling pathways, many of which involve tyrosine kinases. Inhibition can impair the production of red blood cells (anemia), platelets (thrombocytopenia), and various white blood cells (neutropenia), increasing risks of bleeding and infection.[31]

## SIDE EFFECTS OF "-AB" DRUGS (MONOCLONAL ANTIBODIES): UNBALANCING THE IMMUNE SYSTEM

Monoclonal antibodies are designed to target specific components of the immune system or cancer cells. While this specificity aims to reduce damage to healthy cells, the immune system is a highly interconnected network. Manipulating one part can have ripple effects throughout the entire system. For example, drugs like ustekinumab and secukinumab target specific interleukins (IL-12, IL-17, IL-23) that play roles in inflammatory pathways.[32]

- **Infusion Reactions (Fever, Chills, Allergic Reactions):** These reactions are often immune-mediated responses to the infused antibody itself, even if it's "humanized." The body can recognize the biologic as foreign, triggering a rapid immune response.

- **Infections (Increased Susceptibility):** This is a primary concern with many biologics that modulate the immune system. By blocking specific inflammatory pathways (e.g., IL-12, IL-17, IL-23), these drugs can inadvertently weaken the body's ability to fight off certain pathogens, leading to an increased risk of infections.[33] The selective blockade creates a specific vulnerability.
- **Gastrointestinal Symptoms (Nausea, Vomiting, Diarrhea):** Similar to TKIs, some mAbs can indirectly affect gastrointestinal function through their immune-modulating effects, leading to inflammation or altered gut motility.[34]
- **Skin Reactions (Rashes, Injection Site Reactions):** Rashes can be part of an allergic reaction or an immune response to the drug. Injection site reactions are localized inflammatory responses to the physical injection and the drug itself.
- **Fatigue:** Chronic inflammation and immune dysregulation contribute to fatigue in many conditions, and while biologics aim to reduce inflammation, their systemic effects can still induce fatigue.[35]
- **Cardiovascular Issues (Heart Failure):** Certain monoclonal antibodies, particularly those targeting specific growth factors or cytokines, can have direct or indirect cardiotoxic effects, sometimes leading to heart failure in susceptible individuals.[36]

## THE "EMERGENT FEATURE" HYPOTHESIS: BIOLOGIC SIDE EFFECTS AS IMMUNE SYSTEM IMBALANCE

The core of the issue with biologic drug side effects, particularly immune-modulating ones, appears to be an emergent feature due to the manipulation of an isolated component of the immune system compared to side-effect-free holistic immune system control by vitamin D. The immune system is a dynamic, tightly regulated network in which multiple pathways and cell types constantly interact to maintain balance, known as homeostasis. When a biologic drug selectively blocks one specific cytokine (like IL-12 or IL-17) or one specific enzyme, it's akin to removing a single pillar from a multi-pillar bridge. The bridge might not collapse entirely, but the load distribution shifts, creating stress and instability elsewhere. This "piecemeal" targeting, while precise, can lead to:

1. **Compensatory Pathways:** The immune system is resilient. If one pathway is blocked, others may become overactive to compensate, potentially leading to unintended inflammation or immune suppression in different areas.[37]
2. **Loss of Redundancy and Balance:** Many immune functions have redundant pathways, meaning several different mechanisms can

achieve the same goal. Blocking one can remove an important layer of protection without necessarily replacing it, making the system more vulnerable.[38]

3. **Off-Target Effects (Even with "On-Target" Specificity):** Even if a biologic drug binds only to its intended target, that target itself might have a broader physiological role than initially understood. Manipulating it can thus have widespread effects.[39]

Therefore, the side effects seen with biologics are not necessarily "bugs" in the design of the drug in the sense of being poorly understood. Rather, they can be seen as design features—unavoidable consequences of intensely selective intervention in a complex, interconnected biological system like the immune system. The selective blockade of one cytokine by the drug, by creating an imbalance, effectively makes the side effect symptoms an emergent property of the system's re-equilibration and/or calibration in the face of that targeted disruption. In other words, affecting just one or two components of the immune system creates compensatory actions that result in immune-mediated side effects. Hint: If one wanted to reduce the side effects of any "-ib" or "-ab" drug the solution would be to ensure the subject is vitamin D replete . . . just like what is being found with immune checkpoint–inhibiting cancer drugs.[40, 41] Vitamin D would compensate in response to the perturbed immune system caused by the "-ib" or "-ab" drug and restore balance. However, obviously a vitamin D–replete subject would probably not ever need the "-ib" or "-ab" drug in the first place.

## VITAMIN D: THE HOLISTIC MAESTRO OF IMMUNE REGULATION

In stark contrast to the targeted, isolated interventions of biologic drugs, vitamin D operates as a holistic, integrative regulator of the immune system. Rather than selectively blocking one cytokine or one enzyme, vitamin D influences a vast array of immune cells and pathways, simultaneously maintaining overall immune balance and function without causing similar adverse side effects at physiological doses. Vitamin D's mechanism of action is far more pervasive, expert, and nuanced:

- **Ubiquitous Receptors:** Vitamin D receptors (VDRs) are found on nearly all immune cells, including T cells, B cells, macrophages, and dendritic cells.[42] This widespread presence allows vitamin D to exert broad, systemic control upregulating and downregulating to maintain balance.
- **Gene Transcription Modulation:** When activated, vitamin D binds to VDRs, forming a complex that directly influences the transcription of hundreds of genes involved in immune responses. This includes

genes related to cell proliferation, differentiation, apoptosis, and the production of various cytokines and antimicrobial peptides.[43]

- **Balancing Pro- and Anti-Inflammatory Responses:** Vitamin D doesn't simply suppress the immune system; it helps to fine-tune it. It can reduce the production of pro-inflammatory cytokines (like IL-1, IL-6, TNF-alpha) while promoting the production of anti-inflammatory cytokines (like IL-10). It also influences the differentiation of T cells, favoring regulatory T cells (Tregs) that help keep immune responses in check.[44]
- **Maintaining Barrier Integrity:** Vitamin D also plays a role in maintaining the integrity of physical barriers, such as the skin and gut lining, which are the body's first line of defense against pathogens. This further contributes to its holistic immune-supportive role.[45]

Vitamin D's management and control of the immune system has been perfected over eons. Modern pharmaceuticals may be able to mimic one or two aspects of the immune system but they are unlikely to ever be able to mimic the sophisticated, integrated, and balanced control that good old vitamin D provides.

## WHY VITAMIN D HAS NO SIDE EFFECTS AT PHYSIOLOGICAL DOSES

The absence of significant adverse side effects with physiological doses of vitamin D, compared to biologics, stems from its integrative and homeostatic role:

- **Natural Regulator:** Vitamin D is the naturally occurring hormone that the body evolved with. Its actions are part of the body's inherent regulatory mechanisms, designed to maintain balance, not disrupt it.
- **Synergistic Action:** Instead of targeting one isolated component, vitamin D works synergistically with multiple pathways, nudging the immune system toward a balanced and appropriate response rather than a drastic alteration of one specific axis. It promotes overall immune competence without creating specific vulnerabilities.
- **Physiological Dosing:** The body has mechanisms to tightly regulate vitamin D levels. The amounts of vitamin D obtained from sunlight exposure or reasonable supplementation are well within the body's natural regulatory capacity, allowing it to exert its broad, beneficial effects without overwhelming specific pathways.

The adverse side effects observed with modern biologic drugs, particularly the "-ib" and "-ab" varieties, can largely be understood as an emergent feature of their highly targeted, piecemeal approach to manipulating complex biological systems when we have the ideal, natural, integrative, synergistic and highly sophisticated model of how vitamin D controls the immune system as a reference. By selectively blocking isolated components of the immune system or critical cellular pathways, these "-ib" and "-ab" drugs can inadvertently create imbalances, leading to a cascade of unintended consequences. These side effects, rather than being "bugs" in the drugs, can be seen as actually design features inherent in such "primitive" ham-handed drugs—an inherent trade-off of intense specificity in a system that is based on sophisticated and advanced interconnectedness.

## SUNLIGHT AND VITAMIN D SCARE THE LIVING DAYLIGHTS OUT OF BIG PHARMA

Biologics treat the symptoms of chronic vitamin D deficiency that manifest as autoimmune disease, whereas adequate vitamin D, from sensible sun exposure, diet, and supplementation, is highly likely to fix or prevent immune system dysfunction and autoimmune disease. This perspective is not meant to diminish the perceived value of these drugs for many. However, it challenges us to consider a broader, more preventative approach involving a healthier lifestyle that includes sensible sun exposure and vitamin D. If optimal vitamin D status could reduce the incidence or severity of these conditions, the implications for public health and health-care costs would be profound. It compels us to reevaluate our understanding of autoimmune disease, shifting the focus from simply managing symptoms with side-effect-ridden pharmaceuticals to exploring the fundamental nutritional and environmental factors that underpin immune health. The stark difference in incidence in autoimmune disease between black Africans in the tropics (very low) and African Americans in a temperate climate (very high) shouts environmental cause,[46] which is vitamin D. A holistic approach with a robust emphasis on achieving and maintaining adequate vitamin D levels may represent the most comprehensive and sustainable path forward in the fight against autoimmune disease.

In stark contrast to biologic drugs, vitamin D exemplifies a holistic and integrative approach to immune regulation. Its widespread vitamin D receptor–mediated influence on various immune cells and genes, its ability to balance pro- and anti-inflammatory responses, and its role as a natural, synergistic regulator of the immune system explain why it rarely causes any adverse side effects at physiological doses. The body is equipped to incorporate and utilize vitamin D's broad effects to maintain overall immune balance and health, and in the light of this understanding that the profound differences between a natural, systemic modulator like vitamin D and a highly specific, artificial intervention "-ib" or "-ab" drug can be seen and understood.

The choice is clear: Optimize your vitamin D intake to optimize and balance immune system function and likely avoid autoimmune disease, or you can continue to avoid the sun and its vitamin D and assume your place among the eight out of ten Americans currently afflicted with one or more of the chronic diseases and rely on "miracle" drugs to treat your symptoms that are caused by chronic vitamin D deficiency.

## CHAPTER 32

# FINAL THOUGHTS ON SUNLIGHT AND VITAMIN D

This chapter covers some important topics and issues related to all things vitamin D that didn't rise to the level of their own chapter or section within any given chapter. Many of the following items were originally questions or comments that came into the All Things Vitamin D Substack publication (StarPower.Substack.com).

### ESSENTIAL COFACTORS FOR OPTIMAL VITAMIN D FUNCTION

While vitamin D is a powerhouse for health, it doesn't work in isolation. For optimal absorption, utilization, and to unlock its full potential, several key cofactors must be present in adequate amounts. Think of these cofactors as the supporting cast that ensures vitamin D can perform its starring role effectively. Ignoring these important partners can limit the benefits of vitamin D supplementation.

> **Magnesium** is perhaps the most critical cofactor for vitamin D. It's involved in over three hundred enzymatic reactions in the body, including those that activate vitamin D. Without sufficient magnesium, vitamin D remains in its inactive form, unable to exert its beneficial effects. Studies have shown that magnesium deficiency can lead to vitamin D resistance.[1]
>
> General Guidance: The recommended daily allowance (RDA) for magnesium for adult men is 400–420 mg, and for adult women, it's 310–320 mg.[2] Many people don't get enough magnesium from their diet, making supplementation a wise consideration. Common forms include magnesium citrate, glycinate, and malate.

**Zinc** plays a vital role in immune function, and it also contributes to vitamin D receptor expression.[3] Adequate zinc levels are essential for the cellular machinery that responds to vitamin D, further enhancing its immune-modulating properties.

General Guidance: The RDA for zinc for adult men is 11 mg, and for adult women, it's 8 mg.[4] Zinc can be found in various forms, including zinc picolinate, gluconate, and citrate.

**Calcium** and vitamin D are inextricably linked, especially concerning bone health. Vitamin D's primary role in calcium metabolism is to enhance calcium absorption from the gut. However, supplementing with vitamin D without adequate calcium intake is counterproductive, as the body will simply draw calcium from bones to maintain blood calcium levels.[5]

General Guidance: The RDA for calcium for most adults aged nineteen to fifty years is 1,000 mg per day.[6] Dairy products, leafy green vegetables, and fortified foods are excellent dietary sources. If supplementing, calcium carbonate and calcium citrate are common forms.

**Vitamin K**, particularly K2, is important for directing calcium to the bones and preventing its deposition in soft tissues like arteries, where it can contribute to arterial stiffness and cardiovascular disease. Vitamin K2 activates proteins like osteocalcin, which integrates calcium into bone, and matrix GLA protein (MGP), which inhibits calcium buildup in arteries.[7]

Vitamin K is an interesting substance. The human body can make some forms of vitamin K, specifically vitamin K2 (menaquinones), but not vitamin K1 (phylloquinone). Vitamin K2 is produced by certain types of gut bacteria in the large intestine, which synthesize various menaquinones that can be absorbed by the body. Additionally, the human body has the ability to convert vitamin K1, which is obtained from plant sources, into MK-4 (a subtype of vitamin K2) via an enzymatic process in animal tissues, independent of bacterial action.[8]

General Guidance: The adequate intake (AI) for vitamin K for adult men is 120 μg, and for adult women, it's 90 μg.[9] While vitamin K1 is abundant in leafy greens, vitamin K2 (menaquinone) is found in fermented foods, certain cheeses, and natto.

**Vitamin A** (retinol) and vitamin D share a complex and often synergistic relationship, particularly in regulating gene expression and immune function. Both vitamins act as nuclear receptor ligands, meaning they bind to specific receptors within cells to influence gene activity. A balanced intake of both is necessary, as excessively high levels of one can potentially interfere with the other's function.[10]

General Guidance: The RDA for vitamin A for adult men is 900 μg, and for adult women, it's 700 μg.[11] Excellent sources of vitamin A include liver, fish oil, and dairy products. Beta-carotene, a precursor to vitamin A, is found in colorful fruits and vegetables.

Optimizing your vitamin D status requires a holistic approach that acknowledges the critical roles of these cofactors. By ensuring adequate intake of magnesium, zinc, calcium, and vitamin K and maintaining a balanced relationship with vitamin A, you empower your body to fully leverage the profound health benefits of vitamin D. Consult with a health-care professional or, better yet, a dietician, to determine your individual needs and the most appropriate supplementation strategy.

## TATTOOS AND VITAMIN D SYNTHESIS

The presence of tattoos on the skin can indeed have an impact on the body's ability to produce vitamin D from solar exposure. Understanding this effect requires examining how UV radiation interacts with the skin and how tattoos alter this interaction.

### TATTOOS AND UV RADIATION ABSORPTION

Tattoos involve the permanent insertion of ink pigments into the dermis layer of the skin. These pigments, by their very nature, are designed to absorb and reflect light to create the desired visual effect.[12] When sunlight, including UVB radiation, strikes tattooed skin, the ink acts as a physical barrier and absorber. Research indicates that tattoo inks can significantly block UV radiation from reaching the underlying skin cells. The darker and denser the tattoo, the greater its capacity to absorb or scatter UV light.[13] This phenomenon is similar to how sunscreen works, albeit with different mechanisms and intentions. While sunscreen is formulated to filter specific wavelengths to prevent sunburn and DNA damage, tattoo inks are simply light-absorbing substances permanently embedded in the skin.

### IMPACT ON VITAMIN D SYNTHESIS

The primary effect of tattoo ink absorbing UVB radiation is a reduction in the amount of UVB light that reaches the 7-dehydrocholesterol in the epidermal layer. Consequently, the conversion of this precursor into pre-vitamin D3 is diminished in tattooed areas. For individuals with extensive tattoo coverage, particularly over large surface areas of the body that are typically exposed to the sun (e.g., arms, legs, back), this could lead to a decreased capacity for overall vitamin D production through solar exposure.[14] It is important to note that the extent of this reduction is directly proportional to the size, density, and darkness of the tattooed area. A small, lightly colored tattoo will likely have a negligible impact, whereas a full sleeve or a heavily tattooed back could significantly impede vitamin D synthesis in those specific regions.

### COMPENSATORY MECHANISMS AND CONSIDERATIONS

The human body is remarkably adaptable. If large portions of the skin are tattooed, the body can still produce vitamin D from non-tattooed areas. Therefore, individuals with extensive tattoos are not necessarily destined for vitamin D deficiency. However, they may need to be more mindful of ensuring adequate sun exposure on untattooed skin or consider alternative sources of vitamin D, such as diet and supplements, especially if their sun exposure is otherwise limited. Furthermore, the impact of tattoos on vitamin D synthesis is part of a broader discussion about skin health and sun exposure. Tattoos can also affect the skin's ability to tan or show signs of sunburn, potentially masking early warning signs of excessive sun exposure.

Tattoos can indeed reduce the solar-generated production of vitamin D in the skin due to the light-absorbing properties of tattoo inks. The degree of this effect is dependent on the size, density, and darkness of the tattooed areas. While individuals with extensive tattoos may experience a localized reduction in vitamin D synthesis, this does not automatically lead to systemic deficiency. Awareness of this interaction allows individuals to make informed choices regarding sun exposure, diet, and supplementation to maintain optimal vitamin D levels. Finally, since tattoos appear to be risk factors for some cancers (such as a 200 percent increase in rare lymphomas), ensuring optimal immune system function and vitamin D status is important.[15, 16]

## VITAMIN D STATUS AS UNCONTROLLED VARIABLE IN MEDICAL RESEARCH

Uncontrolled variables pose a significant threat to the validity of medical research, often leading to misleading or inaccurate conclusions. One pertinent example is the unacknowledged vitamin D status of study participants. Given the widespread vitamin D deficiency across most demographics, if researchers are investigating the effects of a new drug without first assessing and controlling for subjects' baseline vitamin D levels, any observed outcomes could be confounded by interactions with varying vitamin D statuses.[17] This is because vitamin D plays a critical role in numerous physiological processes, including immune function, bone health, and even gene expression, meaning its deficiency or sufficiency can independently influence disease progression or drug efficacy.[18] For instance, a drug might appear less effective in a group with widespread vitamin D deficiency, simply because the deficiency itself is hindering the body's response or exacerbating the condition being treated. On the other hand, a drug's benefits might be over-attributed to the drug when, in reality, subjects with optimal vitamin D levels are responding better due to their robust physiological state. Such confounding makes it nearly impossible to isolate the true effect of the intervention, undermining the integrity of the research and potentially leading to ineffective or even harmful clinical recommendations.[19, 20]

To mitigate this pervasive artifact, several remedies can be implemented. First and foremost, researchers should routinely measure and record the vitamin D status of all study participants at baseline, the beginning of the study. This allows for parsing of subjects into different groups based on their vitamin D levels, enabling researchers to analyze drug effects within distinct vitamin D groups or to use statistical methods to adjust for baseline differences.[21]

Another robust approach involves standardizing vitamin D levels across the study population, either by supplementing all participants to achieve a target range or by excluding individuals outside a narrow, predefined range. While this might limit the generalizability of findings to broader populations, it significantly enhances internal validity by removing vitamin D as a confounding factor. Furthermore, reporting guidelines for medical research should be strengthened to mandate the disclosure of vitamin D status and any measures taken to control for it. This transparency allows for better interpretation and meta-analysis of study results across different investigations, ultimately leading to a more accurate understanding of drug effects in diverse populations.

## HOW TO READ VITAMIN D STUDIES LIKE A PRO

Did you know that not everyone is thrilled with the idea of free sunlight and vitamin D ameliorating or curing most of the nation's ills? Yes, shocking, isn't it? Joking aside, there are entities that live off the status quo of perpetual disease and expensive, marginally effective side-effect-ridden treatments. So we have to be on the lookout for vitamin D studies that are actually designed to fail. By fail, I mean fail to find a health-saving or health-improving effect of a sunlight or vitamin D intervention. That is not to say that every physiological system or behavior studied is affected by vitamin D, but here is a primer to help you be an educated consumer of vitamin D science, so you can separate the legitimate science from the BS.

A recent study actually found that vitamin D did not improve bone mineral density or structure. Vitamin D was discovered as a cure for rickets, the bone deforming disease, remember? This study found that taking 2,000 IU vitamin D3 daily did not strengthen bones in sixty-four-year-old women (n=687).[22] The 2,000 IU vitamin D did increase serum 25(OH)D levels from 27.64 ng.mL to 39.44 ng/mL. So what's going on here?

First, obviously the 2,000 IU dose is too low to affect bone mineral density and a serum level of 39 ng/mL is too low to affect bone health in a group of sixty-four-year-old women. One flaw with this study is that it did not vary the dose of vitamin D. They picked 2,000 IU as a safe upper limit based on US RDA values, which we've already shown to be flawed and orders of magnitude too low to satisfy daily needs. So, there is no surprise that the study failed to find an effect. The title of the paper should have been "2000 IU Vitamin D3 Daily is Too Low to Affect Bone Mineral Density: Why Is the RDA Still Only 600 IU?"

Second, any drug study, including vitamin D studies, must vary the dose studied to obtain a dose-response measure.[23] Usually in a drug study there is a threshold dosage below which there is no effect and, intermediate doses that are effectual, and then a ceiling either due to toxicity concerns or practicality. Any drug study that does not vary dose should be rejected. A high school student conducting any drug study would know to do this.

What is shocking about the Manson study is that these scientists are not high school students, they are at Harvard. This is a study that was designed to fail from the start. It was designed to find no effect of vitamin D on bones.

The Manson study was singled out because it was a huge study that cost us taxpayers big, and it should have never been approved without the dose-response component in the design of the study and it should have never passed peer review to make it to publication. Studies like this are dangerous because the know-nothing mockingbird media takes the bait and spreads the nonsense in the form of headlines that read "Vitamin D Study Finds No Effect on Bone Health!" This observation also addresses the motivation to conduct a flawed study on vitamin D to find no effect in the first place. To mislead and confuse the public.

Unfortunately there are hundreds of vitamin D studies published and on the books like this that were designed to fail from the start. Questions to ask to determine if any vitamin D study is legitimate:

- What was the dose? (Doses below 5,000 IU per day are likely too low)
- Did they vary the dose? (Doses of 500, 1,000 and 2,000 IU are all below a reasonable therapeutic range and won't work. A study that has a 2,000 IU group, a 5,000 IU group and a 10,000 IU group or more will likely find an effect and a dose-response effect as well)
- What type of vitamin D did they use, D2 or D3? D2 (ergocalciferol) is the expensive prescription-based form of vitamin D. D3 (cholecalciferol) is what the sun makes in skin and is available over the counter for pennies. D3 is 87 percent more effective in raising blood levels of 25(OH)D than is D2. Any study that uses D2 is unlikely to find an effect.[24]

- How long did they give vitamin D to work? (A study that has a thirty-day study period will likely not find any effects of vitamin D. Depending on the condition, a study period of at least one year is a minimum). Recall the noted complex phasic vs. chronic effects of vitamin D on traumatic brain injury that Stein found that are not understood.[25]
- Did the vitamin D that was administered actually raise serum 25(OH) D levels? (Believe it or not, there are published studies that never measured whether the vitamin D they gave was effective in raising vitamin D levels; it was simply assumed it did.)
- What was the vitamin D status of the subjects before the study began? Giving additional vitamin D to a vitamin D–replete subject will encounter a ceiling effect. This means that if the measure of interest is an improvement in a biological value, and the change in that value is evidence of a vitamin D effect, if a subject is already vitamin D optimized, additional vitamin D may not add any benefit. The outcome is the study finds no beneficial effect of the additional vitamin D because a ceiling was reached already.

There is also another form of research that can be used to sway public perception about vitamin D and other off-patent substances called the meta-analysis. A meta-analysis is a fancy way to say we analyzed a bunch of other studies as if they were just one study and are drawing a conclusion from that effort.

As an example, a meta-analysis found that vitamin D supplementation had no effect on cardiovascular disease as measured by heart attack, stroke and cerebrovascular accident and all-cause mortality.[26] There are several flagrant flaws in this meta-analysis, the first of which is the dose of vitamin D studied. The vast majority of studies included used too low a dose of vitamin D (between 800 and 1,000 IU). There were also very few instances of a CVD event in the individual studies, in many cases one group had a single event and the other group had none. There can be no differences found when the variable measured (CVD) doesn't vary between the groups. This is called a floor effect. Looking for a difference when there are no differences in the groups on the measured variable because it did not occur is not a failure to find an effect of vitamin D. It is a failure to find CVD disease in either group.

The most troubling issue with meta-analyses may be in the concept of a meta-analysis itself. Combining a bunch of flawed individual studies into one big study (meta-analysis) just creates one big flawed study with statistical power. Flawed meta-analyses may amplify errors of primary studies, failing to correct for bias, confounding, or poor design.[27]

Combining highly heterogeneous studies can generate results that are statistically significant but clinically irrelevant or even misleading. When separate flawed studies are combined into one larger one as in a meta-analysis what can happen is that methodological errors are transferred and amplified (META). It's like photocopying a blurry page a dozen times and claiming clarity from the stack.

In yet another seemingly absurd course of action, the Endocrine Society, the group that perpetuates the statistical misinterpretation that the US RDA of 600 IU vitamin D is adequate,[28] has come out stating that routine testing of a person's vitamin D status is neither needed nor necessary. Routine vitamin D testing for healthy adults, including those with obesity or darker skin tones, is unnecessary unless specific risk factors or medical conditions impacting vitamin D metabolism are present. The Endocrine Society's 2024 guideline asserts that treating low vitamin D levels in healthy individuals offers no real benefit, and additional supplementation does not alter health outcomes for the majority. Their explicit stance: "We suggest against routine testing for 25-hydroxyvitamin D levels in any of the populations studied, since outcome-specific benefits based on vitamin D levels have not been demonstrated."[29] *Harvard Health*, *BMJ*, and various other US and international sources echo the same advice to avoid routine vitamin D screening in the general population.[30, 31, 32] The *Harvard Health* paper said that "it isn't helpful for most people to know their vitamin D level."

Well, that's a first: a medical diagnostic test that the medical community doesn't like. So what's going on here? Just about every cell in the body has a vitamin D receptor, vitamin D deficiency is epidemic, and many health scourges of modern humankind have a vitamin D connection, yet we don't need to trouble ourselves with knowing our vitamin D status? If one were to get the idea that there is an organized effort to keep the population vitamin D deficient, advising people and their doctors that vitamin D testing is unnecessary coupled with bad advice regarding the RDA values being orders of magnitude too low for daily needs might lend support to that idea.

## PREVAGEN, FOCUS FACTOR, NEURIVA, SUPER BETA PROSTATE, AND OTHER SUPPLEMENTS

Prevagen, a popular memory supplement, contains a dose of vitamin D3. Curiously, other brain pills like Focus Factor, Neuriva (high-dose folic acid, which is a vitamin D enzymatic agonist)[33] and others do as well. Regarding Prevagen, while much attention is given to apoaequorin as the active ingredient, a compelling hypothesis suggests that any observed cognitive benefits might largely stem from the vitamin D3 component.[34] This is particularly relevant because a vast majority of the elderly population, the primary target demographic for such supplements, suffers from widespread vitamin D deficiency. Factors like reduced sun exposure and changes in skin and kidney function contribute to this common insufficiency as people age.

As we've learned, vitamin D plays a critical and multifaceted role in brain health. Receptors for this vitamin are found in key brain areas responsible for learning and memory, indicating its direct involvement in cognitive processes. It acts as a neuroprotectant, shielding neurons from damage, and is involved in neurogenesis (the creation of new brain cells) and synaptic plasticity (the brain's ability to form and strengthen connections).

Vitamin D is also a powerful anti-inflammatory agent. Chronic low-grade neuroinflammation is increasingly recognized as a major contributor to cognitive decline and neurodegenerative diseases. By suppressing pro-inflammatory cytokines and modulating immune cells in the brain, vitamin D can help reduce this harmful inflammation. Therefore, when an individual with a preexisting vitamin D deficiency begins taking Prevagen or any other supplement with vitamin D, the included 2,000 IU of vitamin D3 could be a step in the right direction to correct this deficiency. This repletion of vitamin D could then lead to a reduction in neuroinflammation and a boost in other beneficial brain processes, resulting in improved cognitive function and memory.

In this scenario, the perceived benefits might be more attributable to the fundamental impact of resolving a common vitamin D deficiency rather than the unique properties of apoaequorin or any other listed substance. This is not to imply that the "main ingredient" is ineffective—the science is still out on that. However, the science is in on vitamin D with regard to neuroinflammation, synaptic plasticity, and neurogenesis.

Given these established anti-inflammatory actions, it is plausible that if a person is vitamin D deficient, supplementing with vitamin D could lead to a reduction in neuroinflammation, thereby improving cognitive outcomes.

Future research designs assessing Prevagen's efficacy should meticulously control for baseline vitamin D status and changes in vitamin D levels throughout the study period to disentangle the effects of its individual components. Without such rigorous controls, the observed cognitive improvements could easily be misinterpreted as solely attributable to apoaequorin, when in fact, the resolution of a prevalent and impactful nutritional deficiency could be a major driver. This observation relates to the previous discussion of vitamin D as an uncontrolled factor in drug research. Without knowing the vitamin D status of the subjects, and if the drug operates in the arena where vitamin D does, which is most, then it is impossible to discern whether any observed effect is due to the drug of interest, preexisting vitamin D status, or an interaction of the two. Regardless, that people find these cognitive-function-enhancing drugs useful enough to buy them is testament to their effectiveness. It might be fruitful to explore synergistic effects of high-dose vitamin D with purported nootropic agents like apoaequorin on cognitive function.

Brain supplements are not the only products that include vitamin D without explaining the rationale for its inclusion. Joint support, prostate support, sleep aids, and muscle strength aids include vitamin D in their formulations as well. In a chronically vitamin D–deficient population, adding vitamin D to just about any product may result in a generalized benefit that might effect many systems in addition to the one identified on the label.

## INTERNAL SUNSCREENS

Achieving optimal health necessitates a balanced and sensible approach to sun exposure. The most effective strategy involves regular, brief periods of direct sun exposure to significant portions of your skin, meticulously avoiding sunburn. For prolonged outdoor activities, protective clothing is paramount. Further enhancing your skin's resilience against sun damage can be achieved through a diet rich in antioxidant-dense fruits and vegetables, or by incorporating astaxanthin supplementation.[35, 36, 37] When topical sun protection is necessary, prioritize formulations containing non-nanometer-sized zinc oxide or titanium dioxide, with zinc oxide being the superior choice due to its stability and comprehensive UVA protection.

## PRIORITIZING VITAMIN D PRODUCTION AND SENSIBLE SUN PRACTICES

To ensure adequate vitamin D synthesis while safeguarding your skin, adhere to these essential guidelines:

- Optimize Vitamin D First: Always allow your skin to produce vitamin D before applying sunscreen. Expose at least 40 percent of your body to direct sunlight for short durations daily. Optimal vitamin D levels are important for reducing the risk of numerous internal cancers and even melanoma.
- Mind the Pink: Limit sun exposure to the point where your skin develops only the very lightest shade of pink. Protect your face with a safe sunscreen or a hat, as facial skin is more delicate and prone to sun damage and premature aging. As your skin tans, you'll have more protection.
- Cover Up for Extended Exposure: For longer periods outdoors, utilize clothing or a hat or seek natural shade. An umbrella can also provide effective shade. Topical sunscreen can be applied after you have maximized your daily vitamin D production, though physical barriers like clothing remain the safest method to prevent sunburn and skin damage.

- Consider Internal Sun Protection: Explore the benefits of "internal sunscreens" such as astaxanthin (described below). Consistent daily supplementation for several weeks is typically required to achieve adequate tissue saturation for protective effects. Astaxanthin can also be found in some topical applications.
- Nourish Your Skin from Within: A diet rich in natural antioxidants is a highly effective strategy for preventing sun damage. Fresh, raw, and unprocessed foods provide the essential nutrients, which are critical for defense against sunburn. Vegetables, in particular, supply potent antioxidants that combat free radicals generated by sun exposure, thereby preventing burns and reducing cancer risk.[38]

## ASTAXANTHIN: A POTENT INTERNAL AND TOPICAL PHOTOPROTECTANT

Astaxanthin, a powerful carotenoid pigment, is a significant advancement in photoprotection. Unlike topical sunscreens that primarily block or reflect UV radiation on the skin's surface, internal sunscreens like astaxanthin work from within to bolster the skin's natural defenses.[39]

When ingested, astaxanthin is absorbed into the bloodstream and distributed to various tissues, including the skin. Its protective effects stem from its exceptional antioxidant and anti-inflammatory properties. It is considerably more potent than other well-known antioxidants such as beta-carotene, lycopene, and vitamin E.[40]

- **Antioxidant Powerhouse:** UV radiation generates reactive oxygen species (ROS), or free radicals, which cause oxidative stress and damage to skin cells, DNA, and collagen. Astaxanthin's unique molecular structure allows it to effectively neutralize these free radicals, reducing oxidative damage.[41]
- **Anti-inflammatory Action:** Sunburn is an inflammatory response. Astaxanthin modulates inflammatory pathways, reducing the redness, swelling, and pain associated with sunburn, thereby preventing long-term damage.[42]
- **DNA Protection:** By mitigating oxidative stress, astaxanthin indirectly protects cellular DNA from UV-induced mutations, which are a primary cause of skin aging and cancer.[43]
- **Enhanced Barrier Function:** Research suggests astaxanthin may improve the skin's barrier function, making it more resilient to environmental stressors, including UV radiation.
- **Achieving Protective Benefits:** Consistent, long-term daily supplementation of astaxanthin for several weeks is necessary for it

to accumulate in the skin layers and provide protective benefits. This builds an internal reserve of protection.[44]

- **Role in Topical Sunscreens:** Astaxanthin is also increasingly incorporated into topical sunscreens and skincare products. When applied topically, it delivers potent antioxidant and anti-inflammatory properties directly to the skin, enhancing the sunscreen's ability to neutralize free radicals and calm sun-stressed skin. This creates a synergistic effect with traditional UV filters, offering a more comprehensive defense against sun damage and potentially enhancing the stability of other ingredients.

### NO INTERFERENCE WITH VITAMIN D SYNTHESIS

Importantly, astaxanthin does not negatively affect or inhibit vitamin D synthesis in the skin. Vitamin D synthesis is triggered by UVB radiation converting 7-dehydrocholesterol into vitamin D3. Astaxanthin's mechanism of action involves mitigating the damage caused by UV radiation after it has penetrated the skin, primarily by neutralizing free radicals and reducing inflammation. It does not create a physical or chemical barrier that prevents UVB rays from initiating the vitamin D synthesis pathway. Therefore, you can confidently incorporate astaxanthin into your regimen without compromising your body's natural ability to synthesize vitamin D from sun exposure.[45]

## BEYOND ASTAXANTHIN: OTHER INTERNAL PHOTOPROTECTANTS

Several other compounds act as "internal sunscreens" or photoprotectants, working through antioxidant, anti-inflammatory, and DNA-protective properties to offer additional layers of defense against UV radiation.

- **Polypodium Leucotomos Extract (PLE):** Derived from a tropical fern, PLE is one of the most extensively studied oral photoprotectants. It works through potent antioxidant and anti-inflammatory activity, immunomodulatory effects, and DNA protection. Studies show it can increase the minimal erythema dose (MED), reduce sunburn severity, decrease hyperpigmentation, and may prevent certain skin cancers and polymorphous light eruption.[46]
- **Nicotinamide (Vitamin B3 / Niacinamide):** This form of vitamin B3 enhances DNA repair pathways, boosts the skin's immune response, reduces inflammation, and improves skin barrier function. Research indicates that oral nicotinamide can significantly reduce the incidence of nonmelanoma skin cancers (basal cell carcinoma and squamous cell carcinoma) and actinic keratoses in high-risk individuals.[47]

- **Lycopene:** An abundant red carotenoid in tomatoes and other red fruits, lycopene is a powerful antioxidant that effectively quenches singlet oxygen, a damaging free radical generated by UV exposure. Regular consumption can increase the skin's resistance to UV-induced erythema.[48]
- **Beta-Carotene:** An orange carotenoid found in carrots and other orange/yellow vegetables, beta-carotene is a precursor to vitamin A and an antioxidant. It accumulates in the skin, helping to neutralize free radicals. Long-term supplementation can increase the skin's tolerance to UV exposure, requiring a higher UV dose to cause sunburn.[49]
- **Vitamins C and E:** These powerful antioxidants work synergistically. Vitamin C is water-soluble, neutralizing free radicals in aqueous parts of cells, while vitamin E is fat-soluble, protecting cell membranes. Combined oral supplementation can reduce UV-induced oxidative stress, inflammation, and cellular damage, supporting the skin's natural defenses.[50]
- **Green Tea Extract (EGCG):** Derived from green tea leaves, epigallocatechin gallate (EGCG) is a potent antioxidant with anti-inflammatory and anticarcinogenic properties. It protects DNA, reduces immune suppression, and inhibits pathways involved in skin cancer development. Oral supplementation has shown promise in reducing markers of UV-induced skin damage and inflammation.[51]

**Important Considerations for All Internal Sunscreens:** It is important to understand that internal supplements are not a replacement for mineral-based topical sunscreen, protective clothing, shade, and common sense. They are adjuvant therapies that work with traditional methods to provide an enhanced level of protection. Most internal sunscreens require consistent daily supplementation for several weeks to months to achieve sufficient tissue saturation and measurable benefits. Always choose reputable brands and consult with a health-care professional before starting any new supplement regimen.

## DOES SERUM VITAMIN D STATUS AFFECT MELANIN IN SKIN?

This is an interesting question. Recall the vitamin D intelligence of the lizard. Specifically, time spent in the sun was directly related to vitamin D status.[52] If a lizard was injected with vitamin D it spent less time in the sun. It was as if the lizard had an internal vitamin D meter that influenced how much time it would spend exposing itself to risk in search of vital vitamin D.

We currently don't have an analogous behavior in the human to measure but perhaps melanin content in skin is related. We know that melanin content upregulates in response to UV radiation causing tanning. In a similar manner, does serum vitamin D level in humans affect melanin content in skin in a sort of negative feedback loop? That is, does chronically high (optimal) levels of vitamin D darken the skin?

I say yes because of my personal experience with chronic use of high-dose (8,000–10,000 IU) vitamin D3 over more than twenty years. As a fair-skinned, freckled Caucasian of Irish descent, my skin tone has drastically darkened during this time period. This informal observation was validated when I was recently stopped on my Jet Ski for speeding in a manatee zone (I wasn't, unlike the police officer who sped over in the three-outboard engine speedboat). I did not have any identification on me, and the officer wrote me an official warning. When I got home, I read the citation and he had listed my race as "H" for Hispanic. So the officer thought my complexion was that of a Hispanic.

There is some evidence that vitamin D status can influence melanocyte biology but the evidence is nuanced and complex. Vitamin D has been shown to increase tyrosinase, an enzyme responsible for melanin synthesis.[53] Some cell studies report increased melanocyte survival and proliferation after vitamin D exposure.[54] Perhaps the most relevant research involves topical vitamin D treatments like calcipotriol can facilitate repigmentation of the skin when used with light therapy in vitiligo.[55] Interesting that my wife had vitiligo to her upper arm and it disappeared after her taking high-dose vitamin D for her UC, as mentioned earlier. We didn't track the progress, so we don't know the time course, we just noticed it wasn't there one day.

So, can vitamin D status affect skin color? The science is still out on that. Most of the studies used short-term designs that looked for a more-or-less immediate effect. However my answer is yes, vitamin D does affect skin color but I think the effect is obtained with chronic, long-term use of high-dose vitamin D3. In my case and my wife's, we are in the chronic, high-dose category of vitamin D use. As an aside, I stay in the Florida sun for hours, I don't use any sunscreen, and I don't burn.

With all that sun exposure, I do have regular dermatological skin checks. If I get a basal or squamous cell lesion I treat it topically with either fenbendazole or ivermectin, both safe, over-the-counter antiparasitic medicines.[56] The lesion dries up and flakes off and new skin grows back in about six weeks. No more painful, expensive, disfiguring surgeries for me.

## SUNLIGHT AND VITAMIN D RESEARCH IS IN ITS INFANCY

After reading through these pages you might get the impression that we know just about all there is to know about the effects of sunlight and vitamin D on our health and wellness. In my opinion, we only know the tip of the iceberg, and the greatest discoveries await us. How can I say this? As an example, the near infrared light study on mitochondrial function described in chapter 21, which was the first of its kind, was just published in 2025. NIR light affects visual acuity behavior; what else does it affect? What other frequencies of light are bioreactive? We are at the frontier of an entire new area of study: photobiology or photobiomodulation.

There is the perception among some that science seems to have all the answers to the many problems that plague us. This perception is far from reality. Take vitamin D science, for example. You just read an entire book on all things vitamin D. What have you learned? Hopefully, the main takeaway message is that vitamin D is essential for good health and that we've learned this lesson the hard way by its removal from our lives, and the result is the current epidemic of chronic disease caused by chronic vitamin D starvation. But what do we really know about vitamin D? We know it is essential for the proper function of the immune system. We know it is essential for bone, brain and muscle health. We know some of the mechanisms of action as detailed earlier. But we don't know basic things like what is the optimal serum level of vitamin D and correspondingly how much should we be taking? These glaring gaps in knowledge are due in large part to the corruption of vitamin D science by Big Pharma. Vitamin D deficiency is their golden goose and they have no appetite to give up its secrets.

Another example regarding the primitive state of research into all things vitamin D is our skin. You'd think we would know all there is to know about our skin. It's right there for us to see, no surprises, right? Wrong. Just in 2018 it was discovered that the skin possessed an intricate network of fluid-filled channels and grooves throughout the whole body subsequently named the interstitium.[57] Another entire organ, the largest organ in our body, embedded right under our skin, and it went undiscovered until 2018?[58] The mysteries of the skin don't end it its anatomy, in addition to vitamin D and antimicrobial peptides, the skin produces melatonin, serotonin, endorphins, endocannabinoids, cortisol, oxytocin, leptin, nitric oxide, cis-urocanic acid, itaconate, lumisterol, tachysterol, and a dozen other vitamin D–like compounds that don't even have names yet.[59, 60] The anatomy and physiology of the skin when struck by sunlight, which we should know like the back of our hand, is, relatively speaking, virtually unexplored territory.

## GLASS AND VITAMIN D

No, the skin cannot synthesize vitamin D through glass windows. This is a common misconception. The synthesis of vitamin D in the skin is primarily triggered by ultraviolet B (UVB) radiation from the sun. Standard window glass, even clear glass, effectively blocks almost all UVB radiation.[61] While it allows UVA rays to pass through, UVA rays do not initiate vitamin D synthesis. UVA rays, which do penetrate glass, are primarily responsible for skin aging and can contribute to skin cancer, but they do not help your body produce vitamin D.[62] Therefore, while you might feel the warmth of the sun through a window, and even get a tan from the UVA rays, your body will not produce vitamin D.[63] To synthesize vitamin D, you need direct exposure of your skin to sunlight outdoors.

## WHY DOESN'T THE NFL, OR ANY MAJOR SPORTS LEAGUE, ENDORSE VITAMIN D SUPPLEMENTATION TO REDUCE INJURIES AND CONCUSSIONS?

As we discussed previously, the adverse effects of a traumatic brain injury like a concussion are exacerbated by vitamin D deficiency. This is because the brain's response to the injury is basically an immune response that is dysfunctional and disordered in the vitamin D–deficient brain. A simple, inexpensive, and safe preventative measure would be to systematically raise players' vitamin D levels to optimal ranges. Furthermore, vitamin D–replete football players are better athletes.[64] So if there is such an attractive, low-cost, high-potential-reward treatment, why doesn't the NFL encourage their players to take more vitamin D?

The NFL captures a significant share of pharmaceutical advertising dollars, with the pharma industry heavily investing in advertising during NFL broadcasts. The NFL is pharma's favorite hunting ground, with 8.7 percent of the category's spend, or $442.8 million, finding its way into the coffers of the league's TV partners. By way of comparison, the next-biggest beneficiary of all those drug dollars is TV's top-rated evening news program; *ABC World News Tonight* mopped up 3.2 percent of pharma's national spend, for a haul of some $162.9 million.[65]

Major pharmaceutical companies like Pfizer generated notably large shares of ad impressions during NFL games, reflecting the league's importance as a prime advertising platform for Big Pharma.[66]

This strong financial relationship creates a market environment where pharmaceutical companies prioritize promoting costly, patent-protected medications for chronic illnesses, such as autoimmune disease, diabetes, and weight management, which dominate NFL ad placements. The industry heavily invests in this exposure to sustain and grow demand for their drugs, and this revenue stream is a vested interest tied to the league's media exposure.[67]

If the NFL, or any other major sports league for that matter, were to adopt or promote widespread vitamin D supplementation policies for concussion or general athlete health, and if such policies broadly translated to general population health improvements, it could potentially reduce the prevalence and severity of chronic diseases dependent on pharmaceutical treatments. This in turn might lead to diminished demand for medications, thereby threatening pharmaceutical industry profits.

Given this, the NFL's vested interests in lucrative pharma advertising revenue could present a reluctance or conflict-of-interest barrier to endorsing simple, low-cost interventions like vitamin D supplementation that might disrupt the status quo of chronic illness management reliant on patented drugs.

In short, the combination of massive pharmaceutical ad expenditures during NFL broadcasts and the business incentive to maintain high medication use likely acts as a commercially influenced factor that could inhibit proactive adoption or promotion of vitamin D supplementation as a concussion or health intervention by the NFL or associated stakeholders. However, sports leagues like the NFL should realize that the concussion issue will never be solved by better helmets and that concussions are an existential threat to the sport of football itself. Parents are deciding that the head injury risks are too great and fewer children are playing football.[68] A simple, inexpensive, effective and rational policy of vitamin D repletion among NFL athletes would make for a better and safer game, and may also assuage some parents' concerns regarding the brain safety of their children when playing tackle football.

While waiting for such institutional endorsement, which may or may not come, all is not lost. Players, coaches, and fans can enjoy the sun and supplement with vitamin D without the endorsement of any major sports league.

## WHAT IS THE CURRENT STATE OF THE RESEARCH ON VITAMIN D?

Not good. There has been a notable decline in publication rates and NIH funding for vitamin D research in the United states. Vitamin D–related research publications rose steadily from 1985 to 2000, surged from 2008 to 2021, peaked at 6,019 in 2021, and then drastically declined. NIH funding for vitamin D research peaked at $52.4 million in 2013 but decreased to $10.5 million by 2024.[69] Which is a non sequitur considering the ubiquity of vitamin D receptors on most cells and involvement of vitamin D in virtually all aspects of life from conception to old age.

Despite the wealth of information presented in this book, the state of the knowledge regarding vitamin D and health is really in its beginning stages. This book has basically shown the effects of long-term vitamin D deficiency on just about every physiological system in the body. The solution is simply to get more vitamin D in the form of sensible sun exposure and necessary supplementation. However, significant gaps remain in our understanding of vitamin D, including—but not limited to—its optimal levels and dosages, testing strategies, cofactors, and clinical applications.[70, 71] Emerging research on vitamin D's role in the gut microbiome, cancer, autoimmune disorders, and cardiovascular disease highlights ongoing uncertainties and the evolving nature of the field.[72] The most exciting phase of vitamin D research is ahead in decoding its role in health, disease, and longevity. It is my belief that all things vitamin D will be the foundation of a holistic, preventative, and health-optimization focus in medicine that is imminent.

As an example of what lies ahead is an exciting paper by Zheng et al. on synergistic effects between immune checkpoint inhibitors (ICI) and vitamin D in lung cancer.[73] People who have adequate serum vitamin D respond better to ICI therapy. There are some very intriguing findings regarding the role of vitamin D in the progression of some lung cancers. Specifically, as the cancer progresses it appears to "defend" itself from vitamin D by increasing the amount of the enzyme (CYP24A1) that degrades calcitriol, the active form of vitamin D. Zheng et al. state that by reducing immune suppression and boosting cytotoxic T cell activity, vitamin D may make tumors more sensitive to ICI therapy, which is especially important for patients who show limited response to ICIs alone. Based on what we've covered in this book, it will not be long until these researchers realize that the star in the synergistic relationship is not the ICI but vitamin D, and proceed accordingly.

After having read through thousands of papers on vitamin D over the last thirty years, I can see that US scientists are falling behind in vitamin D research. This is not surprising, given the NIH funding data presented earlier. The cutting-edge research on vitamin D like the Zheng et al. paper, is not being conducted in the United States. We have to ask ourselves a disturbing question: Is the decline in funding and interest in the United States in vitamin D research organic, or is it orchestrated by nefarious interests?

The health revolution that is just around the corner is very likely to proceed with fewer obstacles because, after decades and decades of doing the bidding of interests other than the health interests of the American people, we finally have leadership in Health and Human Services, FDA, NIH, NIMH and CDC that will make a difference. When almost 80 percent of your population has a chronic illness, the current policies have failed miserably and there must be a radical change of course. That change of course includes simple, safe, inexpensive (mostly free) sensible sun exposure and vitamin D supplementation when necessary. The coming health renaissance will pay huge dividends not only in enhancing the well-being and comfort of vitamin D–starved people but also in drastically reducing the cost to the American taxpayer for these preventable chronic diseases currently estimated by HHS Secretary Kennedy at $4 trillion.[74] The return on investment of a sensible sun and vitamin D public health policy could be among the most profound in human history. What is also exciting is that we won't have to wait years and years to see positive results. Public health policies that encourage sensible sun exposure and guided vitamin D supplementation will pay almost immediate health benefits. Providing a starving body with what is needs will restore immune system balance and start us on the road to recovery.

Obviously, sunlight and vitamin D are kryptonite to Big Pharma profits. Casting the sun as a villain to our health and later finding that advice created the health crises of today may not have been the original intent. However, removing the sun from our lives, along with its vitamin D, and not compensating for that loss is inexcusable. Furthermore, the systematic error in RDA guidance repeated by health authorities (IOM, Institute of Medicine, Endocrine Society) to keep the population vitamin D deficient is very troubling. Also, the studies designed to fail to find a beneficial health effect of vitamin D, epitomized by the study that found no beneficial effect of vitamin D on bone health, are not medical science, they are political science. It is interesting that some of the same scientists performing the studies designed to fail are also members of the IOM.[75] Last but not least is the latest advice that people do not need to know their vitamin D status, so don't even bother. This advice is a dog whistle to doctors and, more directly, to health insurance companies to not cover the cost of vitamin D tests. If we are searching for reasons why eight out of ten Americans have a chronic illness, the war against the sun is a major reason.

As we've detailed earlier, Big Pharma has built a large share of its business on treating the symptoms of chronic vitamin D deficiency. The heyday of the effects of a five-decade-long policy of sun avoidance and vitamin D starvation is now as evidenced by eight out of ten of us with a chronic illness. An interesting study found that only 3 percent of their sample was supplementing with at least 4,000 IU vitamin D3 per day.[76] My guess is that 3 percent is strongly represented in the 20 percent of Americans that do not have a chronic disease. Restoration of population-wide vitamin D levels to optimal ranges will ameliorate many of these conditions and prevent future instances in others not yet afflicted. Restoring vitamin D levels to optimal ranges is projected to dramatically increase life expectancy.[77] It is truly a game changer.

Side-effect-ridden biologic drugs are primitive knockoffs of vitamin D and will soon take their rightful place in the back of the medicine cabinet. However, all is not lost for Big Pharma. One suggestion is that instead of developing drugs that you need, please develop drugs that the people need. As mentioned earlier, vitamin D science is in its infancy, and the first-mover advantage will be great. Developing interventions that work and synergize with vitamin D will provide immediate benefit. Developing interventions that extend and improve the biologic actions of vitamin D is a vast and open frontier. Exploring the links between vitamin D and longevity offers science fiction–like possibilities that are readily actionable.

Rather than focusing on the development of interventions to treat conditions in sick people (smaller market), focus on creating interventions that make healthy people healthier by optimizing their well-being and longevity (vast market). Reread what Benjamin Franklin said on this topic, "An ounce of prevention is *worth* more than a pound of cure." Worth more to the individual and also worth more to the business that can facilitate such prevention and enhance worth. Rather than the fostering and perpetuation of disease and treating the results, the prevention of those diseases and optimization of the human condition is a much nobler pursuit.

# NOTES

## Preface

1 Watson, K. B., Wiltz, J. L., Nhim, K., Kaufmann, R. B., Thomas, C. W., & Greenlund, K. J. (2025). Trends in Multiple Chronic Conditions Among US Adults, by Life Stage, Behavioral Risk Factor Surveillance System, 2013–2023. *Prev Chronic Disease* 22, 240539. dx.doi.org/10.5888/pcd22.240539.

## Chapter 1

1 D'Altroy, T. N. (2014). *The Incas* (2nd ed.). Wiley-Blackwell. doi.org/10.1002/9781118610582.

2 Te Velde, H. (1992). The original KERESET. In U. Luft (Ed.), *The Intellectual Heritage of Egypt: Studies Presented to László Kákosy by Friends and Colleagues on the Occasion of His 60th Birthday* (pp. 565–70). Charta.

3 Robinson, J. K. (2005). Sun exposure, sun protection, and vitamin D. *JAMA* 294(12), 1541–43. doi.org/10.1001/jama.294.12.1541.

4 Holick, M. F. (2007). Vitamin D deficiency. *New England Journal of Medicine* 357(3), 266–281. doi.org/10.1056/NEJMra070553.

5 Pike, J. W., & Meyer, M. B. (2010). The vitamin D receptor: New paradigms for the regulation of gene expression by 1,25-dihydroxyvitamin D3. *Endocrinology and Metabolism Clinics of North America* 39(2), 255–69. doi.org/10.1016/j.ecl.2010.02.007.

6 Bidanta, S., Börner, K., Herr II, B.W. et al. Functional tissue units in the Human Reference Atlas. *Nature Communications* 16, 1526 (2025). doi.org/10.1038/s41467-024-54591-6.

7 DeLuca H. F. (2004). Overview of general physiologic features and functions of vitamin D. *The American Journal of Clinical Nutrition* 80(6 Suppl), 1689S–96S. doi.org/10.1093/ajcn/80.6.1689S.

8 van Tienhoven, X. A., Ruiz de Chávez-Gascón, J., Cano-Herrera, G., et al. (2025). Vitamin D in reproductive health disorders: A narrative review focusing on infertility, endometriosis, and polycystic ovarian syndrome. *International Journal of Molecular Sciences* 26(5), 2256. doi.org/10.3390/ijms26052256.

9 Prietl, B., Treiber, G., Pieber, T. R., & Amrein, K. (2013). Vitamin D and immune function. *Nutrients* 5(7), 2502–21. doi.org/10.3390/nu5072502.

10 Dallavalasa, S., Tulimilli, S. V., Bettada, V. G., et al. (2024). Vitamin D in cancer prevention and treatment: A review of epidemiological, preclinical, and cellular studies. *Cancers* 16(18), 3211. doi.org/10.3390/cancers1618321.

11 Norman, P. E., & Powell, J. T. (2014). Vitamin D and cardiovascular disease. *Circulation Research* 114(2), 379–93. doi.org/10.1161/CIRCRESAHA.113.301241.

12 Golan, D., Staun-Ram, E., Glass-Marmor, L., Lavi, I., Rozenberg, O., Dishon, S., Barak, M., Ish-Shalom, S., & Miller, A. (2013). The influence of vitamin D supplementation on melatonin status in patients with multiple sclerosis. *Brain, Behavior, and Immunity* 32, 180–85. doi.org/10.1016/j.bbi.2013.04.010.

13 Annweiler, C., Schott, A. M., Berrut, G., Fantino, B., & Beauchet, O. (2010). Vitamin D and ageing: Neurological issues. *Neuropsychobiology* 62(3), 139–50. doi.org/10.1159/000318570.

14 Annweiler, C., Fantino, B., Parot-Schinkel, E., Thiery, S., Gautier, J., & Beauchet, O. (2012). Alzheimer's disease—input of vitamin D. *Fortschritte der Neurologie-Psychiatrie* 80(4), 213–222. doi.org/10.1055/s-0031-1299406.

15 Ceglia, L., & Harris, S. S. (2013). Vitamin D and its role in skeletal muscle. *Calcified Tissue International* 92(2), 151–62. doi.org/10.1007/s00223-012-9645-y.

16 Bischoff-Ferrari, H. A., Dawson-Hughes, B., Willett, W. C., Staehelin, H. B., Bazemore, M. G., Zee, R. Y., & Wong, J. B. (2004). Effect of vitamin D on falls: A meta-analysis. *JAMA* 291(16), 1999–2006. doi.org/10.1001/jama.291.16.1999.

17 Bouillon, R., Marcocci, C., Carmeliet, G., et al. (2019). Skeletal and extraskeletal actions of vitamin D: Current evidence and outstanding questions. *Endocrine Reviews* 40(4), 1109–51. doi.org/10.1210/er.2018-00126.

18 Jablonski, N. G., & Chaplin, G. (2010). Human skin pigmentation as an adaptation to UV radiation. *Proceedings of the National Academy of Sciences* 107 (Supplement 2), 8962–68. doi.org/10.1073/pnas.0914628107.

19 Jablonski, N. G., & Chaplin, G. (2000). The evolution of human skin coloration. *Journal of Human Evolution 39*(1), 57–106. doi.org/10.1006/jhev.2000.0403.

20 Holick, M. F. (2004). Sunlight and vitamin D for bone health and prevention of autoimmune diseases, cancers, and cardiovascular disease. *The American Journal of Clinical Nutrition 80*(6 Suppl), 1678S–1688S. doi.org/10.1093/ajcn/80.6.1678S.

21 American Academy of Dermatology. (n.d.). Sunscreen FAQs. Retrieved September 3, 2025, from aad.org/media/stats-sunscreen.

22 Robinson, J. K. (2005). Sun exposure, sun protection, and vitamin D. *JAMA* 294(12), 1541–43. doi.org/10.1001/jama.294.12.1541.

23 Te Velde, H. (1992). The original KERESET. In U. Luft (Ed.), *The Intellectual Heritage of Egypt: Studies Presented to László Kákosy by Friends and Colleagues on the Occasion of His 60th Birthday* (pp. 565–70). Charta.

24 D'Altroy, T. N. (2014). *The Incas* (2nd ed.). Wiley-Blackwell. doi.org/10.1002/9781118610582.

25 Atsma, A. J. (n.d.). Helios. *Theoi Project*. Retrieved from theoi.com/Titan/Helios.html.

26 Burkert, W. (1985). *Greek Religion*. Harvard University Press.

27 Halsberghe, G. H. (1972). *The Cult of Sol Invictus*. Brill.

28 Daniell, M. D., & Hill, J. S. (1991). A history of photodynamic therapy. *The Australian and New Zealand Journal of Surgery* 61(5), 340–48. doi.org/10.1111/j.1445-2197.1991.tb00230.x.

29 Pliny the Elder. (77–79 C.E.). *Natural history* (H. Rackham, Trans.).

30 Hobday, R. A. (1999). *The Healing Sun: Sunlight and Health in the 21st Century*. Findhorn Press.

31 Carter, R. (2003). Sunlight and health: The positive and negative effects of the sun on human health (Report OR 23/2003). Norwegian Institute for Air Research.

32 Greenhalgh, I., & Butler, A. R. (2017). Sanatoria revisited: Sunlight and health. *The Journal of the Royal College of Physicians of Edinburgh* 47(3), 276–80. doi.org/10.4997/JRCPE.2017.314.

33 Rollier, A. (1923). *Heliotherapy*. Oxford University Press.

34 Chisholm, H. (Ed.). (1922). Treloar, Sir William Purdie. In *The Encyclopædia Britannica* (12th ed., Vol. 32). The Encyclopædia Britannica Company, Ltd.

35 Huldschinsky, K. (1919). Heilung von Rachitis durch künstliche Höhensonne [Cure of rickets by artificial sunlight]. *Deutsche Medizinische Wochenschrift* 45(26), 712–13. doi.org/10.1055/s-0028-1139960.

36 Chick, H., Dalyell, E. J., Hume, E. M., Mackay, H. M. M., Smith, H. H., & Wimberger, H. (1922). The aetiology of rickets in infants: Prophylactic and curative observations at the Vienna University Kinderklinik. *The Lancet* 200(5157), 7–11. doi.org/10.1016/S0140-6736(01)20839-9.

37 Hobday, R. (2007). *The Light Revolution: Health, Architecture and the Sun*. Findhorn Press.

38 Schatz, A., Bugie, E., & Waksman, S. A. (1944). Streptomycin, a substance exhibiting antibiotic activity against gram-positive and gram-negative bacteria. *Experimental Biology and Medicine* 55(1), 66–69. doi.org/10.3181/00379727-55-14461.

39 Holick, M. F. (2006). Resurrection of vitamin D deficiency and rickets. *The Journal of Clinical Investigation* 116(8), 2062–72. doi.org/10.1172/JCI29449.

40 National Aeronautics and Space Administration. (n.d.). Sun-Earth connection. *NASA Science*. Retrieved from science.nasa.gov/sun-earth-connection/.

41 Cajochen, C. (2007). Alerting effects of light. *Sleep Medicine Reviews* 11(6), 453–64. doi.org/10.1016/j.smrv.2007.07.009.

42 Mead, M. N. (2008). Benefits of sunlight: A bright spot for human health. *Environmental Health Perspectives* 116(4), A160–A167. doi.org/10.1289/ehp.116-a160.

43 Robinson, J. K. (2005). Sun exposure, sun protection, and vitamin D. *JAMA* 294(12), 1541–43. doi .org/10.1001/jama.294.12.1541.

44 American Academy of Dermatology. (n.d.). Sunscreen FAQs. Retrieved September 3, 2025, from aad.org/media/stats-sunscreen.

45 Diffey, B. L. (2009). The historical development of sunscreens. *Sunscreens: Development, evaluation, and regulatory aspects.* In N. J. Lowe, N. A. Shaath, & M. A. Pathak (Eds.), (pp. 1–19). CRC Press.

46 Matsumura, Y., & Ananthaswamy, H. N. (2004). Toxic effects of ultraviolet radiation on the skin. *Toxicology and Applied Pharmacology* 195(3), 298–308. doi.org/10.1016/j.taap.2003.08.019.

47 Holick, M. F. (2007). Vitamin D deficiency. *New England Journal of Medicine* 357(3), 266–81. doi. org/10.1056/NEJMra070553.

48 Annweiler, C., Schott, A. M., Berrut, G., Fantino, B., & Beauchet, O. (2010). Vitamin D and ageing: Neurological issues. *Neuropsychobiology* 62(3), 139–50. doi.org/10.1159/000318570.

49 Aranow, C. (2011). Vitamin D and the immune system. *Journal of Investigative Medicine* 59(6), 881–86. doi.org/10.2310/JIM.0b013e31821b8755.

50 Bischoff-Ferrari, H. A., Dawson-Hughes, B., Willett, W. C., Staehelin, H. B., Bazemore, M. G., Zee, R. Y., & Wong, J. B. (2004). Effect of vitamin D on falls: A meta-analysis. *JAMA* 291(16), 1999–2006. doi.org/10.1001/jama.291.16.1999.

51 Garland, C. F., Garland, F. C., Gorham, E. D., Lipkin, M., Newmark, H., Mohr, S. B., & Holick, M. F. (2006). The role of vitamin D in cancer prevention. *American Journal of Public Health* 96(2), 252–61. doi.org/10.2105/AJPH.2004.045260.

52 Wang, T. J., Pencina, M. J., Booth, S. L., Jacques, P. F., Ingelsson, E., Lanier, K., ... & Vasan, R. S. (2008). Vitamin D deficiency and risk of cardiovascular disease. *Circulation* 117(4), 503–11. doi. org/10.1161/CIRCULATIONAHA.107.706127.

53 American Cancer Society. (2023). Key statistics for melanoma skin cancer. Retrieved September 3, 2025, from cancer.org/cancer/types/melanoma-skin-cancer/about/key-statistics.html.

54 Berwick, M., Armstrong, B. K., Ben-Porat, L., Fine, J., Kricker, A., Eberle, C., & Barnhill, R. (2005). Sun exposure and mortality from melanoma. *Journal of the National Cancer Institute* 97(3), 195–99. doi.org/10.1093/jnci/dji019.

55 Chang, Y. M., Newton-Bishop, J. A., Bishop, D. T., et al. (2010). A pooled analysis of melanocytic nevus phenotype and the risk of cutaneous melanoma at different latitudes. *International Journal of Cancer* 124(2), 420–28. doi.org/10.1002/ijc.23869.

56 Albreski, D., & Sloan, S. B. (2009). Melanoma of the feet: Misdiagnosed and misunderstood. *Clinics in Dermatology* 27(6), 556–63. doi.org/10.1016/j.clindermatol.2008.09.014.

57 Gandini, S., Sera, F., Cattaruzza, M. S., Pasquini, P., Picconi, O., Boyle, P., & Melchi, C. F. (2005). Meta-analysis of risk factors for cutaneous melanoma: II. Sun exposure. *European Journal of Cancer* 41(1), 45–60. doi.org/10.1016/j.ejca.2004.10.016.

58 Autier, P., Boniol, M., Pizot, C., & Mullie, P. (2014). Vitamin D status and ill health: A systematic review. *The Lancet Diabetes & Endocrinology* 2(1), 76–89. doi.org/10.1016/S2213-8587(13)70165-7.

59 Fang, S., Sui, D., Wang, Y., Liu, H., et al. (2016). Association of vitamin D levels with outcome in patients with melanoma after adjustment for C-reactive protein. *Journal of Clinical Oncology* 34(15), 1741–47. doi.org/10.1200/JCO.2015.64.1357.

60 Newton-Bishop, J. A., Beswick, S., Randerson-Moor, J., et al. (2009). Serum 25-hydroxyvitamin D3 levels are associated with Breslow thickness at presentation and survival from melanoma. *Journal of Clinical Oncology* 27(32), 5439–44. doi.org/10.1200/JCO.2009.22.6109.

61 Wimalawansa, S. J. (2023). Physiological basis for using vitamin D to improve health. *Biomedicines* 11(6), 1542. doi.org/10.3390/biomedicines11061542.

62 Antico, A., Tampoia, M., Tozzoli, R., & Bizzaro, N. (2012). Can supplementation with vitamin D reduce the risk or modify the course of autoimmune diseases? A systematic review of the literature. *Autoimmunity Reviews* 12(2), 127–36. doi.org/10.1016/j.autrev.2012.07.007.

63 Dankers, W., Colin, E. M., van Hamburg, J. P., & Lubberts, E. (2017). Vitamin D in autoimmunity: Molecular mechanisms and therapeutic potential. *Frontiers in Immunology* 7, 697. doi.org/10.3389 /fimmu.2016.00697.

64 Pilz, S., Tomaschitz, A., Marz, W., Drechsler, C., Ritz, E., Zittermann, A., . . . & Kienreich, K. (2011). Vitamin D, cardiovascular disease and mortality. *Clinical Endocrinology* 75(5), 575–84. doi.org/10.1111/j.1365-2265.2011.04129.x.

65 Garland, C. F., Garland, F. C., Gorham, E. D., Lipkin, M., Newmark, H., Mohr, S. B., & Holick, M. F. (2006). The role of vitamin D in cancer prevention. *American Journal of Public Health* 96(2), 252–61. doi.org/10.2105/AJPH.2004.045260.

66 Moukayed, M., & Grant, W. B. (2013). Molecular link between vitamin D and cancer prevention. *Nutrients* 5(10), 3993–4021. doi.org/10.3390/nu5103993.

67 Pittas, A. G., Lau, J., Hu, F. B., & Dawson-Hughes, B. (2007). The role of vitamin D and calcium in type 2 diabetes: A systematic review and meta-analysis. *The Journal of Clinical Endocrinology & Metabolism* 92(6), 2017–29. doi.org/10.1210/jc.2007-0298.

68 Annweiler, C., Fantino, B., Parot-Schinkel, E., Thiery, S., Gautier, J., & Beauchet, O. (2012). Alzheimer's disease—input of vitamin D. *Fortschritte der Neurologie-Psychiatrie 80*(4), 213–22. doi.org/10.1055/s-0031-1299406.

69 Bischoff-Ferrari, H. A., Dawson-Hughes, B., Willett, W. C., Staehelin, H. B., Bazemore, M. G., Zee, R. Y., & Wong, J. B. (2004). Effect of vitamin D on falls: A meta-analysis. *JAMA* 291(16), 1999–2006. doi.org/10.1001/jama.291.16.1999.

## Chapter 2

1 Whistler, D. (1645). *De Morbo Puerili Anglorum, Quo Vulgò Vocant The Rickets.* Lugduni Batavorum (Leiden): Ex Officina Wilhelmi Christiani.

2 Glisson, F. (1650). *De Rachitide Sive Morbo Puerili, Qui Vulgo The Rickets Dicitur.* London: Typis Du-Gardianis.

3 Rajakumar, K. (2003). Vitamin D, cod-liver oil, sunlight, and rickets: A historical perspective. *Pediatrics* 112(2), e132–e135. doi.org/10.1542/peds.112.2.e132.

4 Guy, R. A. (1923). The history of cod liver oil as a remedy. *American Journal of Diseases of Children* 26(2), 112–16. doi.org/10.1001/archpedi.1923.04120140003001.

5 Mellanby, E. (1919). An experimental investigation on rickets. *The Lancet* 193(5007), 407–12. doi.org/10.1016/S0140-6736(01)27328-3.

6 McCollum, E. V., Simmonds, N., Becker, J. E., & Shipley, P. G. (1922). Studies on experimental rickets. XXI. An experimental demonstration of the existence of a vitamin which promotes calcium deposition. *Journal of Biological Chemistry* 53(2), 293–312. doi.org/10.1016/S0021-9258(18)86111-9.

7 Huldschinsky, K. (1919). Heilung von Rachitis durch künstliche Höhensonne [Cure of rickets by artificial sunbaths]. *Deutsche Medizinische Wochenschrift* 45(26), 712–13. doi.org/10.1055/s-0028-1139414.

8 Hess, A. F., Rosenheim, O., & Webster, T. A. (1927). The antirachitic value of irradiated cholesterol and phytosterol: V. The non-saponifiable fraction from irradiated cholesterol. *Journal of Biological Chemistry* 73(1), 147–53. doi.org/10.1016/S0021-9258(18)84252-9.

9 Steenbock, H., & Black, A. (1925). Fat-soluble vitamins: XXIII. The induction of growth-promoting and calcifying properties in fats and their unsaponifiable constituents by exposure to light. *Journal of Biological Chemistry* 64, 263–98.

10 Hess, A. F. (1924). The antirachitic activation of foods and of cholesterol by ultraviolet irradiation. *Journal of the American Medical Association* 83(24), 1831–34. doi.org/10.1001/jama.1924.02660240013004.

11 Hess, A. F., Rosenheim, O., & Webster, T. A. (1927). The antirachitic value of irradiated cholesterol and phytosterol: V. The non-saponifiable fraction from irradiated cholesterol. *Journal of Biological Chemistry* 73(1), 147–53. doi.org/10.1016/S0021-9258(18)84252-9.

12 Rosenheim, O., & Webster, T. A. (1927). The parent substance of vitamin D. *The Lancet* 209(5402), 553. doi.org/10.1016/S0140-6736(01)17616-0.

13 Windaus, A., Schenck, F., & von Werder, F. (1936). Über das antirachitisch wirksame Bestrahlungsprodukt aus 7-Dehydro-cholesterin. *Hoppe-Seyler's Zeitschrift für physiologische Chemie* 241(1–3), 100–103. doi.org/10.1515/bchm2.1936.241.1-3.100.

14 Tripkovic, L., Lambert, H., Hart, K., Smith, C. P., Bucca, G., Penson, S., Chope, G., Hyppönen, E., Berry, J., Vieth, R., & Lanham-New, S. (2012). Comparison of vitamin D2 and vitamin D3

supplementation in raising serum 25-hydroxyvitamin D status: A systematic review and meta-analysis. *The American Journal of Clinical Nutrition* 95(6), 1357–64. doi.org/10.3945/ajcn.111.031070.

15 Holick, M. F., MacLaughlin, J. A., & Doppelt, S. H. (1981). Regulation of cutaneous previtamin D3 photosynthesis in man: Skin pigment is not an essential regulator. *Science* 211(4482), 590–93. doi .org/10.1126/science.6256799.

16 Deluca, H. F. (2014). History of the discovery of vitamin D and its active metabolites. *BoneKEy Reports* 3, 479. doi.org/10.1038/bonekey.2013.213.

17 Deluca, H. F. (2014). History of the discovery of vitamin D and its active metabolites. *BoneKEy Reports* 3, 479. doi.org/10.1038/bonekey.2013.213.

18 Haussler, M. R., Whitfield, G. K., Kaneko, I., Haussler, C. A., Hsieh, D., Hsieh, J.-C., & Jurutka, P. W. (2013). Molecular mechanisms of vitamin D action. *Calcified Tissue International* 92(2), 77–98. doi.org/10.1007/s00223-012-9619-0.

19 Hess, A. F., & Unger, L. J. (1921). The cure of infantile rickets by sunlight. *Journal of the American Medical Association* 77(1), 39. doi.org/10.1001/jama.1921.02630270041016.

20 Garland, C. F., Garland, F. C., Gorham, E. D., Lipkin, M., Newmark, H., Mohr, S. B., & Holick, M. F. (2006). The role of vitamin D in cancer prevention. *American Journal of Public Health* 96(2), 252–61. doi.org/10.2105/AJPH.2004.

21 Wang, T. J., Pencina, M. J., Booth, S. L., Jacques, P. F., Ingelsson, E., Lanier, K., Benjamin, E. J., D'Agostino, R. B., Wolf, M., & Vasan, R. S. (2008). Vitamin D deficiency and risk of cardiovascular disease. *Circulation* 117(4), 503–11. doi.org/10.1161/CIRCULATIONAHA.107 .706127.

22 Holick, M. F. (2004). Sunlight and vitamin D for bone health and prevention of autoimmune diseases, cancers, and cardiovascular disease. *The American Journal of Clinical Nutrition* 80(6 Suppl), 1678S–1688S. doi.org/10.1093/ajcn/80.6.1678S.

23 Ginde, A. A., Mansbach, J. M., & Camargo, C. A. (2009). Association between serum 25-hydroxyvitamin D level and upper respiratory tract infection in the Third National Health and Nutrition Examination Survey. *Archives of Internal Medicine* 169(4), 384–90. doi.org/10.1001 /archinternmed.2008.560.

24 Steenbock, H., & Black, A. (1925). Fat-soluble vitamins: XXIII. The induction of growth-promoting and calcifying properties in fats and their unsaponifiable constituents by exposure to light. *Journal of Biological Chemistry* 64, 263–98.

25 Windaus, A., Schenck, F., & von Werder, F. (1936). Über das antirachitisch wirksame Bestrahlungsprodukt aus 7-Dehydro-cholesterin. *Hoppe-Seyler's Zeitschrift für physiologische Chemie* 241(1–3), 100–103. doi.org/10.1515/bchm2.1936.241.1-3.100.

26 Tripkovic, L., Lambert, H., Hart, K., Smith, C. P., Bucca, G., Penson, S., Chope, G., Hyppönen, E., Berry, J., Vieth, R., & Lanham-New, S. (2012). Comparison of vitamin D2 and vitamin D3 supplementation in raising serum 25-hydroxyvitamin D status: A systematic review and meta-analysis. *The American Journal of Clinical Nutrition* 95(6), 1357–64. doi.org/10.3945/ajcn.111.031070.

27 Houghton, L. A., & Vieth, R. (2006). The case against ergocalciferol (vitamin D2) as a vitamin for humans. *The American Journal of Clinical Nutrition* 84(4), 694–97. doi.org/10.1093/ajcn/84.4.694.

28 Tripkovic, L., Lambert, H., Hart, K., Smith, C. P., Bucca, G., Penson, S., Chope, G., Hyppönen, E., Berry, J., Vieth, R., & Lanham-New, S. (2012). Comparison of vitamin D2 and vitamin D3 supplementation in raising serum 25-hydroxyvitamin D status: A systematic review and meta-analysis. *The American Journal of Clinical Nutrition* 95(6), 1357–64. doi.org/10.3945/ajcn.111.031070.

29 Heaney, R. P., Robert R. Recker, R. R., Grote, J. et al. (2011). Vitamin D3 is more potent than vitamin D2 in humans, *The Journal of Clinical Endocrinology & Metabolism*, 96(3), E447–E452. doi .org/10.1210/jc.2010-2230.

## Chapter 3

1 Pough, F. H., Janis, C. M., & Heiser, J. B. (2018). *Vertebrate Life* (10th ed.). Sinauer Associates, Oxford University Press.

2 Holick, M. F. (2007). Vitamin D deficiency. *The New England Journal of Medicine*, 357(3), 266–81. doi.org/10.1056/NEJMra070553.

3 Diehl, M. Kik, et al. (2020). The nocturnal leopard gecko (Eublepharis macularius) uses UVb radiation for vitamin D3 synthesis. *Comparative Biochemistry and Physiology Part B: Biochemistry and Molecular Biology*, 250, 110506, ISSN 1096-4959. doi.org/10.1016/j.cbpb.2020.

4 Karsten, K. B., Ferguson, G. W., Chen, T. C., & Holick, M. F. (2009). Panther chameleons, Furcifer pardalis, behaviorally regulate optimal exposure to UV depending on dietary vitamin D3 status. *Physiological and Biochemical Zoology: PBZ*, 82(3), 218–25. doi.org/10.1086/597525.

5 Ferguson, G. W., Gehrmann, W. H., Karsten, K. B., Landwer, A. J., Carman, E. N., Chen, T. C., & Holick, M. F. (2003). Do panther chameleons bask to regulate endogenous vitamin D3 production? *Physiological and Biochemical Zoology* 76(1), 52–59. doi.org/10.1086/367947.

6 Baines, F. M., & Beveridge, C. (2012). The new UV-guide for reptiles and amphibians. *Reptilia: The European Herp Magazine*, 83, 49–55.

7 Courtney-Smith, J. (2017). *The Arcadia Guide to Reptile and Amphibian Lighting.* Arcadia Products PLC.

8 Allen, M. E., Oftedal, O. T., & Ullrey, D. E. (1993). Effect of dietary vitamin D3 on growth and bone development of young iguanas (Iguana iguana). *Journal of Zoo and Wildlife Medicine* 24(1), 34–41.

9 Huey, R. B., & Slatkin, M. (1976). Cost and benefits of lizard thermoregulation. *The Quarterly Review of Biology* 51(3), 363–84. doi.org/10.1086/409470.

10 Cooper, W.E. Jr (2003), Effect of risk on aspects of escape behavior by a lizard, *Holbrookia propinqua*, in relation to optimal escape theory. *Ethology* 109, 617–26. doi.org/10.1046/j.1439-0310.2003.00912.x.

11 Holick, M. F. (2004). Sunlight and vitamin D for bone health and prevention of autoimmune diseases, cancers, and cardiovascular disease. *The American Journal of Clinical Nutrition* 80(6 Suppl), 1678S–1688S. doi.org/10.1093/ajcn/80.6.1678S.

12 C-Span (2025). Health and Human Services Secretary Kennedy Testifies on Health Care Agenda, Part 1. September 4, 2025. https://www.c-span.org/program/senate-committee/health-and-human-services-secretary-kennedy-testifies-on-health-care-agenda-part-1/664946.

13 Watson, K. B., Wiltz, J. L., Nhim, K., Kaufmann, R. B., Thomas, C. W., & Greenlund, K. J. (2025). Trends in Multiple Chronic Conditions Among US Adults, by Life Stage, Behavioral Risk Factor Surveillance System, 2013–2023. *Prev Chronic Disease* 22, 240539. dx.doi.org/10.5888/pcd22.240539.

## Chapter 4

1 Zasloff, M. (2002). Antimicrobial peptides of multicellular organisms. *Nature* 415(6870), 389–95. doi.org/10.1038/415389a.

2 Zanetti, M., Gennaro, R., & Romeo, D. (1997). The cathelicidin family of antimicrobial peptide precursors: a component of the oxygen-independent defense mechanisms of neutrophils. *Annals of the New York Academy of Sciences* 832, 147–62. doi.org/10.1111/j.1749-6632.1997.tb46244.x.

3 Sørensen, O. E., Follin, P., Johnsen, A. H., Calafat, J., Tjabringa, G. S., Hiemstra, P. S., & Borregaard, N. (2001). Human cathelicidin, hCAP-18, is processed to the antimicrobial peptide LL-37 by extracellular cleavage with proteinase 3. *Blood* 97(12), 3951–59. doi.org/10.1182/blood.v97.12.3951.

4 Bals, R., Wang, X., Zasloff, M., & Wilson, J. M. (1998). The peptide antibiotic LL-37/hCAP-18 is expressed in epithelia of the human lung where it has broad antimicrobial activity at the airway surface. *Proceedings of the National Academy of Sciences of the United States of America* 95(16), 9541–46. doi.org/10.1073/pnas.95.16.9541.

5 Schauber, J., Dorschner, R. A., Coda, A. B., et al. (2007). Injury enhances TLR2 function and antimicrobial peptide expression through a vitamin D-dependent mechanism. *The Journal of Clinical Investigation* 117(3), 803–11. doi.org/10.1172/JCI30142.

6 Tecle, T., Tripathi, S., & Hartshorn, K. L. (2010). Review: Defensins and cathelicidins in lung immunity. *Innate Immunity* 16(3), 151–59. doi.org/10.1177/1753425910365734.

7 Charoenngam, N., & Holick, M. F. (2020). Immunologic effects of vitamin D on human health and disease. *Nutrients* 12(7), 2097. doi.org/10.3390/nu12072097.

8 Chromek, M., Slamová, Z., Bergman, P., Kovács, L., Podracká, L., Ehrén, I., Hökfelt, T., Gudmundsson, G. H., Gallo, R. L., Agerberth, B., & Brauner, A. (2006). The antimicrobial peptide cathelicidin protects the urinary tract against invasive bacterial infection. *Nature Medicine* 12 (6), 636–41. doi.org/10.1038/nm1407.

9 Gordon, Y. J., Huang, L. C., Romanowski, E. G., Yates, K. A., Proske, R. J., & McDermott, A. M. (2005). Human cathelicidin (LL-37), a multifunctional peptide, is expressed by ocular surface

epithelia and has potent antibacterial and antiviral activity. *Current Eye Research* 30(5), 385–94. doi .org/10.1080/02713680590934111.

10 Bals, R., Wang, X., Zasloff, M., & Wilson, J. M. (1998). The peptide antibiotic LL-37/hCAP-18 is expressed in epithelia of the human lung where it has broad antimicrobial activity at the airway surface. *Proceedings of the National Academy of Sciences of the United States of America* 95(16), 9541–46. doi.org/10.1073/pnas.95.16.9541.

11 Scott, M. G., Dullaghan, E., Mouncey, N. J., & Ryder, K. (2002). The human antimicrobial peptide LL-37 binds and neutralizes lipopolysaccharide. *The Journal of Immunology* 169(7), 3883–91. doi.org /10.4049/jimmunol.169.7.3883.

12 De Yang, Chen, Q., Schmidt, A. P., Anderson, G. M., Wang, J. M., Wooters, J., Oppenheim, J. J., & Chertov, O. (2000). LL-37, the neutrophil granule- and epithelial cell-derived cathelicidin, utilizes formyl peptide receptor-like 1 (FPRL1) as a receptor to chemoattract human peripheral blood neutrophils, monocytes, and T cells. *The Journal of Experimental Medicine* 192(7), 1069–74. doi.org /10.1084/jem.192.7.1069.

13 Reinholz, M., Ruzicka, T., & Schauber, J. (2012). Cathelicidin LL-37: An antimicrobial peptide with a role in inflammatory skin disease. *Annals of Dermatology* 24(2), 126–35. doi.org/10.5021/ad.2012 .24.2.126.

14 Carretero, M., Escámez, M. J., García, M., Duarte, B., Holguín, A., Retamosa, L., Jorcano, J. L., Río, M. D., & Larcher, F. (2008). In vitro and in vivo wound healing-promoting activities of human cathelicidin LL-37. *The Journal of Investigative Dermatology* 128(1), 223–36. doi.org/10.1038 /sj.jid.5701043.

15 Charoenngam, N., & Holick, M. F. (2020). Immunologic effects of vitamin D on human health and disease. *Nutrients* 12(7), 2097. doi.org/10.3390/nu12072097.

16 Reinholz, M., Ruzicka, T., & Schauber, J. (2012). Cathelicidin LL-37: An antimicrobial peptide with a role in inflammatory skin disease. *Annals of Dermatology* 24(2), 126–35. doi.org/10.5021 /ad.2012.24.2.126.

17 Gudmundsson, G. H., Agerberth, B., Odeberg, J., Bergman, T., Olsson, B., & Salcedo, R. (1996). The human gene FALL39 and processing of the cathelin precursor to the antibacterial peptide LL-37 in granulocytes. *European Journal of Biochemistry* 238 (2), 325–32. doi.org /10.1111/j.1432-1033.1996.0325q.x.

18 Wang, T. T., Nestel, F. P., Bourdeau, V., Nagai, Y., Wang, Q., Liao, J., Tavera-Mendoza, L., Lin, R., Hanrahan, J. W., Mader, S., & White, J. H. (2004). Cutting edge: 1,25-dihydroxyvitamin D3 is a direct inducer of antimicrobial peptide gene expression. *The Journal of Immunology* 173 (5), 2909–12. doi.org/10.4049/jimmunol.173.5.2909.

19 Liu, P. T., Stenger, S., Li, H., et al. (2006). Toll-like receptor triggering of a vitamin D-mediated human antimicrobial response. *Science*, 311 (5768), 1770–73. doi.org/10.1126/science.1123933.

20 Finsen, N. R. (1901). *Phototherapy*. (English translation of original works). Edward Arnold.

21 Holick, M. F. (2004). Sunlight and vitamin D for bone health and prevention of autoimmune diseases, cancers, and cardiovascular disease. *The American Journal of Clinical Nutrition* 80 (6, Suppl), 1678S–1688S. doi.org/10.1093/ajcn/80.6.1678S.

22 Gallo, R. L., & Nakatsuji, T. (2011). Microbial symbiosis with the innate immune defense system of the skin. *The Journal of Investigative Dermatology* 131(10), 1974–80. doi.org/10.1038/jid.2011.182.

23 Gallo, R. L., Kim, K. J., Bernfield, M., Kozak, C. A., Zanetti, M., & Trowbridge, I. S. (1997). Identification of CRAMP, a cathelin-related antimicrobial peptide expressed in the bone marrow and skin of mice. *The Journal of Biological Chemistry* 272(20), 13088–93.

24 Reinholz, M., Ruzicka, T., & Schauber, J. (2012). Cathelicidin LL-37: An antimicrobial peptide with a role in inflammatory skin disease. *Annals of Dermatology* 24(2), 126–35. doi.org/10.5021/ad .2012.24.2.126.

## Chapter 5

1 Holick, M. F. (2004). Sunlight and vitamin D for bone health and prevention of autoimmune diseases, cancers, and cardiovascular disease. *The American Journal of Clinical Nutrition* 80 (6 Suppl), 1678S–1688S. doi.org/10.1093/ajcn/80.6.1678S.

2 MacLaughlin, J., & Holick, M. F. (1985). Aging decreases the capacity of human skin to produce vitamin D3. *The Journal of Clinical Investigation* 76 (4), 1536–38. doi.org/10.1172/JCI112134.

3 Holick, M. F. (1995). Environmental factors that influence the cutaneous production of vitamin D. *The American Journal of Clinical Nutrition*, 61 (3 Suppl), 638S–645S. doi.org/10.1093/ajcn/61.3.638S.

4 Bikle, D. D. (2014). Vitamin D metabolism, mechanism of action, and clinical applications. *Chemistry & Biology* 21 (3), 319–29. doi.org/10.1016/j.chembiol.2013.12.016.

5 Bikle, D. D. (2014). Vitamin D metabolism, mechanism of action, and clinical applications. *Chemistry & Biology* 21 (3), 319–29. doi.org/10.1016/j.chembiol.2013.12.016.

6 Holick, M. F. (1995). Environmental factors that influence the cutaneous production of vitamin D. *The American Journal of Clinical Nutrition* 61 (3 Suppl), 638S–645S. doi.org/10.1093/ajcn/61.3.638S.

7 Bikle, D. D. (2014). Vitamin D metabolism, mechanism of action, and clinical applications. *Chemistry & Biology* 21 (3), 319–29. doi.org/10.1016/j.chembiol.2013.12.016.

8 Bikle, D. D. (2014). Vitamin D metabolism, mechanism of action, and clinical applications. *Chemistry & Biology* 21 (3), 319–29. doi.org/10.1016/j.chembiol.2013.12.016.

9 Jones, G. (2008). Pharmacokinetics of vitamin D toxicity. *The American Journal of Clinical Nutrition* 88 (2), 582S–586S. doi.org/10.1093/ajcn/88.2.582S.

10 Jones, G. (2008). Pharmacokinetics of vitamin D toxicity. *The American Journal of Clinical Nutrition* 88 (2), 582S–586S. doi.org/10.1093/ajcn/88.2.582S.

11 Bikle, D. D. (2014). Vitamin D metabolism, mechanism of action, and clinical applications. *Chemistry & Biology* 21 (3), 319–29. doi.org/10.1016/j.chembiol.2013.12.016.

12 Jones, G. (2008). Pharmacokinetics of vitamin D toxicity. *The American Journal of Clinical Nutrition* 88 (2), 582S–586S. doi.org/10.1093/ajcn/88.2.582S.

13 Aranow, C. (2011). Vitamin D and the immune system. *Journal of Investigative Medicine* 59 (6), 881–86. doi.org/10.2310/JIM.0b013e31821b8755.

14 Hewison, M. (2010). Vitamin D and the immune system: new perspectives on an old theme. *Endocrinology and Metabolism Clinics of North America* 39(2), 365–79. doi.org/10.1016/j.ecl.2010.02.010.

15 Holick, M. F. (2007). Vitamin D deficiency. *The New England Journal of Medicine* 357 (3), 266–81. doi.org/10.1056/NEJMra070553.

16 Hollis, B. W. (2005). Circulating 25-hydroxyvitamin D levels indicative of vitamin D sufficiency: implications for establishing a new effective dietary intake recommendation for vitamin D. *The Journal of Nutrition* 135 (2), 317–22. doi.org/10.1093/jn/135.2.317.

17 Hollis, B. W., & Wagner, C. L. (2004). Vitamin D requirements during lactation: high-dose maternal supplementation as therapy to prevent hypovitaminosis D for both the mother and the nursing infant. *The American Journal of Clinical Nutrition* 80 (6 Suppl), 1752S–1758S. doi.org/10.1093/ajcn/80.6.1752S.

18 Holick, M. F. (2007). Vitamin D deficiency. *The New England Journal of Medicine* 357 (3), 266–81. doi.org/10.1056/NEJMra070553.

19 MacLaughlin, J., & Holick, M. F. (1985). Aging decreases the capacity of human skin to produce vitamin D3. *The Journal of Clinical Investigation* 76 (4), 1536–38. doi.org/10.1172/JCI112134.

20 Clemens, T. L., Adams, J. S., Henderson, S. L., & Holick, M. F. (1982). Increased skin pigment reduces the capacity of skin to synthesise vitamin D3. *The Lancet* 1 (8263), 74–76. doi.org/10.1016/s0140-6736(82)90214-8.

21 Hollis B. W. (2005). Circulating 25-hydroxyvitamin D levels indicative of vitamin D sufficiency: implications for establishing a new effective dietary intake recommendation for vitamin D. *The Journal of Nutrition 135*(2), 317–22. doi.org/10.1093/jn/135.2.317.

22 Institute of Medicine (US) Committee to Review Dietary Reference Intakes for Vitamin D and Calcium. (2011). *Dietary Reference Intakes for Calcium and Vitamin D*. National Academies Press (US). doi.org/10.17226/13050.

23 Veugelers, P. J., & Ekwaru, J. P. (2014). A statistical error in the estimation of the recommended dietary allowance for vitamin D. *Nutrients* 6 (10), 4472–75. doi.org/10.3390/nu6104472.

24 Veugelers, P. J., & Ekwaru, J. P. (2014). A statistical error in the estimation of the recommended dietary allowance for vitamin D. *Nutrients* 6 (10), 4472–75. doi.org/10.3390/nu6104472.

25 Heaney, R. P., & Holick, M. F. (2011). Why the IOM recommendations for vitamin D are deficient. *Journal of Bone and Mineral Research*, 26 (3), 455–57. doi.org/10.1002/jbmr.328.

26 McChesney, C., Singer, A., Duquette, D., Forouhi, N. G., Levinson, W. (2022). Do not routinely test for vitamin D. *BMJ*. 378, e070270. doi.org/10.1136/bmj-2022-070270.

27 Shah,V., Nayfeh, T., Alsawaf, Y. et al. (2024). A Systematic Review Supporting the Endocrine Society Clinical Practice Guidelines on Vitamin D, *The Journal of Clinical Endocrinology & Metabolism* 109(8), 1961–74, doi.org/10.1210/clinem/dgae312.

28 Aranow, C. (2011). Vitamin D and the immune system. *Journal of Investigative Medicine* 59 (6), 881–86. doi.org/10.2310/JIM.0b013e31821b8755.

29 Hewison, M. (2010). Vitamin D and the immune system: new perspectives on an old theme. *Endocrinology and Metabolism Clinics of North America* 39(2), 365–79. doi.org/10.1016/j.ecl.2010.02.010.

30 Holick, M. F. (2007). Vitamin D deficiency. *The New England Journal of Medicine* 357 (3), 266–81. doi.org/10.1056/NEJMra070553.

31 MacLaughlin, J., & Holick, M. F. (1985). Aging decreases the capacity of human skin to produce vitamin D3. *The Journal of Clinical Investigation* 76 (4), 1536–38. doi.org/10.1172/JCI112134.

32 Mayo Clinic Laboratories. International System of Units (SI) Conversion. https://www.mayocliniclabs.com/order-tests/si-unit-conversion.html. Accessed October 1, 2025.

33 National Institutes of Health. Vitamin D: Fact sheet for health professionals. https://ods.od.nih.gov/factsheets/VitaminD-HealthProfessional/. Accessed October 1. 2025.

34 Zhang, Y. C., & Schwarz, N. (2012). How and Why 1 Year Differs from 365 Days: A Conversational Logic Analysis of Inferences from the Granularity of Quantitative Expressions. *Journal of Consumer Research* 39(2), 248–59. doi.org/10.1086/662612.


## Chapter 6


1 Ginde, A. A., Liu, M. C., & Camargo, C. A., Jr (2009). Demographic differences and trends of vitamin D insufficiency in the US population, 1988–2004. *Archives of Internal Medicine* 169(6), 626–32. doi.org/10.1001/archinternmed.2008.604.

2 Ginde, A. A., Liu, M. C., & Camargo, C. A., Jr (2009). Demographic differences and trends of vitamin D insufficiency in the US population, 1988–2004. *Archives of Internal Medicine* 169(6), 626–32. doi.org/10.1001/archinternmed.2008.604.

3 Liu, Hu C., & Yang, M. (2024). Trends of serum 25(OH) vitamin D and association with cardiovascular disease and all-cause mortality: from NHANES survey cycles 2001–2018. *Frontiers in Nutrition* 11, 1328136. doi.org/10.3389/fnut.2024.1328136.

4 Cui A., Peilun, X., & Yuzhuo, M. et al. (2022). Prevalence, trend, and predictor analyses of vitamin D deficiency in the US population, 2001–2018. *Frontiers in Nutrition* 9, doi.org/10.3389/fnut.2022.965376.

5 Ames, B. N., Grant, W. B., & Willett, W. C. (2021). Does the High Prevalence of Vitamin D Deficiency in African Americans Contribute to Health Disparities? *Nutrients* 13(2), 499. doi.org/10.3390/nu13020499.

6 Cui A., Peilun, X., & Yuzhuo, M. et al. (2022). Prevalence, trend, and predictor analyses of vitamin D deficiency in the US population, 2001–2018. *Frontiers in Nutrition* 9, doi.org/10.3389/fnut.2022.965376.

7 Ginde, A. A., Liu, M. C., & Camargo, C. A., Jr (2009). Demographic differences and trends of vitamin D insufficiency in the US population, 1988–2004. *Archives of Internal Medicine* 169(6), 626–32. doi.org/10.1001/archinternmed.2008.604.

8 Brown, L. L., Cohen, B., Tabor, D. et al. (2018). The vitamin D paradox in Black Americans: a systems-based approach to investigating clinical practice, research, and public health - expert panel meeting report. *BMC Proceedings* 12 (Suppl 6), 6 (2018). doi.org/10.1186/s12919-018-0102-4.

9 Ames, B. N., Grant, W. B., & Willett, W. C. (2021). Does the High Prevalence of Vitamin D Deficiency in African Americans Contribute to Health Disparities? *Nutrients* 13(2), 499. doi.org/10.3390/nu13020499.

10 Holick, M. F. (2014). Vitamin D deficiency: A worldwide pandemic. *Dermato-Endocrinology* 6(1), e986877. doi.org/10.4161/19381980.2014.986877.

11 Powe, C. E., et al. (2013). Vitamin D–Binding Protein and Vitamin D Status of Black Americans and White Americans. *New England Journal of Medicine* 369 (21), 1991–2000. doi:10.1056/NEJMoa1306357.

12 Ames, B. N., Grant, W. B., & Willett, W. C. (2021). Does the High Prevalence of Vitamin D Deficiency in African Americans Contribute to Health Disparities? *Nutrients* 13(2), 499. doi.org/10.3390/nu13020499.

13 Holick, M. F. (2014). Vitamin D deficiency: A worldwide pandemic. *Dermato-Endocrinology* 6(1), e986877. doi.org/10.4161/19381980.2014.986877.

14 Powe, C. E., et al. (2013). Vitamin D–Binding Protein and Vitamin D Status of Black Americans and White Americans. *New England Journal of Medicine* 369 (21), 1991–2000. doi:10.1056/NEJMoa1306357.

15 Holick, M. F. (2014). Vitamin D deficiency: A worldwide pandemic. *Dermato-Endocrinology* 6(1), e986877. doi.org/10.4161/19381980.2014.986877.

16 Holick, M. F. (2014). Vitamin D deficiency: A worldwide pandemic. *Dermato-Endocrinology* 6(1), e986877. doi.org/10.4161/19381980.2014.986877.

17 Powe, C. E., et al. (2013). Vitamin D–Binding Protein and Vitamin D Status of Black Americans and White Americans. *New England Journal of Medicine* 369 (21), 1991–2000. doi:10.1056/NEJMoa1306357.

18 Veugelers, P. J., & Ekwaru, J. P. (2014). A statistical error in the estimation of the recommended dietary allowance for vitamin D. *Nutrients* 6 (12), 5122–29. doi.org/10.3390/nu6125122.

19 Kimball, S. M., Mirhosseini, N., & Holick, M. F. (2017). Evaluation of vitamin D3 intakes up to 15,000 international units/day and serum 25-hydroxyvitamin D concentrations up to 300 nmol/L on calcium metabolism in a community setting. *DermatoEndocrinology* 9 (1), e1300213. doi.org/10.1080/19381980.2017.1300213.

20 Kimball, S. M., Mirhosseini, N., & Holick, M. F. (2017). Evaluation of vitamin D3 intakes up to 15,000 international units/day and serum 25-hydroxyvitamin D concentrations up to 300 nmol/L on calcium metabolism in a community setting. *DermatoEndocrinology* 9 (1), e1300213. doi.org/10.1080/19381980.2017.1300213.

21 Rosenstreich, S. J., Rich, C., & Volwiler, W. (1971). Deposition in and release of vitamin D3 from body fat: evidence for a storage site in the rat. *The Journal of Clinical Investigation* 50(3), 679–87. doi.org/10.1172/JCI106538.

22 Martinaityte, I., Kamycheva, E., Didriksen, A., et al. (2017). Vitamin D Stored in Fat Tissue During a 5-Year Intervention Affects Serum 25-Hydroxyvitamin D Levels the Following Year, *The Journal of Clinical Endocrinology & Metabolism* 102 (10), 3731–38. doi.org/10.1210/jc.2017-01187.

23 Janoušek, J., Pilařová, V., Macáková, K., et al. (2022). Vitamin D: sources, physiological role, biokinetics, deficiency, therapeutic use, toxicity, and overview of analytical methods for detection of vitamin D and its metabolites. *Critical Reviews in Clinical Laboratory Sciences* 59(8), 517–54. doi.org/10.1080/10408363.2022.2070595.

24 Bikle, D. D. Vitamin D: Production, Metabolism, and Mechanism of Action. (Updated 2025 Jun 15). In: Feingold, K. R., Ahmed, S. F., Anawalt, B. et al., editors. Endotext [Internet]. South Dartmouth (MA): MDText.com, Inc.; 2000–. https://www.ncbi.nlm.nih.gov/books/NBK278935/.

25 Bikle, D. D. Vitamin D: Production, Metabolism, and Mechanism of Action. (Updated 2025 Jun 15). In: Feingold, K. R., Ahmed, S. F., Anawalt, B. et al., editors. Endotext [Internet]. South Dartmouth (MA): MDText.com, Inc.; 2000–. https://www.ncbi.nlm.nih.gov/books/NBK278935/.

26 Holick, M. F. & Jenkins, M. (2001). *The UV Advantage*. Simon & Schuster. ISBN 0-7434-8647-1.


## Chapter 7


1 Gombart A. F. (2009). The vitamin D-antimicrobial peptide pathway and its role in protection against infection. *Future Microbiology* 4(9), 1151–65. doi.org/10.2217/fmb.09.87.

2 Urrutia, R. P., & Thorp, J. M. (2012). Vitamin D in pregnancy: current concepts. *Current Opinion in Obstetrics & Gynecology* 24(2), 57–64. doi.org/10.1097/GCO.0b013e3283505ab3.

3 Lerchbaum, E., & Obermayer-Pietsch, B. (2012). Vitamin D and fertility: a systematic review. *European Journal of Endocrinology* 166 (5), 765–78. doi.org/10.1530/EJE-11-0984.

4 Adamczewska, D., Słowikowska-Hilczer, J., & Walczak-Jedrzejowska, R. (2023). The association between vitamin D and the components of male fertility: A systematic review. *Biomedicines* 11, 90. doi.org/10.3390/ biomedicines11010090.

5 Blomberg Jensen, M. (2014). Vitamin D and male reproduction. *Nature Reviews Endocrinology* 10 (3), 175–86. doi.org/10.1038/nrendo.2013.262.

6 Cito, G., Cocci, A., Micelli, E., Gabellieri, E., Fucci, R., & Russo, G. I. (2020). Vitamin D and male fertility: An updated review. *The World Journal of Men's Health* 38 (2), 164–77. doi.org/10.5534/wjmh.190058.

7 Chu, J., Gallos, I., Tobias, A., Tan, B., Eapen, A., & Coomarasamy, A. (2018). Vitamin D and assisted reproductive treatment outcome: a systematic review and meta-analysis. *Human Reproduction* 33 (1), 65–80. doi.org/10.1093/humrep/dex326.

8 Lerchbaum, E., & Rabe, T. (2014). Vitamin D and female fertility. *Current Opinion in Obstetrics & Gynecology* 26 (3), 145–50. doi.org/10.1097/GCO.0000000000000065.

9 Anagnostis, P., Karras, S., & Goulis, D. G. (2013). Vitamin D in human reproduction: a narrative review. *International Journal of Clinical Practice* 67 (3), 225–35. doi.org/10.1111/ijcp.12031.

10 Chu, J., Gallos, I., Tobias, A., Tan, B., Eapen, A., & Coomarasamy, A. (2018). Vitamin D and assisted reproductive treatment outcome: a systematic review and meta-analysis. *Human Reproduction* 33 (1), 65–80. doi.org/10.1093/humrep/dex326.

11 Hollis, B. W. (2007). Vitamin D requirement during pregnancy and lactation. *Journal of Bone Mineral Research* 22, V39–V44. doi.org/10.1359/jbmr.07s215.

12 Zanetti, M., Gennaro, R., & Romeo, D. (1995). Cathelicidins: a novel protein family with a common proregion and a variable C-terminal antimicrobial domain. *FEBS Letters* 374(1), 1–5.

13 Zasloff, M. (2002). Antimicrobial peptides of multicellular organisms. *Nature* 415 (6870), 389–95. doi.org/10.1038/415389a.

14 Moutsatsou, P., Oikonomou, G., & Koussoulakos, S. (2018). Cathelicidins in reproduction. *Current Protein & Peptide Science* 19(6), 596–608. doi.org/10.2174/1389203718666170808121039.

15 Dürr, U. H. (2006). LL-37, the only human member of the cathelicidin family of antimicrobial peptides. *Biochimica et Biophysica Acta (BBA) - Biomembranes* 1758(9), 1408–25, doi.org/10.1016/j.bbamem.2006.03.030.

16 Kiattiburut, W., Zhi, R., Lee, S. G., Foo, A. C., Hickling, D. R., Keillor, J. W., Goto, N. K., Li, W., Conlan, W., Angel, J. B., Wang, G., & Tanphaichitr, N. (2018). Antimicrobial peptide LL-37 and its truncated forms, GI-20 and GF-17, exert spermicidal effects and microbicidal activity against Neisseria gonorrhoeae. *Human Reproduction* 33(12), 2175–83. doi.org/10.1093/humrep/dey315.

17 King, A. E., Paltoo, A., Kelly, R. W., Sallenave, J. M., Bocking, A. D., & Challis, J. R. (2007). Expression of natural antimicrobials by human placenta and fetal membranes. *Placenta* 28(2–3), 161–69. doi.org/10.1016/j.placenta.2006.01.006.

18 Yarbrough, V. L., Winkle, S., & Herbst-Kralovetz, M. M. (2015). Antimicrobial peptides in the female reproductive tract: a critical component of the mucosal immune barrier with physiological and clinical implications. *Human Reproduction Update* 21(3), 353–77. doi.org/10.1093/humupd/dmu065.

19 Yoshio, H., Yamada, M., Yoshida, M. et al. (2005). Expression of a Human Cathelicidin Antimicrobial Peptide, LL-37, in Amniotic Fluid with Neonatal or Maternal Infection. *Pediatric Research* 58, 427. doi.org/10.1203/00006450-200508000-00455.

20 Yarbrough, V. L., Winkle, S., & Herbst-Kralovetz, M. M. (2015). Antimicrobial peptides in the female reproductive tract: a critical component of the mucosal immune barrier with physiological and clinical implications. *Human Reproduction Update* 21(3), 353–77. doi.org/10.1093/humupd/dmu065.

21 Moutsatsou, P., Oikonomou, G., & Koussoulakos, S. (2018). Cathelicidins in reproduction. *Current Protein & Peptide Science* 19(6), 596–608. doi.org/10.2174/1389203718666170808121039.

22 Guo, J., Liu, S., Wang, P., Ren, H., & Li, Y. (2020). Characterization of VDR and CYP27B1 expression in the endometrium during the menstrual cycle before embryo transfer: implications for endometrial receptivity. *Reproductive Biology and Endocrinology: RB&E* 18(1), 24. doi.org/10.1186/s12958-020-00579-y.

23 Yoshio, H., Yamada, M., Yoshida, M. et al. (2005). Expression of a Human Cathelicidin Antimicrobial Peptide, LL-37, in Amniotic Fluid with Neonatal or Maternal Infection. *Pediatric Research* 58, 427. doi.org/10.1203/00006450-200508000-00455.

24 Selsted, M. E., Szklarek, D., & Lehrer, R. I. (1984). Purification and antibacterial activity of antimicrobial peptides of rabbit granulocytes. *Infection and Immunity* 45 (1), 150–54. doi.org/10.1128/iai.45.1.150-154.1984.

25 Lehrer, R. I., Lichtenstein, A. K., & Ganz, T. (1993). Defensins: antimicrobial and cytotoxic peptides of mammalian cells. *Annual Review of Immunology* 11, 105–28. doi.org/10.1146/annurev.iy.11.040193.000541.

26 Gombart, A. F., Borregaard, N., & Koeffler, H. P. (2005). Human cathelicidin antimicrobial peptide (CAMP) gene is a direct target of the vitamin D receptor and is strongly up-regulated in myeloid cells by 1,25-dihydroxyvitamin D3. *FASEB journal: Official publication of the Federation of American Societies for Experimental Biology* 19(9), 1067–77. doi.org/10.1096/fj.04-3284com.

27 Liu, P. T., Stenger, S., Li, H., Wenzel, L., et al. (2006). Toll-like receptor triggering of a vitamin D-mediated human antimicrobial response. *Science* 311 (5768), 1770–73. doi.org/10.1126/science.1123933.

28 Com, E., Bourgeon, F., Evrard, B., Ganz, T., Colleu, D., Jégou, B., & Pineau, C. (2003). Expression of antimicrobial defensins in the male reproductive tract of rats, mice, and humans. *Biology of Reproduction* 68(1), 95–104. doi.org/10.1095/biolreprod.102.005389.

29 Tollner, T., Bevins, C. & Cherr, G. (2012). Multifunctional glycoprotein DEFB126—a curious story of defensin-clad spermatozoa. *Nature Reviews Urology* 9(7), 365–75. doi.org/10.1038/nrurol.2012.109.

30 Quayle, A. J. (2002). The innate and early immune response to pathogen challenge in the female reproductive tract and the pivotal role of epithelial cells. *Journal of Reproductive Immunology* 57 (1–2), 61–79. doi.org/10.1016/s0165-0378(02)00019-0.

31 King, A. E., Paltoo, A., Kelly, R. W., Sallenave, J. M., Bocking, A. D., & Challis, J. R. (2007). Expression of natural antimicrobials by human placenta and fetal membranes. *Placenta* 28(2–3), 161–69. doi.org/10.1016/j.placenta.2006.01.006.

32 Romero, R., Espinoza, J., Gonçalves, L. F., Kusanovic, J. P., Friel, L. A., & Nien, J. K. (2006). Inflammation in preterm and term labour and delivery. *Seminars in Fetal & Neonatal Medicine* 11(5), 317–26. doi.org/10.1016/j.siny.2006.05.001.

33 Yarbrough, V. L., Winkle, S., & Herbst-Kralovetz, M. M. (2015). Antimicrobial peptides in the female reproductive tract: a critical component of the mucosal immune barrier with physiological and clinical implications. *Human Reproduction Update* 21(3), 353–77. doi.org/10.1093/humupd/dmu065.

34 Das, S., Vince, G. S., Lewis-Jones, I., Bates, M. D., & Gazvani, R. (2007). The expression of human alpha and beta defensin in the endometrium and their effect on implantation. *Journal of Assisted Reproduction and Genetics* 24(11), 533–39. doi.org/10.1007/s10815-007-9173-2.

35 Com, E., Bourgeon, F., Evrard, B., Ganz, T., Colleu, D., Jégou, B., & Pineau, C. (2003). Expression of antimicrobial defensins in the male reproductive tract of rats, mice, and humans. *Biology of Reproduction* 68(1), 95–104. doi.org/10.1095/biolreprod.102.005389.

36 Quayle, A. J. (2002). The innate and early immune response to pathogen challenge in the female reproductive tract and the pivotal role of epithelial cells. *Journal of Reproductive Immunology* 57 (1–2), 61–79. doi.org/10.1016/s0165-0378(02)00019-0.

37 Tollner, T., Bevins, C. & Cherr, G. (2012). Multifunctional glycoprotein DEFB126—a curious story of defensin-clad spermatozoa. *Nature Reviews Urology* 9(7), 365–75. doi.org/10.1038/nrurol.2012.109.

38 Schröder-Heurich, B., Springer, C. J. P., & von Versen-Höynck, F. (2020). Vitamin D effects on the immune system from periconception through pregnancy. *Nutrients* 12(5), 1432. doi.org/10.3390/nu12051432.

39 Rojansky, N., Brzezinski, A., & Schenker, J. G. (1992). Seasonality in human reproduction: an update. *Human Reproduction* (Oxford, England), 7 (6), 735–45. doi.org/10.1093/oxfordjournals.humrep.a137729.

40 Buckles, K. S. (2008). Understanding the returns to delayed childbearing for working women. *American Economic Review* 98 (2), 403–7. doi.org/10.1257/aer.98.2.403.

41 Holick, M. F. (2004). Sunlight and vitamin D for bone health and prevention of autoimmune diseases, cancers, and cardiovascular disease. *The American Journal of Clinical Nutrition* 80 (6 Suppl), 1678S–1688S. doi.org/10.1093/ajcn/80.6.1678S.

42 Cancho-Candela, R., Andrés-de Llano, J. M., & Ardura-Fernández, J. (2007). Decline and loss of birth seasonality in Spain: analysis of 33,421,731 births over 60 years. *Journal of Epidemiology and Community Health* 61 (8), 713–18. doi.org/10.1136/jech.2006.050211.

43 Holick, M. F. (2004). Sunlight and vitamin D for bone health and prevention of autoimmune diseases, cancers, and cardiovascular disease. *The American Journal of Clinical Nutrition* 80 (6 Suppl), 1678S–1688S. doi.org/10.1093/ajcn/80.6.1678S.

44 Vandermotten, R., & Dessouroux, C. (2024). The decline of fertility in developed countries: a review of current trends and contributing factors. *Journal of Population Research*, 41 (1), 1–25. doi.org/10.1007/s41118-023-00213-3.

## Chapter 8

1 Campbell, J. (1949). *The Hero with a Thousand Faces.* Princeton University Press.

2 Lawrence, D. H. (1928). *Lady Chatterley's Lover.* (Various publishers).

3 Pilz, S., Frisch, S., Koertke, H., Kuhn, J., Dreier, J., Obermayer-Pietsch, B., Wehr, E., & Zittermann, A. (2011). Effect of vitamin D supplementation on testosterone levels in men. *Hormone and Metabolic Research* 43(3), 223–25. doi.org/10.1055/s-0030-1269854.

4 Lerchbaum, E., & Obermayer-Pietsch, B. (2012). Vitamin D and fertility: a systematic review. *European Journal of Endocrinology* 166(5), 765–78. doi.org/10.1530/EJE-11-0984.

5 Lambert, G. W., Reid, C., Kaye, D. M., Jennings, G. L., & Esler, M. D. (2002). Effect of sunlight and season on serotonin turnover in the brain. *The Lancet* 360(9348), 1840–42. doi.org/10.1016/S0140-6736(02)11737-5.

6 Lerchbaum, E., & Obermayer-Pietsch, B. (2012). Vitamin D and fertility: a systematic review. *European Journal of Endocrinology* 166(5), 765–78. doi.org/10.1530/EJE-11-0984.

7 Lewy, A. J., Wehr, T. A., Goodwin, F. K., Newsome, D. A., & Markey, S. P. (1980). Light suppresses melatonin secretion in humans. *Science* 210(4475), 1267–69. doi.org/10.1126/science.7434030.

8 Slominski, J. Y. Chen, Raman, C. & Slominski, A. T. (2024). Photo-neuro-immuno-endocrinology: How the ultraviolet radiation regulates the body, brain, and immune system, *Proc. Natl. Acad. Sci. U.S.A.* 121 (14) e2308374121. doi.org/10.1073/pnas.2308374121.

9 Liu, D., Fernandez, B. O., Hamilton, A., Lang, N. N., Gallagher, J. M., Newby, D. E., Feelisch, M., & Weller, R. B. (2014). UVA irradiation of human skin vasodilates arterial vasculature and lowers blood pressure independently of nitric oxide synthase. *Journal of Investigative Dermatology* 134(7), 1839–46. doi.org/10.1038/jid.2014.27.

10 Canguven, O., & Al Malki, A. H. (2021). Vitamin D and Male Erectile Function: An Updated Review. *World Journal of Men's Health* 39(1), 31–37. doi.org/10.5534/wjmh.190151.

11 Diffey, B. L. (2008). Climate change, ozone depletion and the impact on ultraviolet exposure of human skin. *Physics in Medicine & Biology* 53(12), R1–R11. doi.org/10.1088/0031-9155/53/12/R01.

12 Twenge, J. M., Sherman, R. A., & Wells, B. E. (2017). Declines in sexual frequency among American adults, 1989–2014. *Archives of Sexual Behavior* 46(8), 2389–2401. doi.org/10.1007/s10508-017-0953-1.

13 Parikh, R., et al. (2021). Skin exposure to UVB light induces a skin-brain-gonad axis and sexual behavior. *Cell Reports* 36(8), 2211–47. doi.org/10.1016/j.celrep.2021.109579.

14 United Nations, Department of Economic and Social Affairs, Population Division (2022). World Fertility and Family Planning 2022: Meeting the Changing Needs for Family Planning. (ST/ESA/SER.A/466).

15 Bongaarts, J. (2008). Fertility transitions in developing countries: Progress or stagnation? *Studies in Family Planning* 39(2), 105–10. doi.org/10.1111/j.1728-4465.2008.00157.x.

16 Marazziti, D., Baroni, S., Mucci, F., et al. (2019). Sex-Related Differences in Plasma Oxytocin Levels in Humans. *Clinical Practice and Epidemiology in Mental Health* 15, 58–63. http://dx.doi.org/10.2174/1745017901915010058.

17 Morales, M. (2021). Hormones, Couples' Romantic Passion Levels, May Be Affected by Their Exposure to Sunlight. *Science Times*, https://www.sciencetimes.com/articles/33063/20210825/hormones-couples-romantic-passion-levels-affected-exposure-sunlight.htm. Accessed September 10, 2025.

## Chapter 9

1 Parkin, J., & Cohen, B. (2001). An overview of the immune system. *The Lancet* 357(9270), 1777–89. doi.org/10.1016/S0140-6736(00)04904-7.

2 Janeway, C. A., Jr., & Medzhitov, R. (2002). Innate immune recognition. *Annual Review of Immunology* 20, 197–216. doi.org/10.1146/annurev.immunol.20.083001.084359.

3 Zasloff, M. (2002). Antimicrobial peptides of multicellular organisms. *Nature* 415(6870), 389–95. doi.org/10.1038/415389a.
4 Parkin, J., & Cohen, B. (2001). An overview of the immune system. *The Lancet*, 357(9270), 1777–89. doi.org/10.1016/S0140-6736(00)04904-7.
5 Murphy, K., & Weaver, C. (2017). *Janeway's Immunobiology* (9th ed.). Garland Science.
6 Zhu, J., & Paul, W. E. (2008). CD4 T cells: Fates, functions, and faults. *Blood* 112(5), 1557–69. doi .org/10.1182/blood-2008-05-078154.
7 Russell, J. H., & Ley, T. J. (2002). Lymphocyte-mediated cytotoxicity. *Annual Review of Immunology* 20, 323–70. doi.org/10.1146/annurev.immunol.20.100201.131730.
8 Sakaguchi, S., Yamaguchi, T., Nomura, T., & Ono, M. (2008). Regulatory T cells and immune tolerance. *Cell* 133(5), 775–87. doi.org/10.1016/j.cell.2008.05.009.
9 Janeway, C. A., Jr., & Medzhitov, R. (2002). Innate immune recognition. *Annual Review of Immunology* 20, 197–216. doi.org/10.1146/annurev.immunol.20.083001.084359.
10 Baeke, F., Takiishi, T., Korf, H., Gysemans, C., & Mathieu, C. (2010). Vitamin D: Modulator of the immune system. *Current Opinion in Pharmacology* 10(4), 482–96. doi.org/10.1016/j.coph.2010 .04.001.
11 Adams, J. S., & Hewison, M. (2008). Unexpected actions of vitamin D: New perspectives on the regulation of innate and adaptive immunity. *Nature Clinical Practice Endocrinology & Metabolism* 4(2), 80–90. doi.org/10.1038/ncpendmet0717.
12 Pike, J. W., & Meyer, M. B. (2010). The Vitamin D receptor: New paradigms for the regulation of gene expression by 1,25-dihydroxyvitamin D3. *Endocrinology and Metabolism Clinics of North America* 39(2), 255–69. doi.org/10.1016/j.ecl.2010.02.007.
13 Liu, P. T., Stenger, S., Li, H., Wenzel, L., et al. (2006). Toll-like receptor triggering of a vitamin D-mediated human antimicrobial response. *Science* 311(5768), 1770–73. doi.org/10.1126/science.1123933.
14 Schauber, J., Dorschner, R. A., Coda, et al. (2007). Injury enhances TLR2 function and antimicrobial peptide expression through a vitamin D-dependent mechanism. *The Journal of Clinical Investigation* 117(3), 803–11. doi.org/10.1172/JCI30142.
15 Wang, T. T., Nestel, F. P., Bourdeau, V., et al. (2004). Cutting edge: 1,25-dihydroxyvitamin D3 is a direct inducer of antimicrobial peptide gene expression. *The Journal of Immunology* 173(5), 2909–12. doi.org/10.4049/jimmunol.173.5.2909.
16 Rook, G. A. W., Steele, J., Fraher, L., Barker, S., Karmali, R., O'Riordan, J., & Stanford, J. (1986). Vitamin D3, gamma interferon, and control of proliferation of Mycobacterium tuberculosis by human monocytes. *Immunology* 57(1), 159–63. (PMCID: PMC1453912).
17 Guillot, X., Semerano, L., Saidenberg-Kermanac'h, N., Falgarone, G., & Boissier, M. C. (2010). Vitamin D and inflammation. *Joint Bone Spine* 77(6), 552–57. doi.org/10.1016/j.jbspin.2010.09.018.
18 Penna, G., & Adorini, L. (2000). 1 Alpha,25-dihydroxyvitamin D3 inhibits differentiation, maturation, and activation of human monocyte-derived dendritic cells. *The Journal of Immunology* 164(5), 2405–11. doi.org/10.4049/jimmunol.164.5.2405.
19 Liu, P. T., Stenger, S., Li, H., Wenzel, L., et al. (2006). Toll-like receptor triggering of a vitamin D-mediated human antimicrobial response. *Science* 311(5768), 1770–73. doi.org/10.1126/science. 1123933.
20 Cantorna, M. T., Hayes, C. E., & DeLuca, H. F. (1996). 1,25-Dihydroxyvitamin D3 reversibly blocks the progression of relapsing experimental autoimmune encephalomyelitis in mice. *Proceedings of the National Academy of Sciences* 93(15), 7861–64. doi.org/10.1073/pnas.93.15.7861.
21 Sakaguchi, S., Yamaguchi, T., Nomura, T., & Ono, M. (2008). Regulatory T cells and immune tolerance. *Cell* 133(5), 775–87. doi.org/10.1016/j.cell.2008.05.009.
22 Jeffery, L. E., Burke, F., Mura M., et al. (2009). 1,25-Dihydroxyvitamin D3 and IL-2 combine to inhibit T cell production of IFN-gamma and promote development of regulatory T cells. *The Journal of Immunology* 183(9), 5458–67. doi.org/10.4049/jimmunol.0803217.
23 Chen, S., Sims, G. P., Chen, X. X., Gu, Y. Y., Chen, S., & Lipsky, P. E. (2007). Modulatory effects of 1,25-dihydroxyvitamin D3 on human B cell differentiation. *The Journal of Immunology* 179(3), 1634–47. doi.org/10.4049/jimmunol.179.3.1634.
24 Heine, G., Niesner, U., Chang, H. D., Steinmeyer, A., Zügel, U., Zuberbier, T., & Radbruch, A. (2008). 1,25-dihydroxyvitamin D(3) promotes regulatory T cells by modulating innate immune

signaling. *Journal of Allergy and Clinical Immunology* 122(2), 384–91.e4. doi.org/10.1016/j.jaci.2008.05.017.

25 Coussens, L. M., & Werb, Z. (2002). Inflammation and cancer. *Nature* 420(6917), 860–67. doi.org/10.1038/nature01322.

26 Holick, M. F. (2007). Vitamin D deficiency. *The New England Journal of Medicine* 357(3), 266–81. https:/doi.org/10.1056/NEJMra070553.

27 Watson, K. B., Wiltz, J. L., Nhim, K., Kaufmann, R. B., Thomas, C.W., & Greenlund, K. J. (2025). Trends in multiple chronic conditions among US adults, by life stage, Behavioral Risk Factor Surveillance System, 2013–2023. *Prev Chronic Disease* 22, 240539. dx.doi.org/10.5888/pcd22.240539.

28 Coussens, L. M., & Werb, Z. (2002). Inflammation and cancer. *Nature* 420(6917), 860–67. doi.org/10.1038/nature01322.

## Chapter 10

1 C-Span (2025). Health and Human Services Secretary Kennedy Testifies on Health Care Agenda, Part 1. September 4, 2025. https://www.c-span.org/program/senate-committee/health-and-human-services-secretary-kennedy-testifies-on-health-care-agenda-part-1/664946.

2 Watson, K. B., Wiltz, J. L., Nhim, K., Kaufmann, R. B., Thomas, C. W., & Greenlund, K. J. (2025). Trends in Multiple Chronic Conditions Among US Adults, by Life Stage, Behavioral Risk Factor Surveillance System, 2013–2023. *Prev Chronic Disease* 22, 240539. dx.doi.org/10.5888/pcd22.240539.

3 Koch-Henriksen, N., & Sørensen, P. S. (2010). The changing demographic pattern of multiple sclerosis epidemiology. *The Lancet Neurology* 9 (5), 520–32. doi.org/10.1016/S1474-4422(10)70064-8.

4 Ascherio, A., & Munger, K. L. (2007). Environmental risk factors for multiple sclerosis. Part I: The role of infection. *Annals of Neurology* 61 (4), 288–99. doi.org/10.1002/ana.21117.

5 Bentzen, J., Flachs, E. M., Stenager, E., Brønnum-Hansen, H., & Koch-Henriksen, N. (2010). The incidence of multiple sclerosis in Denmark 1970–2005. *Neuroepidemiology* 35 (1), 18–24. doi.org/10.1159/000289327.

6 Kingwell, E., Marriott, J. J., Jetté, N., Pringsheim, T., Makhani, N., Morrow, S. A., . . . & O'Connor, P. (2013). Incidence and prevalence of multiple sclerosis in Europe: a systematic review. *BMC Neurology* 13 (1), 128. doi.org/10.1186/1471-2377-13-128.

7 Patterson, C. C., Dahlquist, G. G., Gyürüs, E., Green, A., & Soltész, G. (2009). Incidence trends for childhood type 1 diabetes in Europe during 1989–2003 and predicted new cases 2005–20: a multicentre prospective registration study. *The Lancet* 373 (9680), 2027–33. doi.org/10.1016/S0140-6736(09)60568-7.

8 Hyppönen, E., Läärä, E., Reunanen, A., Järvelin, M. R., & Virtanen, S. M. (2001). Intake of vitamin D and risk of type 1 diabetes: a birth-cohort study. *The Lancet* 358 (9292), 1500–1503. doi.org/10.1016/S0140-6736(01)06580-1.

9 Ng, S. C., Shi, H. Y., Hamidi, N., Underwood, F. E., Tang, W., Benchimol, E. I., . . . & Kaplan, G. G. (2017). Worldwide incidence and prevalence of inflammatory bowel disease in the 21st century: a systematic review of population-based studies. *The Lancet* 390 (10114), 2769–78. doi.org/10.1016/S0140-6736(17)32448-0.

10 Crowson, C. S., Matteson, E. L., Myasoedova, E., Michet, C. J., Ernste, F. C., Warrington, K. J., . . . & Gabriel, S. E. (2011). The lifetime risk of adult-onset rheumatoid arthritis and other inflammatory polyarthritis. *Arthritis & Rheumatism* 63 (3), 633–39. doi.org/10.1002/art.30155.

11 Rubio-Tapia, A., Kyle, R. A., Kaplan, E. L., Johnson, D. R., Page, W., Erdtmann, F., . . . & Murray, J. A. (2009). Increased prevalence and mortality in undiagnosed celiac disease. *Gastroenterology* 137 (1), 88–93. doi.org/10.1053/j.gastro.2009.03.059.

12 Lerner, A., Jeremias, P., & Matthias, T. (2015). The world incidence and prevalence of autoimmune diseases is increasing. *International Journal of Celiac Disease* 3 (4), 151–55. doi.org/10.12691/ijcd-3-4-8.

13 Lin, J., Liu, J., Davies, M. L., & Chen, W. (2016). Serum vitamin D level and systemic lupus erythematosus disease activity: a meta-analysis. *Lupus* 25 (11), 1267–75. doi.org/10.1177/0961203316632616.

14 Kivity, S., Agmon-Levin, N., Zisappl, M., Shapira, Y., Nagy, E. V., Dankó, K., . . . & Shoenfeld, Y. (2011). Vitamin D and autoimmune thyroid diseases. *Cellular & Molecular Immunology* 8 (3), 243–47. doi.org/10.1038/cmi.2010.73.
15 McInnes, I. B., & Schett, G. (2011). The pathogenesis of rheumatoid arthritis. *New England Journal of Medicine* 365 (23), 2205–19. doi.org/10.1056/NEJMra1004965.
16 Lowes, M. A., Suárez-Fariñas, M., & Krueger, J. G. (2014). Immunology of psoriasis. *Annual Review of Immunology* 32 , 227–55. doi.org/10.1146/annurev-immunol-032713-120225.
17 Dendrou, C. A., Fugger, L., & Friese, M. A. (2015). Immunopathology of multiple sclerosis. *Nature Reviews Immunology* 15 (9), 545–58. doi.org/10.1038/nri3871.
18 Strober, W., & Fuss, I. J. (2011). Proinflammatory cytokines in the pathogenesis of inflammatory bowel diseases. *Gastroenterology* 140 (6), 1756–67. doi.org/10.1053/j.gastro.2011.02.004.
19 Tsokos, G. C. (2011). Systemic lupus erythematosus. *New England Journal of Medicine* 365 (22), 2110–21. doi.org/10.1056/NEJMra1100359.
20 Kivity, S., Agmon-Levin, N., Zisappl, M., Shapira, Y., Nagy, E. V., Dankó, K., . . . & Shoenfeld, Y. (2011). Vitamin D and autoimmune thyroid diseases. *Cellular & Molecular Immunology* 8 (3), 243–47. doi.org/10.1038/cmi.2010.73.
21 Aranow, C. (2011). Vitamin D and the immune system. *Journal of Investigative Medicine* 59 (6), 881–86. doi.org/10.2310/JIM.0b013e31821b8755.
22 Baeke, F., Takiishi, T., Korf, H., Gysemans, C., & Mathieu, C. (2010). Vitamin D: modulator of the immune system. *Current Opinion in Pharmacology* 10 (4), 482–96. doi.org/10.1016/j.coph.2010.04.001.
23 Aranow, C. (2011). Vitamin D and the immune system. *Journal of Investigative Medicine* 59 (6), 881–86. doi.org/10.2310/JIM.0b013e31821b8755.
24 Aranow, C. (2011). Vitamin D and the immune system. *Journal of Investigative Medicine* 59 (6), 881–86. doi.org/10.2310/JIM.0b013e31821b8755.
25 Aranow, C. (2011). Vitamin D and the immune system. *Journal of Investigative Medicine* 59 (6), 881–86. doi.org/10.2310/JIM.0b013e31821b8755.
26 Baeke, F., Takiishi, T., Korf, H., Gysemans, C., & Mathieu, C. (2010). Vitamin D: modulator of the immune system. *Current Opinion in Pharmacology* 10 (4), 482–96. doi.org/10.1016/j.coph.2010.04.001.
27 Baeke, F., Takiishi, T., Korf, H., Gysemans, C., & Mathieu, C. (2010). Vitamin D: modulator of the immune system. *Current Opinion in Pharmacology* 10 (4), 482–96. doi.org/10.1016/j.coph.2010.04.001.

## Chapter 11

1 Haider, F., Ghafoor, H., Hassan, O. F., Farooqui, K., Bel Khair, A. O. M., & Shoaib, F. (2023). Vitamin D and Cardiovascular Diseases: An Update. *Cureus* 15 (11), e49734. doi.org/10.7759/cureus.49734.
2 Henein, M. Y., Vancheri, S., Longo, G., & Vancheri, F. (2022). The Role of Inflammation in Cardiovascular Disease. *International Journal of Molecular Sciences* 23 (21), 12906. doi.org/10.3390/ijms232112906.
3 Haider, F., Ghafoor, H., Hassan, O. F., Farooqui, K., Bel Khair, A. O. M., & Shoaib, F. (2023). Vitamin D and Cardiovascular Diseases: An Update. *Cureus* 15 (11), e49734. doi.org/10.7759/cureus.49734.
4 Henein, M. Y., Vancheri, S., Longo, G., & Vancheri, F. (2022). The Role of Inflammation in Cardiovascular Disease. *International Journal of Molecular Sciences* 23 (21), 12906. doi.org/10.3390/ijms232112906.
5 Tsao, C. W., Aday, A. W., Almarzooq, Z. I., et al. (2022). Heart Disease and Stroke Statistics—2022 Update: A Report From the American Heart Association. *Circulation* 145 (8), e153–e639. doi.org/10.1161/CIR.0000000000001052.
6 Haider, F., Ghafoor, H., Hassan, O. F., Farooqui, K., Bel Khair, A. O. M., & Shoaib, F. (2023). Vitamin D and Cardiovascular Diseases: An Update. *Cureus* 15 (11), e49734. doi.org/10.7759/cureus.49734.

7 Tsao, C. W., Aday, A. W., Almarzooq, Z. I., et al. (2022). Heart Disease and Stroke Statistics—2022 Update: A Report From the American Heart Association. *Circulation* 145 (8), e153–e639. doi.org/10.1161/CIR.0000000000001052.

8 Khan, A., Dawoud, H., & Malinski, T. (2018). Nanomedical studies of the restoration of nitric oxide/peroxynitrite balance in dysfunctional endothelium by 1,25-dihydroxy vitamin D3—clinical implications for cardiovascular diseases. *International Journal of Nanomedicine* 13, 455–66. doi.org/10.2147/IJN.S152822.

9 Sijbrands, E. J. G., Westendorp, J., Defesche, J. C., et al. (2001). Mortality over two centuries in large pedigree with familial hyper-cholesterolaemia: family tree mortality study. *BMJ* 322,1019–23.

10 Haider, F., Ghafoor, H., Hassan, O. F., Farooqui, K., Bel Khair, A. O. M., & Shoaib, F. (2023). Vitamin D and Cardiovascular Diseases: An Update. *Cureus* 15 (11), e49734. doi.org/10.7759/cureus.49734.

11 American College of Cardiology (2013). Cholesterol levels rise, fall with changing seasons. https://www.acc.org/about-acc/press-releases/2013/03/11/19/01/seasonal-cholesterol. Accessed September 15, 2025.

12 Crescioli, C. (2021). The Role of Estrogens and Vitamin D in Cardiomyocyte Protection: A Female Perspective. *Biomolecules* 11(12), 1815. doi.org/10.3390/biom11121815.

13 Zhaojun, M., Hong, H., Yi , Z. & Dandan, L. (2023). The role of vitamin D in menopausal women's health. *Frontiers in Physiology* 14. doi.org/10.3389/fphys.2023.1211896.

14 Liu, D., Fernandez, B. O., Hamilton, A., et al. (2014). UVA irradiation of human skin vasodilates arterial vasculature and lowers blood pressure independently of nitric oxide synthase. *Journal of Investigative Dermatology* 134 (7), 1839–46. doi.org/10.1038/jid.2014.27.

15 Liu, D., Fernandez, B. O., Hamilton, A., et al. (2014). UVA irradiation of human skin vasodilates arterial vasculature and lowers blood pressure independently of nitric oxide synthase. *Journal of Investigative Dermatology* 134 (7), 1839–46. doi.org/10.1038/jid.2014.27.

16 Weller, R. B. (2020). Does Incident Solar Ultraviolet Radiation Lower Blood Pressure? *Journal of the American Heart Association* 9(5), e013837. doi.org/10.1161/JAHA.119.013837.

17 Zasloff, M. (2002). Antimicrobial peptides of multicellular organisms. *Nature* 415 (6870), 389–95. doi.org/10.1038/415389a.

18 Liccardo, D., Cannavo, A., Spagnuolo, G., et al. (2019). Periodontal Disease: A Risk Factor for Diabetes and Cardiovascular Disease. *International Journal of Molecular Sciences* 20 (6), 1414. doi.org/10.3390/ijms20061414.

19 Grimes, D. S. (2012). Are statins beneficial or harmful? *The Journal of the Royal College of Physicians of Edinburgh* 42 (3), 262–65. doi.org/10.4997/JRCPE.2012.316.

20 Mensah, G, Arnold, N, Prabhu, S. et al. (2025). Inflammation and Cardiovascular Disease: ACC Scientific Statement: A Report of the American College of Cardiology. *Journal of the American College of Cardiology*. doi.org/10.1016/j.jacc.2025.08.047.

## Chapter 12

1 Phillips, C. (2025). As Rates of Some Cancers Increase in Younger People, Researchers Search for Answers. National Cancer Institute, https://www.cancer.gov/news-events/cancer-currents-blog/2025/early-onset-cancer-research-environment-genetics-support. Accessed September 14, 2025.

2 Bray, F., Ferlay, J., Soerjomataram, I., Siegel, R. L., Torre, L. A., & Jemal, A. (2018). Global cancer statistics 2018: GLOBOCAN estimates of incidence and mortality worldwide for 36 cancers in 185 countries. *CA: A Cancer Journal for Clinicians* 68 (6), 394–424. doi.org/10.3322/caac.21492.

3 Siegel, R. L., Miller, K. D., & Jemal, A. (2020). Cancer statistics, 2020. *CA: A Cancer Journal for Clinicians* 70 (1), 7–30. doi.org/10.3322/caac.21590.

4 Devesa, S. S., Blot, W. J., Stone, B. J., Miller, B. A., Tarone, R. E., & Fraumeni, J. F., Jr. (1995). Recent cancer trends in the United States. *Journal of the National Cancer Institute* 87 (3), 175–82. doi.org/10.1093/jnci/87.3.175.

5 Grant, W. B. (2002). An estimate of premature cancer mortality in the U.S. due to inadequate doses of solar ultraviolet-B radiation. *Cancer* 94, 1867–75. doi.org/10.1002/cncr.10427.

6 Siegel, R. L., Fedewa, S. A., Anderson, W. F., Miller, K. D., Ma, J., Rosenberg, P. S., & Jemal, A. (2017). Colorectal Cancer Incidence Patterns in the United States, 1974–2013. *Journal of the National Cancer Institute* 109 (8), djw322. doi.org/10.1093/jnci/djw322.

7 Garland, C., & Garland, F. (1980). Do sunlight and vitamin D reduce the likelihood of colon cancer? *International Journal of Epidemiology* 9 (3), 227–31. doi.org/10.1093/ije/9.3.227.

8 Garland, C. F., Garland, F. C., Gorham, E. D., Lipkin, M., Newmark, H., Mohr, S. B., & Holick, M. F. (2006). The role of vitamin D in cancer prevention. *American Journal of Public Health* 96 (2), 252–61. doi.org/10.2105/AJPH.2004.045260.

9 Garland, C. F., Comstock, G. W., Garland, F. C., Helsing, K. J., Shaw, E. K., & Gorham, E. D. (1989). Serum 25-hydroxyvitamin D and colon cancer: eight-year prospective study. *Lancet* 2 (8673), 1176–78. doi.org/10.1016/s0140-6736(89)91789-3.

10 Lowe, L. C., Guy, M., Mansi, J. L., & Colston, K. W. (2005). Vitamin D and breast cancer. *Recent Results in Cancer Research* 164, 223-241. doi.org/10.1007/3-540-26980-3_16.

11 McDonnell, S. L., Baggerly, C. A., French, C. B., Baggerly, L. L., Garland, C. F., Gorham, E. D., Lappe, J. M., & Heaney, R. P. (2018). Breast cancer risk markedly lower with serum 25-hydroxyvitamin D concentrations ≥60 vs <20 ng/ml (150 vs <50 nmol/L): Pooled analysis of two randomized trials and a prospective cohort. *PLoS ONE* 13 (6), e0199265. doi.org/10.1371/journal.pone.0199265.

12 Garland, C. F., Gorham, E. D., Mohr, S. B., Grant, W. B., Giovannucci, E. L., Lipkin, M., Newmark, H., Holick, M. F., & Garland, F. C. (2007). Vitamin D and prevention of breast cancer: pooled analysis. *The Journal of Steroid Biochemistry and Molecular Biology* 103(3–5), 708–11. doi .org/10.1016/j.jsbmb.2006.12.007.

13 Murphy, A. B., Nyame, Y., Martin, I. K., Catalona, W. J., & Hollowell, C. M. P. (2014). Vitamin D deficiency in a multiethnic cohort of men with prostate cancer. *The Journal of Steroid Biochemistry and Molecular Biology* 144, 240–44. doi.org/10.1016/j.jsbmb.2013.06.009.

14 Kanaan, Y., Copeland, R.L. (2022). The link between vitamin D and prostate cancer. *Nature Reviews Cancer* 22, 435. doi.org/10.1038/s41568-022-00493-y.

15 Berwick, M., Armstrong, B. K., Ben-Porat, L., Fine, J., Kricker, A., Eberle, C., & Barnhill, R. (2005). Sun exposure and mortality from melanoma. *Journal of the National Cancer Institute* 97 (3), 195–99. doi.org/10.1093/jnci/dji019.

16 van der Pols, J. C., Williams, G. M., Pandeya, N., Logan, V., & Green, A. C. (2006). Prolonged sun exposure and the risk of developing cutaneous melanoma. *Cancer Epidemiology, Biomarkers & Prevention* 15 (12), 2539–41. doi.org/10.1158/1055-9965.EPI-06-0563.

17 Shiratsuchi, H. Wang, Z. et al. (2017). Oncogenic Potential of CYP24A1 in Lung Adenocarcinoma. *Journal of Thoracic Oncolology* 12, 269–80.

18 Piotrowska, A., Zaucha, R., & Żmijewski, M. A. (2023). Vitamin D modulates the response of patient-derived metastatic melanoma cells to anticancer drugs. *International Journal of Molecular Sciences* 24(9), 8037. https:/doi.org/10.3390/ijms24098037.

19 Brunner, A. S., Haddad, S., Weise, J. J., Wagenpfeil, S., Vogt, T., & Reichrath, J. (2025). Malignant melanoma: The relationship between sunscreen use and cancer risk—A systematic review and meta-analysis. *Anticancer Research* 45(9), 3595–3603. https:/doi.org/10.21873/anticanres.17724.

20 Lapides, R., Saravi, B., Mueller, A., Wang-Evers, M., Maul, L. V., Németh, I., Navarini, A., Manstein, D., & Roider, E. (2023). Possible explanations for rising melanoma rates despite increased sunscreen use over the past several decades. *Cancers* 15(24), 5868. https:/doi.org/10.3390/cancers15245868.

21 Haddad, S., Weise, J. J., Wagenpfeil, S., Vogt, T., & Reichrath, J. (2025). Malignant melanoma: Vitamin D status as a risk and prognostic factor—Meta-analyses and systematic review. *Anticancer Research* 45(1), 27–37. https:/doi.org/10.21873/anticanres.17390.

22 Slominski, R. M., Kim, T.-K., Janjetovic, Z., et al. (2024). Malignant melanoma: An overview, new perspectives, and vitamin D signaling. *Cancers* 16(12), 2262. https:/doi.org/10.3390/cancers 16122262.

23 Dallavalasa, S., Tulimilli, S. V., Bettada, V. G., et al. (2024). Vitamin D in cancer prevention and treatment: A review of epidemiological, preclinical, and cellular studies. *Cancers* 16(18), 3211. https: /doi.org/10.3390/cancers16183211.

24 Colston, K., Colston, M. J., & Feldman, D. (1981). 1,25-dihydroxyvitamin D3 and malignant melanoma: The presence of receptors and inhibition of cell growth in culture. *Endocrinology* 108(3), 1083–86. https:/doi.org/10.1210/endo-108-3-1083.

25 Lapides, R., Saravi, B., Mueller, A., Wang-Evers, M., Maul, L. V., Németh, I., Navarini, A., Manstein, D., & Roider, E. (2023). Possible explanations for rising melanoma rates despite increased sunscreen use over the past several decades. *Cancers* 15(24), 5868. https:/doi.org/10.3390/cancers15245868.

26 Nicholson, L. B. (2016). The immune system. *Essays in Biochemistry* 60 (3), 275–301. doi.org/10.1042/EBC20160017.

27 Medzhitov, R. (2008). Origin and physiological roles of inflammation. *Nature* 454 (7203), 428–35. doi.org/10.1038/nature07201.

28 Taniguchi, K., & Karin, M. (2022). Chronic inflammation, cancer development and immunotherapy. *Frontiers in Pharmacology* 13, 1040163. doi.org/10.3389/fphar.2022.1040163.

29 Aranow, C. (2011). Vitamin D and the immune system. *Journal of Investigative Medicine* 59 (6), 881–86. doi.org/10.231/JIM.0b013e31821b8755.

30 Grant W. B. (2018). A Review of the Evidence Supporting the Vitamin D-Cancer Prevention Hypothesis in 2017. *Anticancer Research* 38(2), 1121–36. doi.org/10.21873/anticanres.12331.

31 Cantorna, M. T., Snyder, L., Lin, Y. D., & Yang, L. (2015). Vitamin D and 1,25(OH)2D regulation of T cells. *Nutrients* 7 (4), 3011–21. doi.org/10.3390/nu7043011.

32 Daryabor, G., Gholijani, N & Kahmini, F. (2023). A review of the critical role of vitamin D axis on the immune system, *Experimental and Molecular Pathology* 132–33, 104866. doi.org/10.1016/j.yexmp.2023.104866.

33 Campbell, M. J. & Trump, D. L. (2017). Vitamin D Receptor Signaling and Cancer. *Endocrinol Metab Clin North Am.* 46(4):1009–38. doi.org/10.1016/j.ecl.2017.07.007.

34 Zhang, Y., Xu, Y., Zhong, W., et al. (2025). Vitamin D and Immune Checkpoint Inhibitors in Lung Cancer: A Synergistic Approach to Enhancing Treatment Efficacy. *International Journal of Molecular Sciences* 26(10), 4511. doi.org/10.3390/ijms26104511.

35 Cantorna, M. T., Snyder, L., Lin, Y. D., & Yang, L. (2015). Vitamin D and 1,25(OH)2D regulation of T cells. *Nutrients* 7 (4), 3011–21. doi.org/10.3390/nu7043011.

36 Khazan, N., Quarato, E. R., Singh, N. A., et al. (2023). Vitamin D Receptor Antagonist MeTC7 Inhibits PD-L1. *Cancers* 15(13), 3432. doi.org/10.3390/cancers15133432.

37 Bersanelli, M., Cortellini, A., Leonetti, A., et al. (2023). Systematic vitamin D supplementation is associated with improved outcomes and reduced thyroid adverse events in patients with cancer treated with immune checkpoint inhibitors: results from the prospective PROVIDENCE study. *Cancer Immunology, Immunotherapy: CII* 72(11), 3707–16. doi.org/10.1007/s00262-023-03522-3.

38 You, W., Liu, X., Tang, H. et al. (20253). Vitamin D Status Is Associated With Immune Checkpoint Inhibitor Efficacy and Immune-related Adverse Event Severity in Lung Cancer Patients: A Prospective Cohort Study. *Journal of Immunotherapy* 46 (6), 236–43. doi.org/ 10.1097/CJI.0000000000000469.

39 Zhang, Y., Xu, Y., Zhong, W., Zhao, J., Liu, X., Gao, X., Chen, M., & Wang, M. (2025). Vitamin D and Immune Checkpoint Inhibitors in Lung Cancer: A Synergistic Approach to Enhancing Treatment Efficacy. *International Journal of Molecular Sciences* 26(10), 4511. doi.org/10.3390/ijms26104511.

40 Galus, Ł., Michalak, M., Lorenz, M. et al (2023).Vitamin D Supplementation Increases Objective Response Rate and Prolongs Progression-Free Time in Patients with Advanced Melanoma Undergoing Anti–PD-1 Therapy. *Cancer* 129, 2047–55.

41 Keum, N., Chen, Q. Y., Lee, D. H., Manson, J. E., & Giovannucci, E. (2022). Vitamin D supplementation and total cancer incidence and mortality by daily vs. infrequent large-bolus dosing strategies: a meta-analysis of randomised controlled trials. *British Journal of Cancer* 127(5), 872–78. doi.org/10.1038/s41416-022-01850-2.

42 Medzhitov, R. (2008). Origin and physiological roles of inflammation. *Nature* 454 (7203), 428–35. doi.org/10.1038/nature07201.

43 Grover, S., Dougan, M., Tyan, K., et al. (2020). Vitamin D intake is associated with decreased risk of immune checkpoint inhibitor-induced colitis. *Cancer* 126(16), 3758–67. doi.org/10.1002/cncr.32966.

44 Wu, X., Hu, W., Lu, L., et al. (2019). Repurposing Vitamin D for Treatment of Human Malignancies via Targeting Tumor Microenvironment. *Acta. Pharm. Sin. B.* 9, 203–19.

45 Makis, W., Baghli, I., & Martinez, P. (2025). Fenbendazole as an anticancer agent? A case series of self-administration in three patients. *Case Reports in Oncology* 18, 1, 856–63. doi.org/10.1159/000546362.

46 Supple, W. F. (2026). *Cancer is a Parasite: Kill It with the Safe, Over-the-Counter Antiparasitic Fenbendazole*. Skyhorse Publishing.

47 Chiang, K. C., & Chen, T. C. (2013). The anti-cancer actions of vitamin D. *Anti-cancer Agents in Medicinal Chemistry* 13(1), 126–39. doi.org/10.2174/1871520611307010126.

48 Muñoz, A., & Grant, W. B. (2022). Vitamin D and Cancer: An Historical Overview of the Epidemiology and Mechanisms. *Nutrients* 14(7), 1448. doi.org/10.3390/nu14071448.

## Chapter 13

1 World Health Organization. (2024, March 1). Obesity and overweight. WHO. https://www.who.int/news-room/fact-sheets/detail/obesity-and-overweight.

2 Afzal, S., Bojesen, S. E., & Nordestgaard, B. G. (2013). Low 25-hydroxyvitamin D and risk of type 2 diabetes: A prospective cohort study and metaanalysis. *Clinical Chemistry* 59(2), 381–91. doi.org/10.1373/clinchem.2012.193004.

3 Pittas, A. G., Lau, J., Hu, F. B., & Dawson-Hughes, B. (2007). The role of vitamin D and calcium in type 2 diabetes. A systematic review and meta-analysis. *The Journal of Clinical Endocrinology and Metabolism* 92(6), 2017–29. doi.org/10.1210/jc.2007-0298.

4 Szymczak-Pajor, I., & Śliwińska, A. (2019). Analysis of the relationship between vitamin D deficiency and insulin resistance. *Nutrients* 11(5), 969. doi.org/10.3390/nu11050969.

5 Kolb, R., Sutterwala, F. S., & Zhang, W. (2016). Obesity and cancer: inflammation bridges the two. *Current Opinion in Pharmacology* 29, 77–89. doi.org/10.1016/j.coph.2016.07.005.

6 Wyatt M, Choudhury A, Von Dohlen G, et al. (2024). Randomized control trial of moderate dose vitamin D alters microbiota stability and metabolite networks in healthy adults. *Microbiology Spectrum* 12, e00083-24. doi.org/10.1128/spectrum.00083-24.

7 Singh, P., Rawat, A., Alwakeel, M. et al. (2020). The potential role of vitamin D supplementation as a gut microbiota modifier in healthy individuals. *Scientific Reports* 10, 21641 (2020). doi.org/10.1038/s41598-020-77806-4.

8 Tangestani, H., Boroujeni, H. K., Djafarian, K., Emamat, H., & Shab-Bidar, S. (2021). Vitamin D and The Gut Microbiota: a Narrative Literature Review. *Clinical Nutrition Research* 10(3), 181–91. doi.org/10.7762/cnr.2021.10.3.181/

9 Wang, H., Tian, G., Pei, Z., Yu, X., Wang, Y., Xu, F., Zhao, J., Lu, S., & Lu, W. 2025. *Bifidobacterium longum* increases serum vitamin D metabolite levels and modulates intestinal flora to alleviate osteoporosis in mice. *mSphere* 10, e01039-24. doi.org/10.1128/msphere.01039-24.

10 Huang, F.-C., & Huang, S.-C. (2021). The Cooperation of Bifidobacterium longum and Active Vitamin D3 on Innate Immunity in Salmonella Colitis Mice via Vitamin D Receptor. *Microorganisms* 9(9), 1804. doi.org/10.3390/microorganisms9091804.

11 Lauby-Secretan, B., Scoccianti, C., Loomis, D., Grosse, Y., Bianchini, F., & Straif, K. (2016). Body fatness and cancer–viewpoint of the IARC Working Group. *The New England Journal of Medicine* 375(8), 794–98. doi.org/10.1056/NEJMsr1606602.

12 Sung, H., Siegel, R. L., Torre, L. A., Pearson-Stuttard, J., Islami, F., Fedewa, S. A., Goding Sauer, A., Shu-Hong, L., & Jemal, A. (2019). Global patterns in excess body weight and the associated cancer burden. *CA: A Cancer Journal for Clinicians* 69(2), 88–112. doi.org/10.3322/caac.21556.

13 Petrelli, F., Cortellini, A., Indini, A., Tomasello, G., Ghidini, A., Nigro, O., Salati, M., Dottorini, L., Iaculli, A., Bersanelli, M., & Ghidini, M. (2021). Association of obesity with survival outcomes in patients with cancer: a systematic review and meta-analysis. *JAMA Network Open* 4(3), e213520. doi.org/10.1001/jamanetworkopen.2021.3520.

14 Avgerinos, K. I., Spyrou, N., Mantzoros, C. S., & Dalamaga, M. (2019). Obesity and cancer risk: Emerging biological mechanisms and perspectives. *Metabolism* 92, 121–35. doi.org/10.1016/j.metabol.2018.11.001.

15 Martinez, P., & Grant, W. B. (2025). Vitamin D: What role in obesity-related cancer? *Seminars in Cancer Biology* 112, 135–49. https:/doi.org/10.1016/j.semcancer.2025.03.007.

16 Furukawa, S., Fujita, T., Shimabukuro, M., Iwaki, M., Yamada, Y., Nakajima, Y., Nakayama, O., Makishima, M., Matsuda, M., & Shimomura, I. (2004). Increased oxidative stress in obesity and its impact on metabolic syndrome. *The Journal of Clinical Investigation* 114(12), 1752–61. doi.org/10.1172/JCI21625.

17 Hopkins, B. D., Goncalves, M. D., & Cantley, L. C. (2016). Obesity and cancer mechanisms: cancer metabolism. *Journal of Clinical Oncology* 34(35), 4277–83. doi.org/10.1200/JCO.2016.67.9712.

18 Key, T. J., Appleby, P. N., Reeves, G. K., et al. (2003). Body mass index, serum sex hormones, and breast cancer risk in postmenopausal women. *Journal of the National Cancer Institute* 95(16), 1218–26. doi.org/10.1093/jnci/djg022.

19 Renehan, A. G., Zwahlen, M., & Egger, M. (2015). Adiposity and cancer risk: new mechanistic insights from epidemiology. *Nature Reviews Cancer* 15(8), 484–98. doi.org/10.1038/nrc3967.

20 Deshayes, F., & Nahmias, C. (2005). Angiotensin receptors: a new role in cancer? *Trends in Endocrinology and Metabolism* 16(7), 293–99. doi.org/10.1016/j.tem.2005.07.009.

21 Pereira-Santos, M., Costa, P. R., Assis, A. M., Santos, C. A., & Santos, D. B. (2015). Obesity and vitamin D deficiency: a systematic review and meta-analysis. *Obesity Reviews* 16(4), 341–49. doi.org /10.1111/obr.12239.

22 Wortsman, J., Matsuoka, L. Y., Chen, T. C., Lu, Z., & Holick, M. F. (2000). Decreased bioavailability of vitamin D in obesity. *The American Journal of Clinical Nutrition* 72(3), 690–93. doi.org /10.1093/ajcn/72.3.690.

23 Drincic, A. T., Armas, L. A., Van Diest, E. E., & Heaney, R. P. (2012). Volumetric dilution, rather than sequestration, best explains the low vitamin D status of obesity. *Obesity* 20(7), 1444–48. doi.org /10.1038/oby.2011.404.

24 Bikle, D. D. (2016). Extraskeletal actions of vitamin D. *Annals of the New York Academy of Sciences* 1376(1), 29–52. doi.org/10.1111/nyas.13129.

25 Zhang, Y., Leung, D. Y., Richers, B. N., Liu, Y., Remigio, L. K., Riches, D. W., & Goleva, E. (2012). Vitamin D inhibits monocyte/macrophage proinflammatory cytokine production by targeting MAPK phosphatase-1. *Journal of Immunology* 188(5), 2127–35. doi.org/10.4049/jimmunol.1102415.

26 Nakai, K., Fujii, H., Kono, K., Goto, S., Kitazawa, R., Kitazawa, S., Hirata, M., & Nishi, S. (2014). Vitamin D activates the Nrf2-Keap1 antioxidant pathway and ameliorates nephropathy in diabetic rats. *American Journal of Hypertension* 27(4), 586–95. doi.org/10.1093/ajh/hpt142.

27 Ameri, P., Giusti, A., Boschetti, M., Murialdo, G., Minuto, F., & Ferone, D. (2013). Interactions between vitamin D and IGF-I: from physiology to clinical practice. *Clinical Endocrinology* 79(4), 457–63. doi.org/10.1111/cen.12208.

28 Li, Y. C. (2011). Vitamin D and the renin-angiotensin system. In D. Feldman, J. W. Pike, & J. S. Adams (Eds.), *Vitamin D* (Third Edition, pp. 707–723). Academic Press. doi.org/10.1016/B978-0 -12-381978-9.10040-5.

29 Dougherty, U., Mustafi, R., Sadiq, F., Almoghrabi, A., Mustafi, D., Khare, S., Hart, J., Joseph, L., Pekow, J., Fichera, A., Li, Y. C., & Bissonnette, M. (2014). The renin-angiotensin system mediates EGF receptor-vitamin D receptor cross-talk in colitis-associated colon cancer. *Clinical Cancer Research* 20(22), 5848–59. doi.org/10.1158/1078-0432.CCR-14-1180.

30 Krishnan, A. V., Swami, S., & Feldman, D. (2010). Vitamin D and breast cancer: inhibition of estrogen synthesis and signaling. *The Journal of Steroid Biochemistry and Molecular Biology* 121(1–2), 343–48. doi.org/10.1016/j.jsbmb.2010.02.019.

31 Giampazolias, E., Pereira da Costa, M., Lam, K. C., Mlecnik, B., Zlobec, I., Bindea, G., Angell, H. K., Galon, J., & Vousden, K. H. (2024). Vitamin D regulates microbiome-dependent cancer immunity. *Science* 384(6694), 428–37. doi.org/10.1126/science.adj9213.

32 Su, D., Nie, Y., Zhu, A., Chen, Z., Wu, P., Zhang, L., Luo, M., Sun, Q., Cai, L., & Lai, Y. (2016). Vitamin D signaling through induction of paneth cell defensins maintains gut microbiota and improves metabolic disorders and hepatic steatosis in animal models. *Frontiers in Physiology* 7, 498. doi.org/10.3389/fphys.2016.000498.

33 Chandler, P. D., Chen, W. Y., Ajala, O. N., Hazra, A., Cook, N., Buring, J. E., Lee, I.-M., Giovannucci, E. L., & Manson, J. E. (2020). Effect of Vitamin D3 supplements on development of advanced cancer: A secondary analysis of the VITAL Randomized Clinical Trial. *JAMA Network Open* 3(11), e2025850. doi.org/10.1001/jamanetworkopen.2020.25850.

34 Ekwaru, J. P., Zwicker, J. D., Holick, M. F., Giovannucci, E., & Veugelers, P. J. (2014). The importance of body weight for the dose response relationship of oral vitamin D supplementation and serum 25-hydroxyvitamin D in healthy volunteers. *PLoS One* 9(11), e111265. doi.org/10.1371/journal.pone.0111265.

35 Kennel, K. A., Drake, M. T., & Hurley, D. L. (2010). Vitamin D deficiency in adults: when to test and how to treat. *Mayo Clinic Proceedings* 85(8), 752–58. doi.org/10.4065/mcp.2010.0138.

36 Mason, C., Xiao, L., Imayama, I., Duggan, C., Wang, C. Y., Korde, L., & McTiernan, A. (2011). Effects of weight loss on serum vitamin D in postmenopausal women. *The American Journal of Clinical Nutrition* 94(1), 95–103. doi.org/10.3945/ajcn.110.005971.

## Chapter 14

1 Buell, J. S., & Dawson-Hughes, B. (2008). Vitamin D and neurocognitive dysfunction: preventing "D"ecline? *Molecular Aspects of Medicine* 29(6), 415–22. doi.org/10.1016/j.mam.2008.05.001.

2 Nichols, E., et al. (2022). Global, regional, and national incidence, prevalence, and years lived with disability for 354 diseases and injuries for 204 countries and territories, 1990–2019: a systematic analysis for the Global Burden of Disease Study 2019. *The Lancet* 396(10258), 1204-22.

3 Dorsey, E. R., Sherer, T., & Bloem, B. R. (2018). The Parkinson Pandemic: A Call to Action. *Journal of Parkinson's Disease* 8(s1), S1–S3.

4 Ascherio, A., & Munger, K. L. (2016). Environmental risk factors for multiple sclerosis. Part I: the role of infection, tobacco smoking, and socioeconomic status. *Annals of Neurology* 79(2), 220–28.

5 Zhang, W., Xiao, D., Mao, Q., et al. (2023). Role of neuroinflammation in neurodegeneration development. *Signal Transduction and Targeted Therapy* 8, 267. doi.org/10.1038/s41392-023-01486-5.

6 Dias-Carvalho, A., Sá, S. I., Carvalho, F., Fernandes, E., & Costa, V. M. (2024). Inflammation as common link to progressive neurological diseases. *Archives of Toxicology* 98(1), 95–119. doi.org/10.1007/s00204-023-03628-8.

7 American Brain Foundation. (n.d.). What is neuroinflammation? Retrieved September 7, 2025, from https://www.americanbrainfoundation.org/what-is-neuroinflammation/.

8 Afridi, R., Tsuda, M., Ryu, H., & Suk, K. (2022). The function of glial cells in the neuroinflammatory and neuroimmunological responses. *Cells* 11(4), 659. doi.org/10.3390/cells11040659.

9 Afridi, R., Tsuda, M., Ryu, H., & Suk, K. (2022). The function of glial cells in the neuroinflammatory and neuroimmunological responses. *Cells* 11(4), 659. doi.org/10.3390/cells11040659.

10 Dias-Carvalho, A., Sá, S. I., Carvalho, F., Fernandes, E., & Costa, V. M. (2024). Inflammation as common link to progressive neurological diseases. *Archives of Toxicology* 98(1), 95–119. doi.org/10.1007/s00204-023-03628-8.

11 Zhang, W., Xiao, D., Mao, Q., et al. (2023). Role of neuroinflammation in neurodegeneration development. *Signal Transduction and Targeted Therapy* 8, 267. doi.org/10.1038/s41392-023-01486-5.

12 Zhang, W., Xiao, D., Mao, Q., et al. (2023). Role of neuroinflammation in neurodegeneration development. *Signal Transduction and Targeted Therapy* 8, 267. doi.org/10.1038/s41392-023-01486-5.

13 Dias-Carvalho, A., Sá, S. I., Carvalho, F., Fernandes, E., & Costa, V. M. (2024). Inflammation as common link to progressive neurological diseases. *Archives of Toxicology* 98(1), 95–119. doi.org/10.1007/s00204-023-03628-8.

14 Afridi, R., Tsuda, M., Ryu, H., & Suk, K. (2022). The function of glial cells in the neuroinflammatory and neuroimmunological responses. *Cells* 11(4), 659. doi.org/10.3390/cells11040659.

15 Menéndez, S. G., & Manucha, W. (2024). Vitamin D as a modulator of neuroinflammation: Implications for brain health. *Current Pharmaceutical Design* 30(5), 323–32. doi.org/10.2174/13816 12829666231219113942.

16 Mirarchi, A., Albi, E., Beccari, T., & Arcuri, C. (2023). Microglia and brain disorders: The role of vitamin D and its receptor. *International Journal of Molecular Sciences* 24(15), 11892. doi.org/10.3390/ijms241511892.

17 Afridi, R., Tsuda, M., Ryu, H., & Suk, K. (2022). The function of glial cells in the neuroinflammatory and neuroimmunological responses. *Cells* 11(4), 659. doi.org/10.3390/cells11040659.

18 Afridi, R., Tsuda, M., Ryu, H., & Suk, K. (2022). The function of glial cells in the neuroinflammatory and neuroimmunological responses. *Cells* 11(4), 659. doi.org/10.3390/cells11040659.

19 Mirarchi, A., Albi, E., Beccari, T., & Arcuri, C. (2023). Microglia and brain disorders: The role of vitamin D and its receptor. *International Journal of Molecular Sciences* 24(15), 11892. doi.org/10.3390/ijms241511892.

20 Ascherio, A., & Munger, K. L. (2016). Environmental risk factors for multiple sclerosis. Part I: the role of infection, tobacco smoking, and socioeconomic status. *Annals of Neurology* 79(2), 220–28.

21 Sultan, S., Taimuri, U., Basnan, S. A., et al. (2020). Low vitamin D and its association with cognitive impairment and dementia. *Journal of Aging Research* 2020, 6097820. doi.org/10.1155/2020/6097820.

22 Li, D., Ma, X., Zhang, W., et al. (2025). Impact of vitamin D3 supplementation on motor functionality and the immune response in Parkinson's disease patients with vitamin D deficiency. *Scientific Reports* 15, 25154. doi.org/10.1038/s41598-025-10821-5.

23 Buell, J. S., & Dawson-Hughes, B. (2008). Vitamin D and neurocognitive dysfunction: preventing "D"ecline? *Molecular Aspects of Medicine* 29(6), 415–22. doi.org/10.1016/j.mam.2008.05.001.

24 Menéndez, S. G., & Manucha, W. (2024). Vitamin D as a modulator of neuroinflammation: Implications for brain health. *Current Pharmaceutical Design* 30(5), 323–32. doi.org/10.2174/13816 12829666231219113942.

25 Mirarchi, A., Albi, E., Beccari, T., & Arcuri, C. (2023). Microglia and brain disorders: The role of vitamin D and its receptor. *International Journal of Molecular Sciences* 24(15), 11892. doi.org/10.3390 /ijms241511892.

26 Mirarchi, A., Albi, E., Beccari, T., & Arcuri, C. (2023). Microglia and brain disorders: The role of vitamin D and its receptor. *International Journal of Molecular Sciences* 24(15), 11892. doi.org/10.3390 /ijms241511892.

27 Lu'o'ng, K. V., & Nguyên, L. T. (2011). The beneficial role of vitamin D in Alzheimer's disease. *American Journal of Alzheimer's Disease and Other Dementias* 26(7), 511–20. doi.org/10.1177 /1533317511429321.

28 Mirarchi, A., Albi, E., Beccari, T., & Arcuri, C. (2023). Microglia and brain disorders: The role of vitamin D and its receptor. *International Journal of Molecular Sciences* 24(15), 11892. doi.org /10.3390/ijms241511892.

29 Verkman, A. S., Binder, D. K., Bloch, O., Papadopoulos, M. C., & Hamilton, S. A. (2006). Three faces of AQP4 in brain edema. *Translational Stroke Research* 37(6), 1145–55.

30 Cekic, M., & Stein, D. G. (2010). Traumatic brain injury and aging: Is a combination of progesterone and vitamin D hormone a simple solution to a complex problem? *Neurotherapeutics* 7(1), 81–90. doi.org/10.1016/j.nurt.2009.10.017.

31 Mirarchi, A., Albi, E., Beccari, T., & Arcuri, C. (2023). Microglia and brain disorders: The role of vitamin D and its receptor. *International Journal of Molecular Sciences* 24(15), 11892. doi.org /10.3390/ijms241511892.

32 Zhang, W., Xiao, D., Mao, Q., et al. (2023). Role of neuroinflammation in neurodegeneration development. *Signal Transduction and Targeted Therapy* 8, 267. doi.org/10.1038/s41392-023-01486-5.

33 Menéndez, S. G., & Manucha, W. (2024). Vitamin D as a modulator of neuroinflammation: Implications for brain health. *Current Pharmaceutical Design* 30(5), 323–32. doi.org/10.2174/13816 12829666231219113942.

34 Boontanrart, M., Hall, S. D., Spanier, J. A., Hayes, C. E., & Olson, J. K. (2016). Vitamin D3 alters microglia immune activation by an IL-10 dependent SOCS3 mechanism. *Journal of Neuroimmunology* 292, 126–36. doi.org/10.1016/j.jneuroim.2016.01.015.

35 Luciano, M. (2025). Immune suppression proposed as way to slow Parkinson's progression: Researchers tested azathioprine to see if it reduced brain inflammation. Parkinsonsnewstoday. Retrieved September 7, 2025, from https://parkinsonsnewstoday.

36 Nehls, M. (2023). *The indoctrinated brain: How to successfully fend off the global attack on your mental freedom*. Skyhorse Publishing.

## Chapter 15

1 Kinney, J. W., Bemiller, S. M., Murtishaw, A. S., Leisgang, A. M., Salazar, A. M., & Lamb, B. T. (2018). Inflammation as a central mechanism in Alzheimer's disease. *Alzheimer's & Dementia: Translational Research & Clinical Interventions* 4, 575–90. doi.org/10.1016/j.trci.2018.06.014.

2 Eratne, D., Loi, S. M., & Farrand, S. (2020). The history of Alzheimer's disease: A journey of scientific and clinical discovery. *History of Psychiatry* 31 (2), 202–24. doi.org/10.1177/0957154X20905187.

3 Alzheimer's Association. (2024). 2024 Alzheimer's disease facts and figures. *Alzheimer's & Dementia* 20 (5), 1598–1695. doi.org/10.1002/alz.13698.

4 World Health Organization. (2023, March 15). Dementia. https://www.who.int/news-room/fact -sheets/detail/dementia.

5 You, W. (2025). The protective role of ambient ultraviolet radiation against dementia: An ecological analysis of global data. *Health Science Reports* 8 (1), e70302. doi.org/10.1002/hsr2.70302.

6 Van der Flier, W. M. (2022). The amyloid cascade hypothesis: are we at a watershed moment? *The Lancet Neurology* 21 (11), 963–65. doi.org/10.1016/S1474-4422(22)00346-6.

7 Heneka, M. T., van der Flier, W. M., Jessen, F., et al. (2025). Neuroinflammation in Alzheimer disease. *Nature Reviews Immunology* 25, 321–52. doi.org/10.1038/s41577-024-01104-7.

8 Leng, F., & Edison, P. (2021). Neuroinflammation and microglial activation in Alzheimer's disease: where are we at? *Biological Psychiatry* 89 (1), 4–11. doi.org/10.1016/j.biopsych.2020.09.006.

9 Leng, F., & Edison, P. (2021). Neuroinflammation and microglial activation in Alzheimer's disease: where are we at? *Biological Psychiatry* 89 (1), 4–11. doi.org/10.1016/j.biopsych.2020.09.006.

10 Heneka, M. T., van der Flier, W. M., Jessen, F., et al. (2025). Neuroinflammation in Alzheimer disease. *Nature Reviews Immunology* 25, 321–52. doi.org/10.1038/s41577-024-01104-7.

11 Gáll, Z., & Székely, O. (2021). The role of vitamin D in the prevention of dementia and Alzheimer's disease. *Nutritional Neuroscience* 24 (11), 925–37. doi.org/10.1080/1028415X.2019.1683933.

12 Dursun, E., Gezen-Ak, D., & Yilmazer, S. (2011). A novel role for vitamin D in controlling amyloid-β-induced-inflammation. *Journal of Alzheimer's Disease* 23 (1), 7–12. doi.org/10.3233/JAD-2010-101131.

13 Bivona, G., Lo Sasso, B., Gambino, C. M., Giglio, R. V., Scazzone, C., Agnello, L., & Ciaccio, M. (2021). The Role of Vitamin D as a Biomarker in Alzheimer's Disease. *Brain Sciences* 11(3), 334. doi.org/10.3390/brainsci11030334.

14 Cantorna, M. T., Snyder, L., & Arora, J. (2019). Vitamin D and 1,25(OH)2D regulation of T-cells. *Nutrients* 11 (9), 2053. doi.org/10.3390/nu11092053.

15 Boontanrart, M., Hall, S. D., Spanier, J. A., Hayes, C. E., & Olson, J. K. (2016). Vitamin D3 alters microglia immune activation by an IL-10 dependent SOCS3 mechanism. *Journal of Neuroimmunology* 292, 126–36. doi.org/10.1016/j.jneuroim.2016.01.015.

16 Bivona, G., Lo Sasso, B., Gambino, C. M., Giglio, R. V., Scazzone, C., Agnello, L., & Ciaccio, M. (2021). The role of vitamin D as a biomarker in Alzheimer's disease. *Brain Sciences* 11 (3), 334. doi.org/10.3390/brainsci11030334.

17 Raha, S., & Shardell, M. D. (2021). Vitamin D and tau in dementia: A review of the literature. *Journal of Alzheimer's Disease Reports* 5 (1), 183–95. doi.org/10.3233/ADR-200277.

18 Jansen, W. J., Ossenkoppele, R., Knol, D. L., et al. (2015). Prevalence of cerebral amyloid pathology in persons without dementia: a meta-analysis. *JAMA* 313 (19), 1924–38. doi.org/10.1001/jama.2015.4668.

19 You, W. (2025). The protective role of ambient ultraviolet radiation against dementia: An ecological analysis of global data. *Health Science Reports* 8 (1), e70302. doi.org/10.1002/hsr2.70302.

20 Dobson, R., & Giovannoni, G. (2019). Multiple sclerosis—a review. *European Journal of Neurology* 26 (1), 27–40. doi.org/10.1111/ene.13819.

21 Laursen, J. H., Søndergaard, H. B., Sørensen, P. S., Sellebjerg, F., & Oturai, A. B. (2016). Association between age at onset of multiple sclerosis and vitamin D level-related factors. *Neurology* 86 (1), 88–93. doi.org/10.1212/WNL.0000000000002075.

22 Jayedi, A., Rashidy-Pour, A., & Shab-Bidar, S. (2020). Vitamin D status and risk of dementia and Alzheimer's disease: A meta-analysis of dose-response. *Nutritional Neuroscience* 23 (12), 933–43. doi.org/10.1080/1028415X.2019.1587331.

23 Bivona, G., Lo Sasso, B., Gambino, C. M., Giglio, R. V., Scazzone, C., Agnello, L., & Ciaccio, M. (2021). The role of vitamin D as a biomarker in Alzheimer's disease. *Brain Sciences* 11 (3), 334. doi.org/10.3390/brainsci11030334.

24 Ghahremani, M., Smith, E. E., Chen, H. Y., Creese, B., Goodarzi, Z., & Ismail, Z. (2023). Vitamin D supplementation and incident dementia: Effects of sex, APOE, and baseline cognitive status. *Alzheimer's & Dementia: Diagnosis, Assessment & Disease Monitoring* 15 (3), e12404. doi.org/10.1002/dad2.12404.

25 Grant, W. B., & Holick, M. F. (2005). Benefits and requirements of vitamin D for optimal health: a review. *Alternative Medicine Review* 10 (2), 94–111.

26 Heaney, R. P. (2008). Vitamin D in health and disease. *Clinical Journal of the American Society of Nephrology* 3 (5), 1535–41. doi.org/10.2215/CJN.01160308/.

27 You, W. (2025). The protective role of ambient ultraviolet radiation against dementia: An ecological analysis of global data. *Health Science Reports* 8 (1), e70302. doi.org/10.1002/hsr2.70302.

28 Heneka, M. T., van der Flier, W. M., Jessen, F., et al. (2025). Neuroinflammation in Alzheimer disease. *Nature Reviews Immunology* 25, 321–52. doi.org/10.1038/s41577-024-01104-7.

## Chapter 16

1 Holick, M. F. (2006). Resurrection of vitamin D deficiency and rickets. *The Journal of Clinical Investigation* 116 (8), 2062–72. doi.org/10.1172/JCI29454.

2 Christakos, S., Dhawan, P., Verstuyf, A., Verlinden, L., & Carmeliet, G. (2016). Vitamin D: Metabolism, molecular mechanism of action, and clinical application. *Physiological Reviews* 96 (1), 365–408. doi.org/10.1152/physrev.00014.2015.

3 Uday, S., & Högler, W. (2017). Nutritional Rickets and Osteomalacia in the 21st Century. *Endocrinology and Metabolism Clinics of North America* 46 (4), 867–91. doi.org/10.1016/j.ecl.2017.07.004.

4 Johnell, O., & Kanis, J. A. (2006). An estimate of the worldwide prevalence and disability associated with osteoporotic fractures. *Osteoporosis International* 17 (12), 1726–33. doi.org/10.1007/s00198-006-0172-4.

5 Bischoff-Ferrari, H. A., Dietrich, T., Orav, E. J., & Dawson-Hughes, B. (2005). Positive association between 25-hydroxy vitamin D levels and bone mineral density: A population-based study of younger and older adults. *The American Journal of Medicine* 118 (6), 637–40. doi.org/10.1016/j.amjmed.2005.01.035.

6 Paz-Zulueta, M., Lledías-López, F., Lázaro-García, A., Abella-Gamazo, A., Calvo-Alegre, C., Cimas-Hernando, M., & de Cos-Blanco, A. I. (2021). Vitamin D and bisphosphonates: A narrative review of the therapeutic alliance in osteoporosis. *Journal of Osteoporosis* 2021, 5580228. doi.org/10.1155/2021/5580228.

7 Fukumoto, S., & Martin, T. J. (2009). Bone as an endocrine organ. *Trends in Endocrinology and Metabolism* 20 (5), 230–36. doi.org/10.1016/j.tem.2009.02.001.

8 Ginaldi, L., Di Benedetto, M. C., & De Martinis, M. (2005). Osteoporosis, inflammation and ageing. *Immunity & Ageing* 2 (1), 14. doi.org/10.1186/1742-4933-2-14.

## Chapter 17

1 National Center for Injury Prevention and Control. (2020). Falls are a leading cause of injury and death in older Americans. *Centers for Disease Control and Prevention*. Retrieved from https://www.cdc.gov/injury/features/older-adult-falls/index.html September 10, 2025.

2 Beaudart, C., Buckinx, F., Rabenda, V., Gillain, S., Cavalier, E., Slomian, J., Petermans, J., Reginster, J. Y., & Bruyère, O. (2014). The effects of vitamin D on skeletal muscle strength, muscle mass, and muscle power: a systematic review and meta-analysis of randomized controlled trials. *Journal of Clinical Endocrinology & Metabolism* 99 (11), 4336–45. doi.org/10.1210/jc.2014-1742.

3 Ceglia, L., & Harris, S. S. (2013). Vitamin D and its role in skeletal muscle. *Calcified Tissue International* 92 (2), 151–62. doi.org/10.1007/s00223-012-9645-y.

4 Lexell, J. (1995). Human aging, muscle mass, and fiber type composition. *The Journals of Gerontology Series A: Biological Sciences and Medical Sciences* 50 (Special Issue), 11–16. doi.org/10.1093/gerona/50A.Special_Issue.11.

5 Ceglia, L., Niramitmahapanya, S., da Silva Morais, M., Rivas, D. A., Harris, S. S., Bischoff-Ferrari, H., & Fielding, R. A. (2013). A randomized study on the effect of vitamin D3 supplementation on skeletal muscle morphology and vitamin D receptor concentration in older women. *Journal of Clinical Endocrinology & Metabolism* 98 (12), E1927–E1935. doi.org/10.1210/jc.2013-2820.

6 Hamilton, B. (2010). Vitamin D and athletic performance: the potential role of muscle. *Asian Journal of Sports Medicine* 1 (4), 211–19. doi.org/10.5812/asjsm.34736.

7 Bischoff-Ferrari, H. A., Dawson-Hughes, B., Willett, W. C., Staehelin, H. B., Bazemore, M. G., Zee, R. Y., & Wong, J. B. (2004). Effect of vitamin D on falls: a meta-analysis. *JAMA* 291 (16), 1999–2006. doi.org/10.1001/jama.291.16.1999.

8 Autier, P., Mullie, P., Macacu, A., Dragomir, M., Boniol, M., Coppens, K., Pizot, C., & Boniol, M. (2014). Effect of vitamin D supplementation on non-skeletal disorders: A systematic review of meta-analyses and randomised trials. *The Lancet Diabetes & Endocrinology* 2 (1), 76–89. doi.org/10.1016/S2213-8587(13)70165-3.

9 Agergaard, J., Trøstrup, J., Uth, J. et al. Does vitamin-D intake during resistance training improve the skeletal muscle hypertrophic and strength response in young and elderly men?—a randomized controlled trial. *Nutrition & Metabolism* 12, 32 (2015). doi.org/10.1186/s12986-015-0029-y.

10 Long, C., Tara, Z., Casella, A. et al. (2022). High dose dietary vitamin D allocates surplus calories to muscle and growth instead of fat via modulation of myostatin and leptin signaling. *bioRxiv* 2022.05.19.492715. doi.org/10.1101/2022.05.19.492715.

## Chapter 18

1 Grant, W. B. (2011). A review of the role of solar ultraviolet-B irradiance and vitamin D in reducing risk of dental caries. *Dermato-Endocrinology* 3(3), 193–98. https:// 10.4161/derm.3.3.15841.

2 Grant, W. B. (2011). A review of the role of solar ultraviolet-B irradiance and vitamin D in reducing risk of dental caries. *Dermato-Endocrinology* 3(3), 193–98. https:// 10.4161/derm.3.3.15841.

3 Grant, W. B. (2011). A review of the role of solar ultraviolet-B irradiance and vitamin D in reducing risk of dental caries. *Dermato-Endocrinology* 3(3), 193–98. https:// 10.4161/derm.3.3.15841.

4 Hujoel, P. P. (2013). Vitamin D and dental caries in controlled clinical trials: Systematic review and meta-analysis. *Nutrition Reviews* 71(2), 88–97. https:/doi.org/10.1111/j.1753-4887.2012.00544.x.

5 Mahmood, M. K., Tassery, H., Tardivo, D., & Lan, R. (2023). Association between vitamin D levels and dental caries: A systematic review and dose-response meta-analysis of cross-sectional studies. *Applied Sciences* 13(17), 9883. https:/doi.org/10.3390/app13179883.

6 Li, Z., Wei, X., Shao, Z., et al. (2023). Correlation between vitamin D levels in serum and the risk of dental caries in children: A systematic review and meta-analysis. *BMC Oral Health* 23, 768. https: /doi.org/10.1186/s12903-023-03422-z.

7 Buzatu, R., Luca, M. M., & Bumbu, B. A. (2024). A systematic review of the relationship between serum vitamin D levels and caries in the permanent teeth of children and adolescents. *Dentistry Journal* 12(4), 117. https:/doi.org/10.3390/dj12040117.

8 Mohajeri, A., Abouei Mehrizi, A., & Amini, S. (2024). The influence of vitamin D levels on dental caries: A retrospective study of the United States population. *Nutrients* 16(11), 1572. https:/doi.org /10.3390/nu16111572.

9 Díaz-Zúñiga, J., & Godoy-Gienger, F. (2024). Dental caries in children and vitamin D deficiency: A narrative review. *BMC Oral Health* 24, 247. https:/doi.org/10.1186/s12903-024-03993-3.

10 Botelho, J., Machado, V., Proença, L., Delgado, A. S., & Mendes, J. J. (2020). Vitamin D deficiency and oral health: A comprehensive review. *Nutrients* 12(5), 1471. https:/doi.org/10.3390/nu12051471.

11 Botelho, J., Machado, V., Proença, L., Delgado, A. S., & Mendes, J. J. (2020). Vitamin D deficiency and oral health: A comprehensive review. *Nutrients* 12(5), 1471. https:/doi.org/10.3390/nu12051471.

12 Botelho, J., Machado, V., Proença, L., Delgado, A. S., & Mendes, J. J. (2020). Vitamin D deficiency and oral health: A comprehensive review. *Nutrients* 12(5), 1471. https:/doi.org/10.3390/nu12051471.

13 Ziada, S., Wishahe, A., Mabrouk, N., & Sahtout, S. (2025). Vitamin D deficiency and oral health: A systematic review of literature. *BMC Oral Health* 25, 468. https:/doi.org/10.1186 /s12903-025-05883-w.

14 Botelho, J., Machado, V., Proença, L., Delgado, A. S., & Mendes, J. J. (2020). Vitamin D deficiency and oral health: A comprehensive review. *Nutrients* 12(5), 1471. https:/doi.org/10.3390/nu12051471.

15 Machado, V., Lobo, S., Proença, L., Mendes, J. J., & Botelho, J. (2020). Vitamin D and periodontitis: A systematic review and meta-analysis. *Nutrients* 12(8), 2177. https:/doi.org/10.3390/nu12082177.

16 Lu, E. M. C. (2023). The role of vitamin D in periodontal health and disease. *Journal of Periodontal Research* 58(2), 213–24. https:/doi.org/10.1111/jre.13083.

17 Díaz-Zúñiga, J., & Godoy-Gienger, F. (2024). Dental caries in children and vitamin D deficiency: A narrative review. *BMC Oral Health* 24, 247. https:/doi.org/10.1186/s12903-024-03993-3.

18 Lu, E. M. C. (2023). The role of vitamin D in periodontal health and disease. *Journal of Periodontal Research* 58(2), 213–24. https:/doi.org/10.1111/jre.13083.

19 Lu, E. M. C. (2023). The role of vitamin D in periodontal health and disease. *Journal of Periodontal Research* 58(2), 213–24. https:/doi.org/10.1111/jre.13083.

20 Jagelavičienė E, Vaitkevičienė I, Šilingaitė D, et al. (2018). The Relationship between Vitamin D and Periodontal Pathology. *Medicina*. 54(3):E45. https://10.3390/medicina54030045.

21 Lu, E. M. C. (2023). The role of vitamin D in periodontal health and disease. *Journal of Periodontal Research* 58(2), 213–24. https:/doi.org/10.1111/jre.13083.

22 Shah, D., Patel, K., & Shah, A. (2023). Vitamin D and periodontal health: A systematic review. *Cureus* 15(10), e47771. https:/doi.org/10.7759/cureus.47771.

## Chapter 19

1 MacLaughlin, J., & Holick, M. F. (1985). Aging decreases the capacity of human skin to produce vitamin D3. *The Journal of Clinical Investigation*, 76 (4), 1536–38. doi.org/10.1172/JCI112134.

2 Franceschi, C., Bonafè, M., Valensin, S., Olivieri, F., De Luca, M., Ottaviani, E., & De Benedictis, G. (2000). Inflamm-aging: An evolutionary perspective on immunosenescence. *Annals of the New York Academy of Sciences* 908 (1), 244–54. doi.org/10.1111/j.1749-6632.2000.tb06651.x.

3 Childs, B. G., Durik, M., Baker, D. J., & van Deursen, J. M. (2017). Cellular senescence in aging and age-related disease: from mechanism to therapy. *Nature Medicine* 21 (12), 1424–35. doi.org/10.1038/nm.4000.

4 Epel, E. S., Blackburn, E. H., Lin, J., Dhabhar, F. S., Adler, N. E., Morrow, J. D., & Cawthon, R. M. (2004). Accelerated telomere shortening in response to life stress. *Proceedings of the National Academy of Sciences of the United States of America* 101 (49), 17312–15. doi.org/10.1073/pnas.0407162101.

5 Richards, J. B., Valdes, A. M., Gardner, J. P., Paximadas, D., Kimura, M., Nessa, A., Lu, X., Surdulescu, G. L., Swaminathan, R., Spector, T. D., & Aviv, A. (2007). Higher serum vitamin D concentrations are associated with longer leukocyte telomere length in women. *The American Journal of Clinical Nutrition* 86 (5), 1420–25. doi.org/10.1093/ajcn/86.5.1420.

6 Zhu, H., Manson, J. E., Cook, N. R., Bekele, B. B., Chen, L., Kane, K. J., Huang, Y., Li, W., Christen, W., Lee, I. M., & Dong, Y. (2025). Vitamin D3 and marine ω-3 fatty acids supplementation and leukocyte telomere length: 4-year findings from the VITamin D and OmegA-3 TriaL (VITAL) randomized controlled trial. *The American Journal of Clinical Nutrition* 122(1), 39–47. doi.org/10.1016/j.ajcnut.2025.05.003.

7 Vaidya, A., Sun, B., Larson, M., et al. (2012). Vitamin D, parathyroid hormone, and risk of incident cardiovascular disease: the Framingham Offspring Study. *Arteriosclerosis, Thrombosis, and Vascular Biology* 32 (11), 2748–54.

8 Zarei, M., Zarezadeh, M., Hamedi Kalajahi, F., & Javanbakht, M. H. (2021). The relationship between vitamin D and telomere/telomerase: A comprehensive review. *The Journal of Frailty & Aging* 10(1), 2–9. doi.org/10.14283/jfa.2020.33.

9 Pearl, R. (1928). *The rate of living: Being an account of some experimental studies on the biology of life duration*. Alfred A. Knopf. https://archive.org/details/rateoflivingbein0000pearl.

10 Kleiber, M. (1961). *The fire of life: An introduction to animal energetics*. John Wiley & Sons. https://www.google.com/books/edition/The_Fire_of_Life/XW5RAAAAMAAJ.

11 Haussmann, M. F., Winkler, D. W., O'Reilly, K. M., Huntington, C. E., Nisbet, I. C. T., & Vleck, C. M. (2003). Telomeres shorten more slowly in long-lived birds and mammals than in short-lived ones. *Proceedings of the Royal Society B: Biological Sciences* 270 (1522), 1387–92. doi.org/10.1098/rspb.2003.2385.

12 Haussmann, M. F., Winkler, D. W., Huntington, C. E., Nisbet, I. C., Vleck, C. M. (2004). Telomerase expression is differentially regulated in birds of differing life span. *Annals of the New York Academy of Sciences.* 1019, 186–90. doi.org/10.1196/annals.1297.029. PMID: 15247011.

13 Bikle D. D. (2011). Vitamin D: an ancient hormone. *Experimental Dermatology* 20(1), 7–13. doi.org/10.1111/j.1600-0625.2010.01202.x

14 Hayflick, L., & Moorhead, P. S. (1961). The serial cultivation of human diploid cell strains. *Experimental Cell Research* 25, 585–621. doi.org/10.1016/0014-4827(61)90192-6.

## Chapter 20

1 Bals, R., & Wilson, J. M. (2003). Cathelicidins—a family of multifunctional antimicrobial peptides. *Cellular and Molecular Life Sciences* 60 (4), 711–20. doi.org/10.1007/s00018-003-2159-5.

2 Liu, P. T., Stenger, S., Li, H., et al. (2006). Toll-like receptor triggering of a vitamin D-mediated human antimicrobial response. *Science* 311 (5768), 1770–73. doi.org/10.1126/science.1123933

3 Gombart, A. F. (2009). The vitamin D-antimicrobial peptide pathway and its role in protection against infection. *Future Microbiology* 4 (9), 1151–65. doi.org/10.2217/fmb.09.78.

4 Holick, M. F. (2004). Sunlight and vitamin D for bone health and prevention of autoimmune diseases, cancers, and cardiovascular disease. *The American Journal of Clinical Nutrition* 80 (6 Suppl), 1678S–1688S. doi.org/10.1093/ajcn/80.6.1678S.

5 Tamerius, J. D., Shaman, J., Alonso, W. J., Bloom-Feshbach, K., Uejio, C. K., Comrie, A., & Viboud, C. (2013). Environmental predictors of seasonal influenza epidemics across temperate and tropical climates. *PLoS Pathogens* 9 (3), e1003194. doi.org/10.1371/journal.ppat.1003194.

6 Chen, S., Prettner, K., Kuhn, M., Geldsetzer, P., Wang, C., Bärnighausen, T., & Bloom, D. E. (2021). COVID-19 and climate: global evidence from 117 countries. *Scientific Reports* 11 (1), 8616. doi.org/10.1038/s41598-021-87692-z.

7 Tushabe F. (2020). Comparison of COVID-19 Severity Between Tropical and Non-Tropical Countries. *International Journal of Infection* 7(3):e104142. doi.org/10.5812/iji.104142.

8 Supple, W. F. (2020). Preventing a Possible Second Deadlier Wave of COVID-19 in Fall. April, 27, 2020. (accessed August 18, 2025). https://www.theepochtimes.com/health/preventing-a-possible-second-deadlier-wave-of-covid-19-in-fall-3312731.

9 Nielsen, N. M., Brix, S., Rostgaard, K., et al. (2022). Vitamin D status and severity of COVID-19. *Scientific Reports* 12 (1), 19823. doi.org/10.1038/s41598-022-21513-9.

10 Bae, J. H., & Kim, Y. (2022). Vitamin D and COVID-19: a narrative review. *Reviews in Endocrine & Metabolic Disorders* 23 (3), 579–99. doi.org/10.1007/s11154-021-09705-6.

11 Alessandria, M., Malatesta, G. M., Berrino, F., & Donzelli, A. (2024). A Critical Analysis of All-Cause Deaths during COVID-19 Vaccination in an Italian Province. *Microorganisms* 12(7), 1343. doi.org/10.3390/microorganisms12071343.

12 Zywiec, A., Hulscher, N., Thorp, J. et al. (2025). COVID-19 Injections: Harms and damages, a non-exhaustive conclusion. *Journal of American Physicians and Surgeons* 30(3), 80–89. https://jpands.org/vol30no3/zywiec.pdf.

13 Centers for Disease Control and Prevention (CDC). (2023). Past Seasons Vaccine Effectiveness Estimates. U.S. Department of Health & Human Services. Retrieved from https://www.cdc.gov/flu/vaccines-work/past-seasons-estimates.html.

14 Shrestha, N. K., Burke, P. C., Nowacki, A. S. & Gordon, S. M. (2025). Effectiveness of the Influenza Vaccine During the 2024–2025 Respiratory Viral Season: A Prospective Cohort Study.*medRxiv* 2025.01.30.25321421. doi.org/10.1101/2025.01.30.25321421.

15 Muir, S. W., & Montero-Odasso, M. (2011). Effect of vitamin D supplementation on muscle strength, gait and balance in older adults: a systematic review and meta-analysis. *Journal of the American Geriatrics Society* 59 (12), 2291–2300. doi.org/10.1111/j.1532-5415.2011.03733.x.

## Chapter 21

1 Cannell, J. J., Hollis, B. W., Sorenson, M. B., Taft, T. N., & Anderson, J. J. (2009). Athletic performance and vitamin D. *Medicine and Science in Sports and Exercise* 41(5), 1102–10. doi.org/10.1249/MSS.0b013e3181930c2b.

2 Cannell, J. J., Hollis, B. W., Sorenson, M. B., Taft, T. N., & Anderson, J. J. (2009). Athletic performance and vitamin D. *Medicine and Science in Sports and Exercise* 41(5), 1102–10. doi.org/10.1249/MSS.0b013e3181930c2b.

3 Cannell, J. J., Hollis, B. W., Sorenson, M. B., Taft, T. N., & Anderson, J. J. (2009). Athletic performance and vitamin D. *Medicine and Science in Sports and Exercise* 41(5), 1102–10. doi.org/10.1249/MSS.0b013e3181930c2b.

4 Holway, John B. *The Baseball Astrologer: And Other Weird Tales*. Total/Sports Illustrated, 2000.

5 Spira, G. (2008). The Boys of Late Summer: Why do so many pro baseball players have August birthdays? *Slate*, April 16, 2008. (Accessed August 17, 2025). https://slate.com/culture/2008/04/why-do-so-many-pro-baseball-players-have-august-birthdays.html.

6 Joyner, M. J., Carter, R. E., & Löllgen, H. (2020). Born versus made: a new look at the nature vs nurture debate in athletes. *The Journal of Physiology* 598(12), 2311–13. doi.org/10.1113/JP279761.

7 Farrokhyar, F., Tabasinejad, R., Dao, D., Peterson, D., Ayeni, O. R., Hadioonzadeh, R., & Bhandari, M. (2015). Prevalence of vitamin D inadequacy in athletes: a systematic review and meta-analysis. *Sports Medicine* 45(3), 365–78. doi.org/10.1007/s40279-014-0267-6.

8 Bischoff, H. A., Borchers, M., Gudat, F., Duermueller, U., Theiler, R., Stähelin, H. B., & Dick, W. (2001). In situ detection of 1,25-dihydroxyvitamin D3 receptor in human skeletal muscle tissue. *Histochemical Journal* 33(1), 19–24. doi.org/10.1023/a:1011018602603.

9 Sato, Y., Iwamoto, J., Kanoko, T., & Satoh, K. (2005). Low-dose vitamin D prevents muscular atrophy and reduces falls and hip fractures in women after stroke: a randomized controlled trial. *Cerebrovascular Diseases* 20(3), 187–92. doi.org/10.1159/000087201.

10 Gollnick, P. D., Armstrong, R. B., Saubert, C. W., 4th, Piehl, K., & Saltin, B. (1972). Enzyme activity and fiber composition in skeletal muscle of untrained and trained men. *Journal of Applied Physiology* 33(3), 312–19. doi.org/10.1152/jappl.1972.33.3.312.

11 Gollnick, P. D., Armstrong, R. B., Saltin, B., Saubert, C. W., 4th, Sembrowich, W. L., & Shepherd, R. E. (1973). Effect of training on enzyme activity and fiber composition of human skeletal muscle. *Journal of Applied Physiology* 34(1), 107–11. doi.org/10.1152/jappl.1973.34.1.107.

12 Olsson, K., Saini, A., Strömberg, A., Alam, S., Lilja, M., Rullman, E., & Gustafsson, T. (2016). Evidence for Vitamin D Receptor Expression and direct effects of 1α,25(OH)2D3 in human skeletal muscle precursor cells. *Endocrinology* 157(1), 98–111. doi.org/10.1210/en.2015-1661.

13 Garcia, L. A., King, K. K., & Ferrini, M. G. (2011). 1,25(OH)2D3 stimulates mechanistically-distinct pathways of protein synthesis in C2C12 skeletal muscle cells. *The Journal of Steroid Biochemistry and Molecular Biology* 127(3-5), 331–36. doi.org/10.1016/j.jsbmb.2011.07.009.

14 Dhesi, J. K., Jackson, S. H., Bearne, L. M., Moniz, C., Hurley, M. V., Swift, C. G., & Allain, T. J. (2004). Vitamin D supplementation improves neuromuscular function in older people who fall. *Age and Ageing* 33(6), 589–95. doi.org/10.1093/ageing/afh178.

15 Grant, W. B., Lahore, H., & Rockwell, M. S. (2020). The Benefits of Vitamin D Supplementation for Athletes: Better Performance and Reduced Risk of COVID-19. *Nutrients* 12(12), 3741. doi.org/10.3390/nu12123741.

16 Forney, L. A., Earnest, C. P., Henagan, T. M., Johnson, L. E., Castleberry, T. J., & Stewart, L. K. (2014). Vitamin D and skeletal muscle: a review of molecular mechanisms. *Journal of the American College of Nutrition* 33(2), 143–52. doi.org/10.1080/07315724.2013.844353.

17 Sikora-Klak, J., Narvy, S. J., Yang, J., Makhni, E., Kharrazi, F. D., & Mehran, N. (2018). The Effect of Abnormal Vitamin D Levels in Athletes. *The Permanente Journal* 22, 17–216. doi.org/10.7812/TPP/17-216.

18 Aranow, C. (2011). Vitamin D and the immune system. *Journal of Investigative Medicine* 59(6), 881–86. doi.org/10.2310/JIM.0b013e31821b8755.

19 Sikora-Klak, J., Narvy, S. J., Yang, J., Makhni, E., Kharrazi, F. D., & Mehran, N. (2018). The Effect of Abnormal Vitamin D Levels in Athletes. *The Permanente Journal* 22, 17–216. doi.org/10.7812/TPP/17-216.

20 Grant, W. B., Lahore, H., & Rockwell, M. S. (2020). The Benefits of Vitamin D Supplementation for Athletes: Better Performance and Reduced Risk of COVID-19. *Nutrients* 12(12), 3741. doi.org/10.3390/nu12123741.

21 Vitamin D Council. (2010). The Chicago Blackhawks are the first vitamin D team in modern professional sports history. https://www.prnewswire.com/news-releases/the-chicago-blackhawks-are-the-first-vitamin-d-team-in-modern-professional-sports-history-95041864.html. Accessed September 10, 2025.

## Chapter 22

1 Harman, D. (1972). The biologic clock: the mitochondria? *Journal of the American Geriatrics Society* 20 (4), 145–47. doi.org/10.1111/j.1532-5415.1972.tb00787.x.

2 Jeffery, G., Fosbury, R., Barrett, E., Hogg, C., Carmona, M. R., & Powner, M. B. (2025). Longer wavelengths in sunlight pass through the human body and have a systemic impact which improves vision. *Scientific Reports* 15 (1), 24435. doi.org/10.1038/s41598-025-09785-3.

3 Jeffery, G., Fosbury, R., Barrett, E., Hogg, C., Carmona, M. R., & Powner, M. B. (2025). Longer wavelengths in sunlight pass through the human body and have a systemic impact which improves vision. *Scientific Reports* 15 (1), 24435. doi.org/10.1038/s41598-025-09785-3.

4 Wider, J. M., Gruley, E., Morse, P. T., Wan, J., Lee, I., Anzell, A. R., Fogo, G. M., Mathieu, J., Hish, G., O'Neil, B., Neumar, R. W., Przyklenk, K., Hüttemann, M., & Sanderson, T. H. (2023).

Modulation of mitochondrial function with near-infrared light reduces brain injury in a translational model of cardiac arrest. *Critical Care* 27 (1), 491. doi.org/10.1186/s13054-023-04745-7.

5 Wider, J. M., Gruley, E., Morse, P. T., Wan, J., Lee, I., Anzell, A. R., Fogo, G. M., Mathieu, J., Hish, G., O'Neil, B., Neumar, R. W., Przyklenk, K., Hüttemann, M., & Sanderson, T. H. (2023). Modulation of mitochondrial function with near-infrared light reduces brain injury in a translational model of cardiac arrest. *Critical Care* 27 (1), 491. doi.org/10.1186/s13054-023-04745-7.

6 Matta Reddy, A., Iqbal, M., Chopra, H., Urmi, S., Junapudi, S., Bibi, S., Kumar Gupta, S., Nirmala Pangi, V., Singh, I., & Abdel-Daim, M. M. (2022). Pivotal role of vitamin D in mitochondrial health, cardiac function, and human reproduction. *EXCLI Journal* 21, 967–90. doi.org/10.17179/excli2022-4935.

7 Latham, C. M., Brightwell, C. R., et al. (2021). Vitamin D Promotes Skeletal Muscle Regeneration and Mitochondrial Health. *Frontiers in Physiology*, 12, 660498. doi.org/10.3389/fphys.2021.660498.

## Chapter 23

1 Brody, J. E. (2013). Cycling Is the Top Sport for Head Injuries. *The New York Times Well Blog*, June 3, 2013. https://archive.nytimes.com/well.blogs.nytimes.com/2013/06/03/really-the-claim-cycling-is-the-top-sport-for-head-injuries/ Accessed September 15, 2025.

2 Storelli Sports. (n.d.). Soccer concussion rates vs. other sports. *The Storelli Blog.* https://storelli.com/blogs/the-storelli-blog/soccer-concussion-rates-vs-other-sports.

3 Ferdman, R. (2023). Diagnosis of CTE increases with each year of ice hockey play. *Neurology Advisor.* https://www.neurologyadvisor.com/news/diagnosis-of-cte-increases-with-each-year-of-ice-hockey-play/.

4 Maroon, J. C., Mathyssek, C. M., Bost, J. W., Amos, A., Winkelman, R., Yates, A. P., Duca, M. A., & Norwig, J. A. (2015). Vitamin D profile in National Football League players. *The American Journal of Sports Medicine* 43 (5), 1241–45. doi.org/10.1177/0363546514567297.

5 Scuderi, G. (2012, March 25). Significantly lower levels of vitamin D found in NFL players with muscle injuries. *Healio.* https://www.healio.com/news/orthopedics/20120325/significantly-lower-levels-of-vitamin-d-found-in-nfl-players-with-muscle-injuries.

6 Giza, C. & Hovda, D. (2014). The new neurometabolic cascade of concussion. *Neurosurgery* 75(04), S24–S33, 10.1227/NEU.0000000000000505.

7 Weber J. T. (2012). Altered calcium signaling following traumatic brain injury. *Frontiers in Pharmacology* 3, 60. doi.org/10.3389/fphar.2012.00060.

8 Karve, I. P., Taylor, J. M., & Crack, P. J. (2016). The contribution of astrocytes and microglia to traumatic brain injury. *British Journal of Pharmacology* 173(4), 692–702. https:/doi.org/10.1111/bph.13125.

9 Nguyen, R. H., Newton, M., Kratofil, R. M., et al. (2025). Imaging a concussion and the ensuing immune response at the blood-brain barrier. *Proc. Natl. Acad. Sci. U.S.A.* 122 (21) e2414316122, doi.org/10.1073/pnas.2414316122.

10 Chahin, M., Mutschler, J., Dzhuleva, S. P., Dieterle, C., Jimenez, L. R., Bhattarai, S. R., Van Steenbergen, V., & Bareyre, F. M. (2025). Repetitive concussions promote microglia-mediated engulfment of presynaptic excitatory input associated with cognitive dysfunction. *Communications Biology* 8(1), 335.

11 Cekic, M., & Stein, D. G. (2010). Traumatic brain injury and aging: is a combination of progesterone and vitamin D hormone a simple solution to a complex problem? *Neurotherapeutics : The Journal of the American Society for Experimental NeuroTherapeutics* 7 (1), 81–90. doi.org/10.1016/j.nurt.2009.10.017.

12 Sailike, B., Onzhanova, Z., Akbay, B., Tokay, T., & Molnár, F. (2024). Vitamin D in Central Nervous System: Implications for Neurological Disorders. *International Journal of Molecular Sciences* 25(14), 7809. doi.org/10.3390/ijms25147809.

13 Cekic, M., Sayeed, I., & Stein, D. G. (2009). Combination treatment with progesterone and vitamin D hormone may be more effective than monotherapy for nervous system injury and disease. *Frontiers in Neuroendocrinology* 30 (2), 158–72. doi.org/10.1016/j.yfrne.2009.03.004.

14 Cekic, M., Sayeed, I., & Stein, D. G. (2009). Combination treatment with progesterone and vitamin D hormone may be more effective than monotherapy for nervous system injury and disease. *Frontiers in Neuroendocrinology* 30 (2), 1572. doi.org/10.1016/j.yfrne.2009.03.004.

15 Vitamin D Council. (n.d.). Concussion. Vitamin D Wiki. Retrieved from https://vitamindwiki.com/tiki-index.php?page_id=3031. Accessed September 10, 2025.

16 Stein, D. G., & Cekic, M. (2009). Combination treatment with progesterone and vitamin D hormone may be more effective than monotherapy for nervous system injury and disease. *Frontiers in Neuroendocrinology* 30(2), 158–72. doi.org/10.1016/j.yfrne.2009.03.004.

17 Cekic, M., Sayeed, I., & Stein, D. G. (2009). Combination treatment with progesterone and vitamin D hormone may be more effective than monotherapy for nervous system injury and disease. *Frontiers in Neuroendocrinology* 30 (2), 158–72. doi.org/10.1016/j.yfrne.2009.03.004.

18 Masbough, F., Kouchek, M., Koosha, M., Salarian, S., Miri, M., Raoufi, M., Taherpour, N., Amniati, S., & Sistanizad, M. (2024). Investigating the Effect of High-Dose Vitamin D3 Administration on Inflammatory Biomarkers in Patients with Moderate to Severe Traumatic Brain Injury: A Randomized Clinical Trial. *Iranian Journal of Medical Sciences* 49(10), 643–51. doi.org/10.30476/ijms.2023.99465.3156.

## Chapter 24

1 National Center for Health Statistics. (2016). *Health, United States, 2015: With Special Feature on Racial and Ethnic Health Disparities.* Hyattsville, MD: National Center for Health Statistics. PMID: 27367098.

2 Ramos, P. S., A. M. Shedlock, and C. D. Langefeld. (2015). Genetics of Autoimmune Diseases: Insights from Population Genetics. *Journal of Human Genetics* 60 (11), 657–64. doi.org/10.1038/jhg.2015.94.

3 Williams, D. R. (2012). Miles to Go before We Sleep: Racial Inequities in Health. *Journal of Health and Social Behavior* 53 (3), 279–95. PMID: 22864072.

4 Colen, C. G., D. M. Ramey, E. C. Cooksey, and D. R. Williams. (2018). Racial Disparities in Health among Nonpoor African Americans and Hispanics: The Role of Acute and Chronic Discrimination. *Social Science & Medicine* 199, 167–80. PMID: 28571900.

5 Jablonski, N. G., and G. Chaplin. (2000). The Evolution of Human Skin Coloration. *Journal of Human Evolution* 39 (1), 57–106. PMID: 10896812.

6 Brenner, M., and V. J. Hearing. (2008). The Protective Role of Melanin against UV Damage in Human Skin. *Photochemistry and Photobiology* 84 (3), 539–49. doi.org/10.1111/j.1751-1097.2007.00226.x.

7 Halder, R. M., and K. M. Bang. (1988). Skin Cancer in Blacks in the United States. *Dermatologic Clinics* 6 (3), 397–405. PMID: 3042295.

8 Bianconi, E., A. Piovesan, F. Facchin, A. Beraudi, R. Casadei, F. Frabetti, … S. Canaider. (2013). An Estimation of the Number of Cells in the Human Body. *Annals of Human Biology* 40 (6), 463–71. doi.org/10.3109/03014460.2013.807878.

9 Lucock, M., C. Martin, and B. Tracey. (2015). Vitamin D: Beyond Metabolism. *Journal of Evidence-Based Complementary & Alternative Medicine* 20 (4), 310–22. doi.org/10.1177/2156587215580491.

10 Clemens, T. L., I. K. Henderson, J. S. Adams, and M. F. Holick. (1982). Increased Skin Pigment Reduces the Capacity of Skin to Synthesise Vitamin D3. *The Lancet* 1 (8263), 74–76. PMID: 6119494.

11 Ginde, A. A., M. C. Liu, and C. A. Camargo. (2009). Demographic Differences and Trends of Vitamin D Insufficiency in the US Population, 1988–2004. *Archives of Internal Medicine* 169 (6), 626–32. doi.org/10.1001/archinternmed.2008.604.

12 Weisberg, P., K. S. Scanlon, R. Li, and M. E. Cogswell. (2004). Nutritional Rickets among Children in the United States: Review of Cases Reported between 1986 and 2003. *American Journal of Clinical Nutrition* 80 (6), 1697S–1705S. doi.org/10.1093/ajcn/80.6.1697S.

13 American Heart Association. (2020). Heart Disease Risk Profiles Differ Widely among African Americans, Blacks from the Caribbean and African Immigrants. Abstract 08, *EPI | Lifestyle 2020 Scientific Sessions*, March 3–6, 2020. *Circulation* 141 (Suppl_1). AP008.

14 Wolf, S. T., and W. L. Kenney. (2019). The Vitamin D-Folate Hypothesis in Human Vascular Health. *American Journal of Physiology-Regulatory, Integrative and Comparative Physiology* 317 (3). R491–R501. doi.org/10.1152/ajpregu.00030.2019.

15 Adebajo, A. O. (1997). Low Frequency of Autoimmune Disease in Tropical Africa. *The Lancet* 349 (9048), 361–62. doi.org/10.1016/S0140-6736(05)62867-X.

16 Feairheller, D. L., S. R. Sturgeon, P. Veerabhadrappa, and M. D. Brown. (2011). Racial Differences in Oxidative Stress and Inflammation: In Vitro and In Vivo. *Clinical and Translational Science* 4 (1), 32–37. doi.org/10.1111/j.1752-8062.2011.00264.x.

17 Hansson, G. K. (2005). Inflammation, Atherosclerosis, and Coronary Artery Disease. *New England Journal of Medicine* 352 (16), 1685–95. PMID: 15843673.

18 Harrison, D. G., A. Vinh, H. Lob, and M. S. Madhur. (2010). Role of the Adaptive Immune System in Hypertension. *Current Opinion in Pharmacology* 10 (2), 203–7. doi.org/10.1016/j.coph.2009.11.003.

19 Bischoff-Ferrari, H. A., E. Giovannucci, W. C. Willett, T. Dietrich, and B. Dawson-Hughes. (2006). Estimation of Optimal Serum Concentrations of 25-Hydroxyvitamin D for Multiple Health Outcomes. *American Journal of Clinical Nutrition* 84 (1), 18–28. doi.org/10.1093/ajcn/84.1.18.

20 Holick, M. F. (2007). Vitamin D Deficiency. *New England Journal of Medicine* 357 (3): 266–81. doi.org/10.1056/NEJMra070553.

21 Committee on Understanding and Eliminating Racial and Ethnic Disparities in Health Care, Institute of Medicine. (2002). *Unequal Treatment: Confronting Racial and Ethnic Disparities in Health Care.* Washington, DC: National Academies Press.

22 Perry, T. (2020). Tyler Perry Is Encouraging Black People to Increase Their Vitamin D during the COVID-19 Pandemic. *Black Enterprise*, April 14, 2020. https://www.blackenterprise.com/tyler-perry-is-encouraging-black-people-to-increase-their-vitamin-d-during-the-covid-19-pandemic/.

23 MacDorman, M. F., and T. J. Mathews. (2008). Recent Trends in Infant Mortality in the United States. *NCHS Data Brief* 9, 1–8. PMID: 19388836.

24 Martin, J. A., B. E. Hamilton, P. D. Sutton, S. J. Ventura, F. Menacker, S. Kirmeyer, and T. J. Mathews. (2009). Births: Final Data for 2006. *National Vital Statistics Reports* 57 (7), 1–104. PMID: 19133442.

25 Eskenazi, B., L. Fenster, and S. Sidney. (1991). A Multivariate Analysis of Risk Factors for Preeclampsia. *JAMA* 266 (2), 237–41. PMID: 2056637.

26 MacKay, A. P., C. J. Berg, and H. K. Atrash. (2001). Pregnancy-Related Mortality from Preeclampsia and Eclampsia. *Obstetrics & Gynecology* 97 (4), 533–38. PMID: 11291054

27 Zhang, J., S. Meikle, and A. Trumble. (2003). Severe Maternal Morbidity Associated with Hypertensive Disorders in Pregnancy in the United States. *Hypertension in Pregnancy* 22 (2), 203–12. PMID: 12938743.

28 Diaz, L., N. Noyola-Martinez, D. Barrera, G. Hernandez, E. Avila, A. Halhali, and F. Larrea. (2009). Calcitriol Inhibits TNF-Alpha-Induced Inflammatory Cytokines in Human Trophoblasts. *Journal of Reproductive Immunology* 81 (1), 17–24. PMID: 19410313

29 Gilani, S., & Janssen, P. (2020). Maternal vitamin D levels during pregnancy and their effects on maternal-fetal outcomes: A systematic review. *Journal of Obstetrics and Gynaecology Canada* 42(9), 1129–37. doi.org/10.1016/j.jogc.2019.09.013.

30 Bodnar, L. M., and H. N. Simhan. (2010). Vitamin D May Be a Link to Black-White Disparities in Adverse Birth Outcomes. *Reviews in Obstetrics and Gynecology* 3 (2), 77–81. PMID: 21060938.

31 Benjamin, E. J., S. S. Virani, C. W. Callaway, A. R. Chamberlain, A. R. Chang, S. Cheng, . . . P. Muntner. (2017). Heart Disease and Stroke Statistics—2017 Update: A Report from the American Heart Association. *Circulation* 135 (10). e146–603. doi.org/10.1161/CIR.0000000000000485.

32 Naseem, K. M. (2005). The Role of Nitric Oxide in Cardiovascular Diseases. *Molecular Aspects of Medicine* 26 (1–2), 33–65. doi.org/10.1016/j.mam.2004.09.003.

33 Wolf, S. T., and W. L. Kenney. (2019). The Vitamin D-Folate Hypothesis in Human Vascular Health. *American Journal of Physiology-Regulatory, Integrative and Comparative Physiology* 317 (3). R491–R501. doi.org/10.1152/ajpregu.00030.2019.

34 Forman, J. P., J. B. Scott, K. Ng, B. F. Drake, M. R. Denburg, J. Garry, … M. F. Holick. (2013). Effect of Vitamin D Supplementation on Blood Pressure in Blacks. *Hypertension* 61 (4), 779–85. doi .org/10.1161/HYPERTENSIONAHA.111.00659.

35 Thebault, R. (2020). The Coronavirus Is Infecting and Killing Black Americans at an Alarmingly High Rate. *The Washington Post*, April 7, 2020. https://www.washingtonpost.com/nation/2020/04/07 /coronavirus-is-infecting-killing-black-americans-an-alarmingly-high-rate-post-analysis-shows/.

36 Richardson, S., J. S. Hirsch, M. Narasimhan, J. M. Crawford, T. McGinn, K. W. Davidson, . . . T. P. Zanos. (2020). Presenting Characteristics, Comorbidities, and Outcomes among 5700

Patients Hospitalized with COVID-19 in the New York City Area. *JAMA* 323 (20), 2052–62. doi.org/10.1001/jama.2020.6775.

37 Rhodes, J. M., S. Subramanian, E. Laird, and R. A. Kenny. (2020). Low Population Mortality from COVID-19 in Countries South of Latitude 35 Degrees North Supports Vitamin D as a Factor Determining Severity. *Alimentary Pharmacology & Therapeutics* 51 (10), 1043–49. doi.org/10.1111/apt.15777.

## Chapter 25

1 American Heart Association. (1970). Diet and heart disease. *Circulation* 42(5), 977–81.

2 Keys, A. (1970). Coronary heart disease in seven countries. *Circulation* 41(Suppl 1), 1–211.

3 Jacobson, R. (2019, May 21). Is Sunscreen the New Margarine? *Outside* Magazine. https://www.outsideonline.com/health/wellness/sunscreen-sun-exposure-skin-cancer-science/.

4 Patterson, J. W. (2021). *Weedon's Skin Pathology* (5th ed.). Elsevier.

5 Gracia-Darder, I., Carrera, C., Alamon-Reig, F., Puig, S., Malvehy, J., & Podlipnik, S. (2022). Vitamin D deficiency in melanoma patients is associated with worse overall survival: a retrospective cohort study. *Melanoma Research* 32 (5), 384–87. doi.org/10.1097/CMR.0000000000000842.

6 Timerman, D., McEnery-Stonelake, M., Joyce, C. J., Nambudiri, V. E., Hodi, F. S., Claus, E. B., & Ibrahim, N. (2017). Vitamin D deficiency is associated with a worse prognosis in metastatic melanoma. *Oncotarget* 8 (5), 6873–6882. doi.org/10.18632/oncotarget.14022.

7 Ombra, M. N., Paliogiannis, P., Doneddu, V., Sini, M. C., Colombino, M., Rozzo, C., . . . & Palmieri, G. (2017). Vitamin D status and risk for malignant cutaneous melanoma: recent advances. *European Journal of Cancer Prevention* 26 (6), 532–41. doi.org/10.1097/CEJ.0000000000000334.

8 Lindqvist, P. G., Epstein, E., Nielsen, K., Landin-Olsson, M., Ingvar, C., & Olsson, H. (2016). Avoidance of sun exposure as a risk factor for major causes of death: a competing risk analysis of the Melanoma in Southern Sweden cohort. *Journal of Internal Medicine* 280 (4), 375–87. doi.org/10.1111/joim.12496.

9 Matta, M. K., Florian, J., Zusterzeel, R., Pamer, M., Patel, V., Sarin, L., . . . & Strauss, D. G. (2020). Effect of sunscreen application on plasma concentration of sunscreen active ingredients: A randomized clinical trial. *JAMA* 323 (3), 256–67. doi.org/10.1001/jama.2019.20747.

10 Ruszkiewicz, J. A., Pinkas, A., Ferrer, B., Peres, T. V., Tsatsakis, A., & Aschner, M. (2017). Neurotoxic effect of active ingredients in sunscreen products, a contemporary review. *Toxicology Reports*, 4, 245–59. doi.org/10.1016/j.toxrep.2017.05.006.

11 Hiller, J., Klotz, K. & Meyer, S, (2019). Systemic Availability of Lipophilic Organic UV Filters through Dermal Sunscreen Exposure. *Environment International* 132. 105068. doi.org/10.1016/j.envint.2019.105068.

12 Matsuoka, Y., et al. (2019). Effect of sunscreen application on plasma concentrations of common sunscreen ingredients: a randomized clinical trial. *JAMA* 321 (21), 2088–96. doi.org/10.1001/jama.2019.5232.

13 Matsuoka, Y., et al. (2020). Effect of sunscreen application on plasma concentrations of 12 systemically absorbed active ingredients: A randomized clinical trial. *JAMA* 323 (3), 257–67. doi.org/10.1001/jama.2019.20747.

14 Matsuoka, Y., et al. (2019). Effect of sunscreen application on plasma concentrations of common sunscreen ingredients: a randomized clinical trial. *JAMA* 321 (21), 2088–96. doi.org/10.1001/jama.2019.5232.

15 Calafat, A. M., Ye, X., Wong, L.-Y., Reidy, J. A., & Needham, L. L. (2008). Concentrations of the sunscreen agent benzophenone-3 in urine from the U.S. population: 2003–2004. *Environmental Health Perspectives*, 116 (7), 893–97. doi.org/10.1289/ehp.11261.

16 Klammer, H., Böhme, J., & Witte, I. (2004). Enhancement of genotoxicity of the herbicide 2,4-D by its mixture with sunscreen agent oxybenzone. *Toxicology and Applied Pharmacology* 195 (3), 332–37. doi.org/10.1016/j.taap.2003.11.011.

17 Matsuoka, Y., et al. (2019). Effect of sunscreen application on plasma concentrations of common sunscreen ingredients: a randomized clinical trial. *JAMA* 321 (21), 2088–96. doi.org/10.1001/jama.2019.5232.

18 Matsuoka, Y., et al. (2020). Effect of sunscreen application on plasma concentrations of 12 systemically absorbed active ingredients: A randomized clinical trial. *JAMA* 323 (3), 257–67. doi.org/10.1001/jama.2019.20747.
19 Matsuoka, Y., et al. (2020). Effect of sunscreen application on plasma concentrations of 12 systemically absorbed active ingredients: A randomized clinical trial. *JAMA* 323 (3), 257–67. doi.org/10.1001/jama.2019.20747.
20 Chemical Watch. (2019, May 9). FDA report finds high systemic absorption of sunscreen ingredients.
21 Rastogi, S., Singh, A. K., Singh, A., Srivastava, R., Singh, R. P., & Sinha, R. P. (2016). Sunscreens and their phototoxic effects: A review. *Archives of Environmental Contamination and Toxicology* 70 (2), 265–76. doi.org/10.1007/s00244-015-0210-9.
22 Li, M., Zhang, H., Cui, Y., Cao, H., Li, X., Wu, C., … & Zhu, B. (2017). Oxybenzone induces neurotoxicity in vitro and in vivo. *Toxicology Reports* 4, 245–53. doi.org/10.1016/j.toxrep.2017.04.004.
23 Scinicariello, F., Buser, M. C., & Marr, J. S. (2016). Serum concentrations of ultraviolet filters in adolescent boys and their associations with testosterone. *Environmental Health Perspectives* 124 (8), 1279–85. doi.org/10.1289/ehp.1509612.
24 Rodriguez, E., Valls-Ferrer, F., & Alomar, A. (2004). Effects of oxybenzone on human male reproductive hormones. *Journal of Investigative Dermatology* 123 (1), 57–60. doi.org/10.1111/j.0022-202X.2004.22749.x.
25 Jurewicz, J., Radwan, M., Wielgomas, R., & Hanke, W. (2016). Effects of environmental exposure to endocrine disrupting chemicals on semen quality. *Environmental Health Perspectives* 124 (12), 1779–86. doi.org/10.1289/EHP150.
26 Almstrup, K., et al. (2018). Testicular dysgenesis syndrome: potential role of endocrine disrupting chemicals. *Endocrine Connections* 7 (1), R1–R12. doi.org/10.1530/EC-17-0248.
27 Kunisue, T., Chen, Z., Buck Louis, G. M., Sundaram, R., Hediger, M. L., Sun, L., . . . & Kannan, K. (2012). Urinary concentrations of benzophenone-type UV filters in U.S. women and their associations with endometriosis. *Environmental Science & Technology* 45 (8), 4410–16. doi.org/10.1021/es203491e.
28 Philippat, C., et al. (2017). Exposure to phthalates and phenols during pregnancy and fetal growth: A systematic review. *Reproductive Toxicology* 73, 175–89. doi.org/10.1016/j.reprotox.2017.08.016.
29 Matsuoka, Y., et al. (2020). Effect of sunscreen application on plasma concentrations of 12 systemically absorbed active ingredients: A randomized clinical trial. *JAMA* 323 (3), 257–67. doi.org/10.1001/jama.2019.20747.
30 American Academy of Dermatology. (2020). Sunscreen: Your questions answered. *Journal of the American Academy of Dermatology* 2 (17).
31 Donaldson, K., Stone, V., Clift, C., MacNee, W., & Galea, C. (2007). Nanoparticles: A review of current research and implications for occupational health. *Biointerphases* 2 (4), MRN45–MRN58. doi.org/10.1116/1.2783856.
32 Oberdörster, G., Oberdörster, E., & Oberdörster, J. (2007). Nanotoxicology: An emerging discipline evolving from studies of ultrafine particles. *Biointerphases* 2 (4), MR1–MR24. doi.org/10.1116/1.2778738.
33 Donaldson, K., Stone, V., Clift, C., MacNee, W., & Galea, C. (2007). Nanoparticles: A review of current research and implications for occupational health. *Biointerphases* 2 (4), MRN45–MRN58. doi.org/10.1116/1.2783856.
34 International Agency for Research on Cancer (IARC). (2009, June–July). IARC Monographs Volume 93: Carbon Black, Titanium Dioxide, and Talc.
35 Elsayed, N. M. (2021). Metal fume fever. In *Inorganic Compounds* (pp. 53–56). Springer, Champagne . doi.org/10.1007/978-3-030-58133-1_9.
36 Thomas, T., M. Fat, and G. Kearns. (2024). Sunscreens: Potential Hazards to Environmental and Human Health. *Frontiers in Marine Science* 11, 1471574. doi.org/10.3389/fmars.2024.1471574.
37 National Ocean Service. (2021, April 5). Skincare chemicals and coral reefs. National Oceanic and Atmospheric Administration. https://oceanservice.noaa.gov/news/sunscreen-corals.html.
38 Impacts of sunscreens on coral reefs. Government of Sweden: Ministry of the Environment and Energy. https://icriforum.org/wp content/uploads/2019/12/ICRI_Sunscreen_0.pdf.

39 Therapeutic Goods Administration. 2025. *Freedom of Information Release 25-0104*. Canberra: Australian Government Department of Health. https://www.tga.gov.au/sites/default/files/2025-07/FOI 25-0104.pdf.

40 Wood, R. C. (2018). Hawaii's sunscreen ban: An effective but imperfect tool for protecting coral reefs. *Ecology Law Quarterly 45*, 1039–64.


## Chapter 26


1 Maenner, M. J., Warren, Z., Williams, A. R., Amoakohene, B., Bakian, A. V., Bilder, D. A., . . . & Durkin, M. S. (2023). Prevalence and Characteristics of Autism Spectrum Disorder Among Children Aged 8 Years—Autism and Developmental Disabilities Monitoring Network, 11 Sites, United States, 2020. *MMWR Surveillance Summaries* 72 (2), 1–14. https://www.cdc.gov/mmwr/volumes/72/ss/ss7202a1.htm.

2 Grant, W. B., & Soles, C. M. (2009). Epidemiologic evidence supporting the role of maternal vitamin D deficiency as a risk factor for the development of infantile autism. *Dermato-Endocrinology* 1 (4), 223–28. doi.org/10.4161/derm.1.4.9500.

3 Lee, B. K., Gross, R., Francis, R. W., & Fung, S. (2019). Birth seasonality and risk of autism spectrum disorder. *European Journal of Epidemiology* 34, 785–92. doi.org/10.1007/s10654-019-00506-5.

4 Lee, B. K., Gross, R., Francis, R. W., & Fung, S. (2019). Birth seasonality and risk of autism spectrum disorder. *European Journal of Epidemiology* 34, 785–92. doi.org/10.1007/s10654-019-00506-5.

5 Scientific American. (2015). Vitamin D and Autism. https://www.scientificamerican.com/article/vitamin-d-and-autism/.

6 Grant, W. B., & Soles, C. M. (2009). Epidemiologic evidence supporting the role of maternal vitamin D deficiency as a risk factor for the development of infantile autism. *Dermato-Endocrinology* 1 (4), 223–28. doi.org/10.4161/derm.1.4.9500.

7 Wang, Z., Ding, R., & Wang, J. (2020). The Association between Vitamin D Status and Autism Spectrum Disorder (ASD): A Systematic Review and Meta-Analysis. *Nutrients* 13(1), 86. doi.org/10.3390/nu13010086.

8 Wang, T., Shan, L., Du, L., Feng, J., Xu, Z., Staal, W. G., & Jia, F. (2016). Serum concentration of 25-hydroxyvitamin D in autism spectrum disorder: a systematic review and meta-analysis. *European Child & Adolescent Psychiatry* 25(4), 341–50. doi.org/10.1007/s00787-015-0786-1.

9 Buell, J. S., & Dawson-Hughes, B. (2008). Vitamin D and neurocognitive dysfunction: preventing "D"ecline?. *Molecular Aspects of Medicine* 29 (6), 415–22. doi.org/10.1016/j.mam.2008.05.001.

10 Eyles, D. W., Smith, S., Kinobe, R., Hewison, M., & McGrath, J. J. (2005). Distribution of the vitamin D receptor and 1 alpha-hydroxylase in human brain. *Journal of Chemical Neuroanatomy* 29 (1), 21–30. doi.org/10.1016/j.jchemneu.2004.08.006.

11 Voltas, N., Cendra-Duarte, E., Canals, J., & Hernández-Martínez, C. (2025). Vitamin D status during pregnancy and child neurocognitive functioning at 4 Years. *Pediatric Research*. doi.org/10.1038/s41390-025-04258-9.

12 Eyles, D. W. (2021). Vitamin D: Brain and Behavior. *JBMR Plus* 5 (1), e10419. doi.org/10.1002/jbm4.10419.

13 Ye, X., Zhou, Q., Ren, P., Xiang, W., & Xiao, L. (2023). The Synaptic and Circuit Functions of Vitamin D in Neurodevelopment Disorders. *Neuropsychiatric Disease and Treatment* 19, 1515–30. doi.org/10.2147/NDT.S407731.

14 Sudarov, A. (2013). Defining the role of cerebellar Purkinje cells in autism spectrum disorders. *Cerebellum* 12 (6), 950–55. doi.org/10.1007/s12311-013-0490-y.

15 Supple, W. F., Jr., Fanselow, M. S., Leaton, R. N. (1987). Effects of cerebellar vermal lesions on species-specific fear responses, neophobia, and taste- aversion learning in rats. *Physiology & Behavior* 39. 579–86.

16 Leaton, R. N., & Supple, W. F., Jr (1986). Cerebellar vermis: essential for long-term habituation of the acoustic startle response. *Science* 232(4749), 513–15. doi.org/10.1126/science.3961494.

17 Courchesne, E. (2001). Unusual brain growth patterns in early life in patients with autistic disorder: An MRI study. *Neurology* 57 (2), 245–54. doi.org/10.1212/WNL.57.2.245.

18 Supple, W. F., Jr., Fanselow, M. S., Leaton, R. N. (1987). Effects of cerebellar vermal lesions on species-specific fear responses, neophobia, and taste-aversion learning in rats. *Physiology & Behavior* 39, 579–86.

19 Supple W. F., Jr (1993). Hypothalamic modulation of Purkinje cell activity in the anterior cerebellar vermis. *Neuroreport* 4(7), 979–82. doi.org/10.1097/00001756-199307000-00036.
20 Supple, W. F., Jr., Leaton, R. N. (1990a) Cerebellar vermis: essential for classically conditioned bradycardia in rats. *Brain Research* 509, 17–23.
21 Supple, W. F., Jr, Sebastiani, L., & Kapp, B. S. (1993). Purkinje cell responses in the anterior cerebellar vermis during Pavlovian fear conditioning in the rabbit. *Neuroreport* 4(7), 975–78. doi.org/10.1097/00001756-199307000-00035.
22 Fatemi, S. H., Aldinger, K. A., Ashwood, P., Bauman, M. L., Blaha, C. D., Blatt, G. J., . . . & Welsh, J. P. (2012). Consensus paper: pathological role of the cerebellum in autism. *Cerebellum* 11 (3), 777–807. doi.org/10.1007/s12311-012-0355-9.
23 Webb, S. J., Sparks, B. F., Friedman, S. D., Shaw, D. W., Giedd, J., Dawson, G., & Dager, S. R. (2009). Cerebellar vermal volumes and behavioral correlates in children with autism spectrum disorder. *Psychiatry Research* 172 (1), 61–67. doi.org/10.1016/j.pscychresns.2008.06.001.
24 Sudarov, A. (2013). Defining the role of cerebellar Purkinje cells in autism spectrum disorders. *Cerebellum* 12 (6), 950–55. doi.org/10.1007/s12311-013-0490-y.
25 Eyles, D. W., Smith, S., Kinobe, R., Hewison, M., & McGrath, J. J. (2005). Distribution of the vitamin D receptor and 1 alpha-hydroxylase in human brain. *Journal of Chemical Neuroanatomy* 29 (1), 21–30. doi.org/10.1016/j.jchemneu.2004.08.006.
26 Shi, L., Smith, S. E., Malkova, N., Tse, D., Su, Y., & Patterson, P. H. (2009). Activation of the maternal immune system alters cerebellar development in the offspring. *Brain, Behavior, and Immunity* 23 (1), 116–23. doi.org/10.1016/j.bbi.2008.07.012.
27 Pierce, K., & Courchesne, E. (2001). Evidence for a cerebellar role in reduced exploration and stereotyped behavior in autism. *Biological Psychiatry* 49 (8), 655–64. doi.org/10.1016/s0006-3223(00)01008-8.
28 Supple, W. F., Jr., Fanselow, M. S., Leaton, R. N. (1987). Effects of cerebellar vermal lesions on species-specific fear responses, neophobia, and taste-aversion learning in rats. *Physiology & Behavior* 39. 579–86.
29 Jones, W., Hesselink, J., Courchesne, E., Duncan, T., Matsuda, K., & Bellugi, U. (2002). Cerebellar abnormalities in infants and toddlers with Williams syndrome. *Developmental Medicine & Child Neurology* 44 (10), 688–94. doi.org/10.1017/s0012162201002766.
30 Helt, M., Kelley, E., Kinsbourne, M. et al. (2008). Can Children with Autism Recover? If So, How?. *Neuropsychological Reviews* 18, 339–66. doi.org/10.1007/s11065-008-9075-9.
31 Richler, J. (2013). Is It Possible to Recover from Autism? New research says yes, but how to spark recovery remains a mystery. *Scientific American*, July 1, 2013. https://www.scientificamerican.com/article/is-it-possible-to-recover-from-autism/.
32 Sitholey, P., Agarwal, V., & Pargaonkar, A. (2009). Rapid and spontaneous recovery in autistic disorder. *Indian Journal of Psychiatry* 51(3), 209–11. doi.org/10.4103/0019-5545.55092.
33 Intellistarsaba. (n.d.). Is it possible to recover from autism? Retrieved from https://www.intellistarsaba.com/blog/is-it-possible-to-recover-from-autism. Accessed September 10, 2025.
34 Jia, F., Wang, B., Shan, L., Xu, Z., Staal, W. G., & Du, L. (2015). Core Symptoms of Autism Improved After Vitamin D Supplementation. *Pediatrics* 135 (1), e196–e198. doi.org/10.1542/peds.2014-2121.
35 Tian, P., Zhu, X., Liu, Z., & Gao, J. (2025). Effects of vitamin D on brain function in preschool children with autism spectrum disorder: a resting-state functional MRI study. *BMC Psychiatry* 25, 198. doi.org/10.1186/s12888-025-06534-8.
36 Javadfar, Z., Soltani, S., Khamoushi, F., & Zare, F. (2025). Effect of vitamin D supplementation on inflammatory status and behavioral symptoms in children with autism spectrum disorders: a double-blind randomized clinical trial. *BMC Pediatrics* 25, 615. doi.org/10.1186/s12887-025-05985-y.
37 Burne, T. H., Féron, F., Brown, J., Eyles, D. W., McGrath, J. J., & Mackay-Sim, A. (2004). Combined prenatal and chronic postnatal vitamin D deficiency in rats impairs prepulse inhibition of acoustic startle. *Physiology & Behavior* 81 (4), 651–55. doi.org/10.1016/j.physbeh.2004.03.004.
38 Leaton, R. N., & Supple, W. F., Jr (1986). Cerebellar vermis: essential for long-term habituation of the acoustic startle response. *Science* 232(4749), 513–15. doi.org/10.1126/science.3961494.
39 Supple, W. F., Jr, & Kapp, B. S. (1994). Anatomical and physiological relationships between the anterior cerebellar vermis and the pontine parabrachial nucleus in the rabbit. *Brain Research Bulletin* 33(5), 561–74. doi.org/10.1016/0361-9230(94)90082-5.

40 Supple, W. F. Jr (1993). Hypothalamic modulation of Purkinje cell activity in the anterior cerebellar vermis. *Neuroreport* 4(7), 979–82. doi.org/10.1097/00001756-199307000-00036.

## Chapter 27

1 Krause, M., Klit, A., Jensen, M. B., Søeborg, T., Frederiksen, H., Schlumpf, A., . . . & Nielsen, J. B. (2012). Sunscreens: Are they beneficial for health? An overview of endocrine disrupting properties of UV-filters. *International Journal of Andrology* 35 (3), 424–36. doi.org/10.1111/j.1365-2605.2012.01282.x.

2 Matta, M. K., Zusterzeel, R., Pilli, N. R., Patel, V., Volpe, D. A., Florian, H., . . . & Saraceno, L. L. (2019). Effect of sunscreen application on plasma concentration of active ingredients: A randomized clinical trial. *JAMA* 321 (21), 2082–91. doi.org/10.1001/jama.2019.5232.

3 Ruszkiewicz, J. A., Pinkas, A., Ferrer, B., Peres, T. V., Tsatsakis, A., & Aschner, M. (2017). Neurotoxic effect of active ingredients in sunscreen products, a contemporary review. *Toxicology Reports* 4, 245–59. doi.org/10.1016/j.toxrep.2017.05.006.

4 Matta, M. K., Zusterzeel, R., Pilli, N. R., Patel, V., Volpe, D. A., Florian, H., . . . & Saraceno, L. L. (2019). Effect of sunscreen application on plasma concentration of active ingredients: A randomized clinical trial. *JAMA* 321 (21), 2082–91. doi.org/10.1001/jama.2019.5232.

5 Kharrazian D. (2021). Exposure to environmental toxins and autoimmune conditions. *Integrative Medicine* 20(2), 20–24.

6 Sajdel-Sulkowska, E. M., Xu, M., & Koibuchi, N. (2009). Increase in cerebellar neurotrophin-3 and oxidative stress markers in autism. *Cerebellum* 8 (3), 366–72. doi.org/10.1007/s12311-009-0105-9.

7 Schlumpf, M., Cotton, B., Conscience, M., Haller, N., Steinmann, B., & Lichtensteiger, W. (2004). In vitro and in vivo estrogenicity of UV screens. *Environmental Health Perspectives* 112 (13), 1391–1401. doi.org/10.1289/ehp.7050.

8 Garcion, E., Wion-Barbot, N., Montero-Menei, C. N., Berger, F., & Wion, D. (2004). New data on vitamin D and brain development. *Trends in Endocrinology & Metabolism* 15 (1), 30–35. doi .org/10.1016/j.tem.2003.11.003.

9 Eyles, D. W., Burne, T. H., & McGrath, J. J. (2009). Vitamin D in brain development and adult brain function. *Progress in Neurobiology* 88 (2), 115–33. doi.org/10.1016/j.pneurobio.2009.03.003.

10 Dealberto, M. J. (2011). Is vitamin D deficiency a risk factor for autism spectrum disorders? *Medical Hypotheses* 77 (1), 1–7. doi.org/10.1016/j.mehy.2011.03.016.

11 McGrath, J. J., Frayne, J., Herrmann, D., Castle, D., & Green, T. A. (2010). Vitamin D and mental health: Time to review the evidence. *Journal of Steroid Biochemistry and Molecular Biology* 121 (1–2), 176–79. doi.org/10.1016/j.jsbmb.2010.02.015.

12 Loomes, R., Hull, L., & Mandy, W. P. (2017). What is the male-to-female ratio in autism spectrum disorder? A systematic review and meta-analysis. *Journal of the American Academy of Child & Adolescent Psychiatry* 56 (6), 466–74. doi.org/10.1016/j.jaac.2017.03.013.

13 Schlumpf, M., Cotton, B., Conscience, M., Haller, N., Steinmann, B., & Lichtensteiger, W. (2004). In vitro and in vivo estrogenicity of UV screens. *Environmental Health Perspectives* 112 (13), 1391–1401. doi.org/10.1289/ehp.7050.

14 Di Nisio, A., Rocca, M.S., De Toni, L. et al. (2020). Endocrine disruption of vitamin D activity by perfluoro-octanoic acid (PFOA). *Scientific Reports* 10, 16789. doi.org/10.1038/s41598-020-74026-8.

15 Wang, J., Huang, H., Liu, C., Zhang, Y., Wang, W., Zou, Z., Yang, L., He, X., Wu, J., Ma, J., and Liu, Y. (2022). Research Progress on the Role of Vitamin D in Autism Spectrum Disorder. *Frontiers in Behavioral Neuroscience* 16. 859151. doi.org/10.3389/fnbeh.2022.859151.

16 Sajdel-Sulkowska, E. M., Xu, M., & Koibuchi, N. (2009). Increase in cerebellar neurotrophin-3 and oxidative stress markers in autism. *Cerebellum* 8 (3), 366–72. doi.org/10.1007/s12311-009-0105-9.

17 Sotelo, C. (1990). Morphological correlates of Purkinje cell developmental plasticity. *Brain Research Reviews* 15 (2), 133–47. doi.org/10.1016/0165-0170(90)90008-C.

18 Javadfar, Z., Soltani, S., Khamoushi, F., & Zare, F. (2025). Effect of vitamin D supplementation on inflammatory status and behavioral symptoms in children with autism spectrum disorders: a double-blind randomized clinical trial. *BMC Pediatrics* 25, 615. doi.org/10.1186/s12887-025-05985-y.

19 Leaton, R. N., & Supple, W. F., Jr (1986). Cerebellar vermis: essential for long-term habituation of the acoustic startle response. *Science* 232(4749), 513–15. doi.org/10.1126/science.3961494.

20 Amore, G. et al. (2021). A Focus on the Cerebellum: From Embryogenesis to an Age-Related Clinical Perspective. *Frontiers in Systems Neuroscience* 15. doi.org/10.3389/fnsys.2021.646052.

21 Lyu, W., Thung, K. H., Huynh, K. M. et al. (2025). Functional development of the human cerebellum from birth to age five. *Nature Communications* 16, 6350. doi.org/10.1038/s41467-025-61465-y.

22 Bayin, N. S. et al. (2018). Age-dependent dormant resident progenitors are stimulated by injury to regenerate Purkinje neurons. *eLife* 7.e39879. doi.org/10.7554/eLife.39879.

23 Pose-Méndez S., et al. (2023). Lifelong regeneration of cerebellar Purkinje cells after induced cell ablation in zebrafish. *Elife*.12. e79672. doi: 10.7554/eLife.79672.

24 Chen, B., Chen, Y., & Xu, Y. (2021). Vitamin D deficiency in pregnant women: Influenced by multiple risk factors and increase the risks of spontaneous abortion and small-for-gestational age. *Medicine* 100(41), e27505. https:/doi.org/10.1097/MD.0000000000027505.

25 Cekic, M., Sayeed, I., & Stein, D. G. (2009). Combination treatment with progesterone and vitamin D hormone may be more effective than monotherapy for nervous system injury and disease. *Frontiers in Neuroendocrinology* 30 (2), 158–72. doi.org/10.1016/j.yfrne.2009.03.004.


## Chapter 28


1 Zhilong, C., Shuoyu, R., Nanqu, H. et al. (2025). The role of vitamin D in sleep regulation: mechanisms, clinical advances, and future directions. *Frontiers in Nutrition* 12. doi.org/10.3389/fnut.2025.1595813.

2 Eyles, D. W., Liu, P. Y., Josh, P., & Cui, X. (2014). Intracellular distribution of the vitamin D receptor in the brain: comparison with classic target tissues and redistribution with development. *Neuroscience* 268, 1–9. doi.org/10.1016/j.neuroscience.2014.02.042.

3 Zhilong, C., Shuoyu, R., Nanqu, H. et al. (2025). The role of vitamin D in sleep regulation: mechanisms, clinical advances, and future directions. *Frontiers in Nutrition* 12. doi.org/10.3389/fnut.2025.1595813.

4 Maissan, P., & Carlberg, C. (2025). Circadian Regulation of Vitamin D Target Genes Reveals a Network Shaped by Individual Responsiveness. *Nutrients* 17(7), 1204. doi.org/10.3390/nu17071204.

5 Kaneko, I., Sabir, M. S., Dussik, C. M., et al. (2015). 1,25-Dihydroxyvitamin D regulates expression of the tryptophan hydroxylase 2 and leptin genes: implication for behavioral influences of vitamin D. *FASEB Journal: Official Publication of the Federation of American Societies for Experimental Biology* 29(9), 4023–35. doi.org/10.1096/fj.14-269811.

6 Irwin, M.R. Sleep and inflammation: partners in sickness and in health. *Nature Reviews Immunology* 19, 702–15 (2019). doi.org/10.1038/s41577-019-0190-z.

7 Zhilong, C., Shuoyu, R., Nanqu, H. et al. (2025). The role of vitamin D in sleep regulation: mechanisms, clinical advances, and future directions. *Frontiers in Nutrition* 12. doi.org/10.3389/fnut.2025.1595813.

8 Gominak, S. C. & Stumpf, W. E. (2012).The world epidemic of sleep disorders is linked to vitamin D deficiency. *Medical Hypotheses* 79 (2), 132–35. doi.org/10.1016/j.mehy.2012.03.

9 de Oliveira DL, et al. (2021). Sleep duration as an independent factor associated with vitamin D levels in the EPISONO cohort. *Journal of Clinical Sleep Medicine* 17(12), 2439–49.

10 Gao, Q., Kou, T., Zhuang, B., Ren, Y., Dong, X., & Wang, Q. (2018). The Association between Vitamin D Deficiency and Sleep Disorders: A Systematic Review and Meta-Analysis. *Nutrients* 10(10), 1395. doi.org/10.3390/nu10101395.

11 Muscogiuri, G., Barrea, L., Scannapieco, M., Di Somma, C., Scacchi, M., Aimaretti, G., Savastano, S., Colao, A., & Marzullo, P. (2019). The lullaby of the sun: the role of vitamin D in sleep disturbance. *Sleep Medicine* 54, 262–65. doi.org/10.1016/j.sleep.2018.10.033.

12 Okereke, O. I., Reynolds, C.F., et al. (2020). Effect of long-term vitamin D3 supplementation vs placebo on risk of depression or clinically relevant depressive symptoms and on change in mood scores: a randomized clinical trial. *JAMA* 324, 471–80. doi.org/10.1001/jama.2020.10224.

13 Fu, J., Zhang, Y., Chen, X., et al. (2024). Efficacy of vitamin D supplementation on depressive symptoms in older patients: a meta-analysis of randomized controlled trials. *Frontiers in Medicine* 11, 1467234. doi.org/10.3389/fmed.2024.1467234.

14 Jalali, B. R., Moradi, Z., Farajzadeh, M., Mohammadi, Y., & Moayed, M. (2018). The effect of vitamin D supplementation on sleep quality in individuals with sleep disorders: a meta-analysis

of randomized controlled trials. *Journal of Clinical Sleep Medicine* 14(11), 1883–90. https:/doi.org/10.5664/jcsm.7472.

15 Zhilong, C., Shuoyu, R., Nanqu, H. et al. (2025). The role of vitamin D in sleep regulation: mechanisms, clinical advances, and future directions. *Frontiers in Nutrition* 12. doi.org/10.3389/fnut.2025.1595813.

16 Francis, TC, and Porcu, A. Emotionally clocked out: cell-type specific regulation of mood and anxiety by the circadian clock system in the brain. *Frontiers in Molecular Neuroscience* (2023) 16:1188184. doi.org/10.3389/fnmol.2023.1188184.

17 Mirzaei, B., Kazemifar, A. M., Afzali, M., et al. (2015). The effect of vitamin D supplementation on sleep quality in patients with primary sleep disorders and depression: a randomized, double-blind, placebo-controlled clinical trial. Journal of Clinical Psychopharmacology 35(6), 661–65. doi.org/10.1097/JCP.0000000000000378.

18 Foster, R. G., & Kreitzman, L. (2007). *Rhythms of life: The biological clocks that control the daily lives of every living thing.* Yale University Press.

19 Blume, C., Garbazza, C. & Spitschan, M. (2019). Effects of light on human circadian rhythms, sleep and mood. *Somnologie,* 23, 147–56. doi.org/10.1007/s11818-019-00215-x.

20 Ghareghani, M., Zibara, K. & Rivest, S. (2023). Melatonin and vitamin D, two sides of the same coin, better to land on its edge to improve multiple sclerosis. *Proc. Natl. Acad. Sci. U.S.A.* 120 (14) e2219334120, doi.org/10.1073/pnas.2219334120.

21 Minich, D. M., Henning, M., Darley, C., Fahoum, M., Schuler, C. B., & Frame, J. (2022). Is Melatonin the "Next Vitamin D"?: A Review of Emerging Science, Clinical Uses, Safety, and Dietary Supplements. *Nutrients* 14(19), 3934. doi.org/10.3390/nu14193934.

22 Culver, M. N., Linder, B. A., Lyons, D. E., et al. (2025). Do not sleep on vitamin D: vitamin D is associated with sleep variability in apparently healthy adults. *American Journal of Physiology. Regulatory, Integrative and Comparative Physiology* 328(3), R262–R273. https:/doi.org/10.1152/ajpregu.00168.2024.

23 Culver, M. N., Linder, B. A., Lyons, D. E., Hutchison, Z. J., Garrett, C. L., McNeil, J. N., & Robinson, A. T. (2025). Do not sleep on vitamin D: vitamin D is associated with sleep variability in apparently healthy adults. *American Journal of Physiology. Regulatory, Integrative and Comparative Physiology* 328(3), R262–R273. doi.org/10.1152/ajpregu.00168.2024.

24 Zhu, L & Yao, D (2025). Research advances in children's sleep and vitamin D levels. *Annals of Pediatric Endocrinology & Metabolism* 30(1), 3–10. doi.org/10.6065/apem.2448076.038.

25 Lee, W. H., Chen, Y. H., Wang, T. Y. et al. (2025). Association between vitamin D level and sleep quality in the elderly population: a prospective cohort study. *Sleep & Breathing* 29, 225. doi.org/10.1007/s11325-025-03398-w.

26 Evatt, M. L. (2015). Vitamin D Associations and Sleep Physiology—Promising Rays of Information. *Sleep* 38 (2), 171–72. doi.org/10.5665/sleep.4386.

27 Abad-Santos, M., Moraleda-Cibrián, M. M., & Riera, J. (2017). Vitamin D deficiency and sleep disorders. *Sleep Medicine* 32(Supplement 1), S19–S20. doi.org/10.1016/j.sleep.2017.03.045.

28 Abdul-Razzak, K., & Alkhatatbeh, M. (2021). Nightmares and bad dreams among individuals with musculoskeletal pain: a link to vitamin D and calcium. *Research in Psychotherapy: Psychopathology, Process and Outcome* 24(2). doi.org/10.4081/ripppo.2021.533.

29 Minich, D. M., Henning, M., Darley, C., Fahoum, M., Schuler, C. B., & Frame, J. (2022). Is Melatonin the "Next Vitamin D"?: A Review of Emerging Science, Clinical Uses, Safety, and Dietary Supplements. *Nutrients* 14(19), 3934. doi.org/10.3390/nu14193934.

30 Omidian, H., & Omidian, A. (2025). Clinical Research on Lysergic Acid Diethylamide (LSD) in Psychiatry and Neuroscience. *Pharmaceuticals* 18(4), 499. doi.org/10.3390/ph18040499.

31 Zhilong, C., Shuoyu, R., Nanqu, H. et al. (2025). The role of vitamin D in sleep regulation: mechanisms, clinical advances, and future directions. *Frontiers in Nutrition* 12. doi.org/10.3389/fnut.2025.1595813.

32 Patel, A. K., Reddy, V., & Araujo, J. F. (2025). Physiology, sleep stages. In StatPearls. StatPearls Publishing. https://www.ncbi.nlm.nih.gov/books/NBK526132/.

33 Vaidyanathan, T. V., Collard, M. et al. (2021) Cortical astrocytes independently regulate sleep depth and duration via separate GPCR pathways. eLife 10:e63329. doi.org/10.7554/eLife.63329.

34 Muscogiuri, G., Barrea, L., Scannapieco, M., et al. (2019). The lullaby of the sun: the role of vitamin D in sleep disturbance. *Sleep Medicine* 54, 262–65. doi.org/10.1016/j.sleep.2018.10.033.

35 Gao, Q., Kou, T., Zhuang, B., Ren, Y., Dong, X., & Wang, Q. (2018). The Association between Vitamin D Deficiency and Sleep Disorders: A Systematic Review and Meta-Analysis. *Nutrients* 10(10), 1395. https:/doi.org/10.3390/nu10101395.

36 Bivona, G., Gambino, C. M., Iacolino, G., & Ciaccio, M. (2019). Vitamin D and the nervous system. *Neurological Research*, 41(9), 827–35. doi.org/10.1080/01616412.2019.1622872.

37 Shipton, E. E., & Shipton, E. A. (2015). Vitamin D Deficiency and Pain: Clinical Evidence of Low Levels of Vitamin D and Supplementation in Chronic Pain States. *Pain and Therapy* 4, 67–87.

38 Mengxin, Q., Yujuan,L., Xuan, W. et al. (2023). Role of astrocytes in sleep deprivation: accomplices, resisters, or bystanders? *Frontiers in Cellular Neuroscience* 17. doi.org/10.3389/fncel.2023.1188306.

## Chapter 29

1 Greenblatt, J. M. (2024). Mental Health in the Sun: The Role of Vitamin D Deficiency in Mental Illness. *Psychiatric Times*. Retrieved September 18, 2025 from: https://www.psychiatrictimes.com /view/mental-health-in-the-sun-the-role-of-vitamin-d-deficiency-in-mental-illness.

2 Magnusson, A., & Boivin, D. (2021). Seasonal affective disorder: An update on assessment and treatment. *International Journal of Environmental Research and Public Health*, 18 (9), 4787. doi.org /10.3390/ijerph18094787.

3 Eyles, D. W., Burne, T. H. J., & McGrath, J. J. (2013). Vitamin D, effects on brain development, adult brain function and the links between low levels of vitamin D and neurocognitive disease. *Experimental Gerontology* 48 (8), 652–57. doi.org/10.1016/j.exger.2012.11.002.

4 Rohan, K. J., Roecklein, K. A., Lacy, N., & Vacek, P. (2017). A randomized controlled trial of cognitive-behavioral therapy for seasonal affective disorder and light therapy for seasonal affective disorder. *American Journal of Psychiatry* 174 (1), 58–66. doi.org/10.1176/appi.ajp.2016.16010074.

5 Gloth, F. M., Alam, W., & Hollis, B. (1999). Vitamin D vs broad spectrum phototherapy in the treatment of seasonal affective disorder. *Journal of Nutrition, Health & Aging* 3 (1), 5–7. doi.org/10.1007 /BF02919799.

6 Lansdowne, A. T., & Provost, S. C. (1998). Vitamin D3 enhances mood in healthy subjects during winter. *Psychopharmacology* 135 (4), 319–23. doi.org/10.1007/s002130050517.

7 Kjærgaard, M., Waterloo, K., Wang, C., Ødegård, E., Husøy, T., Schirmer, H., & Jorde, R. (2012). Effect of vitamin D supplement on depression scores in people with low levels of serum 25-hydroxyvitamin D: nested case-control study and randomised clinical trial. *British Journal of Psychiatry* 201 (5), 360–68. doi.org/10.1192/bjp.bp.111.107762.

8 Anglin, R. E., Samaan, Z., Walter, S. D., & McDonald, S. D. (2013). Vitamin D deficiency and depression in adults: A systematic review and meta-analysis. *British Journal of Psychiatry* 202 (2), 100–107. doi.org/10.1192/bjp.bp.111.106666.

9 Jorde, R., Sneve, M., Figenschau, Y., Svartberg, J., & Waterloo, K. (2008). Effects of vitamin D supplementation on symptoms of depression in overweight and obese subjects: randomized double blind trial. *Journal of Internal Medicine* 264 (6), 599–609. doi.org/10.1111/j.1365-2796.2008.02008.x.

10 Khoraminya, N., Tehrani-Doost, M., Jazayeri, S., Hosseini, S. A., Bagheri, M. H., & Eskandari, M. R. (2013). Therapeutic effects of vitamin D as adjunctive therapy to fluoxetine in patients with major depressive disorder. *Australian & New Zealand Journal of Psychiatry* 47 (3), 271–75. doi.org /10.1177/0004867412467262.

11 Ghaemi, S., Zeraattalab-Motlagh, S., Jayedi, A., & Shab-Bidar, S. (2024). The effect of vitamin D supplementation on depression: a systematic review and dose–response meta-analysis of randomized controlled trials. *Psychological Medicine* 54(15), 3999–4008. doi:10.1017/S0033291724001697.

12 Eyles, D. W., Smith, S., Kinobe, R., Hewison, M., & McGrath, J. J. (2005). Distribution of the vitamin D receptor and 1α-hydroxylase in human brain. *Journal of Chemical Neuroanatomy* 29 (1), 21–30. doi.org/10.1016/j.jchemneu.2004.07.001.

13 Annweiler, C., Fantino, B., Klaver, P., Bartha, R., & Beauchet, O. (2013). Vitamin D: A novel neurosteroid. *European Journal of Clinical Nutrition*, 67 (10), 1007–1011. doi.org/10.1038/ejcn.2013.111.

14 Juarez-Rojas, E., Flores-Ramos, M., Castillo-Alarcón, J., Olvera-Reyes, P., González-Chávez, A., & Pérez-Martínez, M. (2022). Vitamin D in major depressive disorder: An inflammatory pathway. *Nutrients* 14 (12), 2415. doi.org/10.3390/nu14122415.

15 Srifuengfung, M., Srifuengfung, S., Pummangura, C., Kanchana, P., Chaythong, P., & Supasitthumrong, T. (2023). Efficacy and acceptability of vitamin D supplements for depressed

patients: a systematic review and meta-analysis of randomized controlled trials. *Nutrition* 108, 111968. doi.org/10.1016/j.nut.2023.111968.

16 Wilczyński, K. M., Chęcińska, K., Kulczyk, K., & Janas-Kozik, M. (2022). Vitamin D deficiency and depressive symptoms: meta-analysis of studies. *Psychiatria Polska* 56 (6), 1327–44. doi.org/10.12740/PP/144949.

17 Novakovic, B., Tofaris, G., & Dissanayake, C. (2015). Vitamin D status in pregnancy: Current concepts and future directions. *Nutrients* 7 (8), 6299–6311. doi.org/10.3390/nu7085299.

18 Sharingar, S., Zafari, M., Aflatoonian, A., & Gholamzadeh, S. (2022). The association between vitamin D status and postpartum depression: A systematic review and meta-analysis. *Journal of Affective Disorders* 300, 233–42. doi.org/10.1016/j.jad.2021.12.062.

19 Abedi, P., Bovayri, M., Fakhri, A., & Jahanfar, S. (2018). The relationship between vitamin D and postpartum depression in reproductive-aged Iranian women. *Journal of Medicine and Life* 11(4), 286–92. doi.org/10.25122/jml-2018-0038.

20 Amini, S., Jafarirad, S., & Amani, R. (2019). Postpartum depression and vitamin D: A systematic review. *Critical Reviews in Food Science and Nutrition* 59(9), 1514–20. https:/doi.org/10.1080/10408398.2017.1423276.

21 Terock, J., Hannemann, A., Van der Auwera, S., Völzke, H., & Grabe, H. J. (2020). Posttraumatic stress disorder is associated with reduced vitamin D levels and functional polymorphisms of the vitamin D binding-protein in a population-based sample. *Progress in Neuro-Psychopharmacology and Biological Psychiatry* 96, 109760. doi.org/10.1016/j.pnpbp.2019.109760.

22 Terock, J., Hannemann, A., Van der Auwera, S., Völzke, H., & Grabe, H. J. (2020). Posttraumatic stress disorder is associated with reduced vitamin D levels and functional polymorphisms of the vitamin D binding-protein in a population-based sample. *Progress in Neuro-Psychopharmacology and Biological Psychiatry* 96, 109760. doi.org/10.1016/j.pnpbp.2019.109760.

23 Greenblatt, J. M. (2024). Mental Health in the Sun: The Role of Vitamin D Deficiency in Mental Illness. *Psychiatric Times.* Retrieved September 18, 2025 from: https://www.psychiatrictimes.com/view/mental-health-in-the-sun-the-role-of-vitamin-d-deficiency-in-mental-illness.

24 Umhau, J. C., George, D. T., Heaney, R. P., Lewis, M. D., Ursano, R. J., & Southwick, S. M. (2013). Low vitamin D status and suicide: a case-control study of active duty military service members. *PLoS One* 8 (1), e51543. doi.org/10.1371/journal.pone.0051543.

25 Grudet, C., Malm, J., Westrin, A., & Brundin, L. (2014). Suicidal patients are deficient in vitamin D, associated with a pro-inflammatory status in the blood. *Psychoneuroendocrinology* 50, 210–19. doi.org/10.1016/j.psyneuen.2014.08.019.

26 Mohammadi, Y., Ansari, N., Daneshi Maskooni, M., & Amiri, M. R. (2023). Association of vitamin D with suicide behaviors: a systematic review and meta-analysis. *Iranian Journal of Psychiatry* 18 (4), 484–92. doi.org/10.33443/JIP.2023.276403.

27 Lavigne, J. E., & Gibbons, J. B. (2023). The association between vitamin D serum levels, supplementation, and suicide attempts and intentional self-harm. *PLoS One* 18 (2), e0279166. doi.org/10.1371/journal.pone.0279166.

28 Greenblatt, J. M. (2024). Mental Health in the Sun: The Role of Vitamin D Deficiency in Mental Illness. *Psychiatric Times.* Retrieved September 18, 2025 from: https://www.psychiatrictimes.com/view/mental-health-in-the-sun-the-role-of-vitamin-d-deficiency-in-mental-illness.

29 Eid, A., Khoja, S., AlGhamdi, S., AlHabeeb, S., AlGhamdi, A., AlZaben, F., & AlGhamdi, M. (2019). Vitamin D supplementation ameliorates severity of generalized anxiety disorder (GAD). *Metabolic Brain Disease* 34 (6), 1781–86. doi.org/10.1007/s11011-019-00465-4.

30 Rajabi-Naeeni, M., Dolatian, M., Qorbani, M., & Vaezi, A. A. (2021). Effect of omega-3 and vitamin D co-supplementation on psychological distress in reproductive-aged women with pre-diabetes and hypovitaminosis D: a randomized controlled trial. *Brain and Behavior* 11(11), e2342. doi.org/10.1002/brb3.2342.

31 Tartagni, M., Cicinelli, M. V., Tartagni, M. V., Alrasheed, H., De Salvia, M. A., & Colaianni, M. (2016). Vitamin D supplementation for premenstrual syndrome-related mood disorders in adolescents with severe hypovitaminosis D. *Journal of Pediatric and Adolescent Gynecology* 29 (4), 357–61. doi.org/10.1016/j.jpag.2016.03.003.

32 Głąbska, D., Kołota, A., Lachowicz, K., Skarżyńska, E., & Włodarek, D. (2021). The influence of vitamin D intake and status on mental health in children: a systematic review. *Nutrients* 13 (3), 952. doi.org/10.3390/nu13030952.

33 Chien, M. C., Huang, C. Y., Wang, J. H., Hsieh, C. J., Hsiao, S. T., & Chen, H. C. (2024). Effects of vitamin D in pregnancy on maternal and offspring health-related outcomes: an umbrella review of systematic review and meta-analyses. *Nutrition & Diabetes* 14 (1), 35. doi.org/10.1038/s41387-024-00275-3.

34 Kotsi, E., & Perrea, D. N. (2019). Vitamin D levels in children and adolescents with attention-deficit hyperactivity disorder (ADHD): a meta-analysis. *Attention Deficit and Hyperactivity Disorders* 11 (3), 221–32. doi.org/10.1007/s12402-018-0284-9.

35 Gan, J., Galer, P., Ma, D., Guo, S., Jiang, W., & Wei, R. (2019). The effect of vitamin D supplementation on attention-deficit/hyperactivity disorder: a systematic review and meta-analysis of randomized controlled trials. *Journal of Child and Adolescent Psychopharmacology* 29 (9), 670–87. doi.org/10.1089/cap.2019.0068.

36 Hemamy, M., Pahlavani, N., Amanollahi, A. et al. (2021). The effect of vitamin D and magnesium supplementation on the mental health status of attention-deficit hyperactive children: a randomized controlled trial. *BMC Pediatrics* 21, 178. doi.org/10.1186/s12887-021-02631-1.

37 Annweiler, C., Allali, G., Allain, P., Maggi, A., Slaughter, J. L., & Herrmann, F. R. (2010). Vitamin D and cognitive performance in healthy adults: A systematic review. *Journal of Alzheimer's Disease* 20 (Suppl 2), S229–S243. doi.org/10.3233/JAD-2010-100236.

38 Llewellyn, D. J., Lang, I. A., Langa, K. M., & Melzer, D. (2010). Vitamin D and risk of cognitive decline in older adults: A systematic review and meta-analysis. *Journal of Geriatric Psychiatry and Neurology* 23 (3), 195–207. doi.org/10.1177/0891988710373992.

39 Buell, J. S., Dawson-Hughes, B., Scott, T. M., Dallal, G. E., Schaefer, E. J., Rosenberg, I. H., & Guss, R. B. (2009). 25-Hydroxyvitamin D, vitamin D receptor gene polymorphisms, and cognitive function in men and women. *Journal of Gerontology: Series A Biological Sciences and Medical Sciences* 64 (2), 273–80. doi.org/10.1093/gerona/gln012.

40 Annweiler, C., Allali, G., Allain, P., Maggi, A., Slaughter, J. L., & Herrmann, F. R. (2010). Vitamin D and cognitive performance in healthy adults: A systematic review. *Journal of Alzheimer's Disease* 20 (Suppl 2), S229–S243. doi.org/10.3233/JAD-2010-100236.

41 Eyles, D. W., Smith, S., Kinobe, R., Hewison, M., & McGrath, J. J. (2005). Distribution of the vitamin D receptor and 1α-hydroxylase in human brain. *Journal of Chemical Neuroanatomy* 29 (1), 21–30. doi.org/10.1016/j.jchemneu.2004.07.001.

42 Eyles, D. W., Burne, T. H. J., & McGrath, J. J. (2013). Vitamin D, effects on brain development, adult brain function and the links between low levels of vitamin D and neurocognitive disease. *Experimental Gerontology* 48 (8), 652–57. doi.org/10.1016/j.exger.2012.11.002.

43 Peterson, A. L., Furlan, J. C., & Fehlings, M. G. (2015). Vitamin D and central nervous system function: Implications for pathophysiology and treatment of neurological disorders. *Neuroscience & Biobehavioral Reviews* 55, 17–27. doi.org/10.1016/j.neubiorev.2015.03.007.

44 Cryan, J. F., O'Riordan, K. J., Cowan, C. S., Sandhu, K. V., Bastiaanssen, T. F., Wiffin, M., . . . & Dinan, T. G. (2020). The microbiota-gut-brain axis. *Physiological Reviews* 100 (4), 1877–2002. doi.org/10.1152/physrev.00031.2019.

45 Bashir, M., Qadir, S., Zafar, A., & Bashir, A. (2020). Vitamin D and the gut microbiome: An emerging link in mental health. *Nutrients* 12 (7), 2097. doi.org/10.3390/nu12072097.

46 Eyles, D. W., Trzaskowski, M., Vinkhuyzen, A.A.E. et al. (2018). The association between neonatal vitamin D status and risk of schizophrenia. *Scientific Reports* 8, 17692. doi.org/10.1038/s41598-018-35418-z.

47 Eyles, D. W., Burne, T. H. J., & McGrath, J. J. (2013). Vitamin D, effects on brain development, adult brain function and the links between low levels of vitamin D and neurocognitive disease. *Experimental Gerontology* 48 (8), 652–57. doi.org/10.1016/j.exger.2012.11.002.

48 Eyles, D. W., Trzaskowski, M., Vinkhuyzen, A. A. E. et al. (2018). The association between neonatal vitamin D status and risk of schizophrenia. *Scientific Reports* 8, 17692. doi.org/10.1038/s41598-018-35418-z.

49 Valipour, G., Saneei, P., Esmaillzadeh, A., & Milajerdi, A. (2019). Vitamin D status and risk of schizophrenia: A systematic review and meta-analysis of observational studies. *Journal of Clinical Psychopharmacology* 39 (3), 205–12. doi.org/10.1097/JCP.0000000000001041.

50 Greenblatt, J. M. (2024). Mental Health in the Sun: The Role of Vitamin D Deficiency in Mental Illness. *Psychiatric Times*. Retrieved September 18, 2025 from: https://www.psychiatrictimes.com/view/mental-health-in-the-sun-the-role-of-vitamin-d-deficiency-in-mental-illness.

## Chapter 30

1 Annweiler, C., Allali, G., Allain, P., Maggi, A., Slaughter, J. L., & Herrmann, F. R. (2010). Vitamin D and cognitive performance in healthy adults: A systematic review. *Journal of Alzheimer's Disease* 20 (Suppl 2), S229–S243. doi.org/10.3233/JAD-2010-100236.

2 Llewellyn, D. J., Lang, I. A., Langa, K. M., Muniz-Terrera, G., Phillips, C. L., Cherubini, A., Ferrucci, L., & Melzer, D. (2010). Vitamin D and risk of cognitive decline in elderly persons. *Archives of Internal Medicine* 170(13), 1135–41. doi.org/10.1001/archinternmed.2010.173.

3 Zugic Soares, J., Pettersen, R., Saltyte Benth, J., Knapskog, A. B., Selbæk, G., & Bogdanovic, N. (2019). Higher Vitamin D Levels Are Associated with Better Attentional Functions: Data from the NorCog Register. *The Journal of Nutrition, Health & Aging* 23(8), 725–31. https:/doi.org/10.1007/s12603-019-1220-z.

4 Buell, J. S., Dawson-Hughes, B., Scott, T. M., et al. (2010). 25-Hydroxyvitamin D, dementia, and cerebrovascular pathology in elders receiving home services. *Neurology* 74(1), 18–26. doi.org/10.1212/WNL.0b013e3181beecb7.

5 Eyles D. W. (2020). Vitamin D: Brain and Behavior. *Journal of Bone and Mineral Research plus* 5(1), e10419. doi.org/10.1002/jbm4.10419.

6 Eyles, D. W., Smith, S., Kinobe, R., Hewison, M., & McGrath, J. J. (2005). Distribution of the vitamin D receptor and 1α-hydroxylase in human brain. *Journal of Chemical Neuroanatomy* 29 (1), 21–30. doi.org/10.1016/j.jchemneu.2004.07.001.

7 Eyles, D. W., Burne, T. H., & McGrath, J. J. (2013). Vitamin D, effects on brain development, adult brain function and the links between low levels of vitamin D and neuropsychiatric disease. *Frontiers in Neuroendocrinology* 34(1), 47–64. doi.org/10.1016/j.yfrne.2012.07.001.

8 Eyles D. W. (2020). Vitamin D: Brain and Behavior. Journal of Bone and Mineral Research plus 5(1), e10419. doi.org/10.1002/jbm4.10419.

9 Formentin, C., Carraro, S., Turco, M., Zarantonello, L., Angeli, P., & Montagnese, S. (2020). Effect of Morning Light Glasses and Night Short-Wavelength Filter Glasses on Sleep-Wake Rhythmicity in Medical Inpatients. *Frontiers in Physiology* 11(5). doi.org/10.3389/fphys.2020.00005Disruptions.

10 Walker, M. (2017). Why we sleep: Unlocking the power of sleep and dreams. Scribner.

11 Eyles, D. W., Smith, S., Kinobe, R., Hewison, M., & McGrath, J. J. (2005). Distribution of the vitamin D receptor and 1α-hydroxylase in human brain. *Journal of Chemical Neuroanatomy* 29 (1), 21–30. doi.org/10.1016/j.jchemneu.2004.07.001.

12 Maissan, P., & Carlberg, C. (2025). Circadian Regulation of Vitamin D Target Genes Reveals a Network Shaped by Individual Responsiveness. *Nutrients* 17(7), 1204. doi.org/10.3390/nu17071204.

13 Cajochen, C., Münch, M., Knoblauch, V., Blatter, K., & Wirz-Justice, A. (2011). High sensitivity of human melatonin suppression to previous light exposure. *Journal of Biological Rhythms* 26 (4), 302–11. doi.org/10.1177/0748730411408092.

14 Lebedev, A. S., Shevlyakov, A. D., Ilyin, N. P. et al. The Neurosteroid Hormone Vitamin D: Modern Prospects. *J Evol Biochem Phys* 60, 2152–71 (2024). https:/doi.org/10.1134/S0022093024060024

15 Eyles D. W. (2020). Vitamin D: Brain and Behavior. *Journal of Bone and Mineral Research plus* 5(1), e10419. doi.org/10.1002/jbm4.10419.

16 Brewer, L. D., Searcy, J. L., et al Vitamin D prevents cognitive decline and enhances hippocampal synaptic function in aging rats, *Proc. Natl. Acad. Sci. U.S.A.* 111 (41) E4359–E4366. doi.org/10.1073/pnas.1404477111 (2014).

17 Eyles D. W. (2020). Vitamin D: Brain and Behavior. *Journal of Bone and Mineral Research plus* 5(1), e10419. https:/doi.org/10.1002/jbm4.10419.

18 Gáll, Z., & Székely, O. (2021). Role of Vitamin D in Cognitive Dysfunction: New Molecular Concepts and Discrepancies between Animal and Human Findings. *Nutrients* 13(11), 3672. doi.org/10.3390/nu13113672.

19 Brewer, L. D., Searcy, J. L., et al Vitamin D prevents cognitive decline and enhances hippocampal synaptic function in aging rats, *Proc. Natl. Acad. Sci. U.S.A.* 111 (41) E4359–E4366. doi.org/10.1073/pnas.1404477111.

20 Chen, H., Pang, X., & Huang, Y. (2025). Higher dietary vitamin D intake influences brain and mental function in elderly Americans: a cross-sectional analysis. *Frontiers in Nutrition* 12, 1564568. doi.org/10.3389/fnut.2025.1564568.

21 Terock, T., Bonk, S., Frenzel, S., et al. (2022).Vitamin D deficit is associated with accelerated brain aging in the general population. *Psychiatry Research: Neuroimaging* 327, 111558. doi.org/10.1016/j.pscychresns.2022.111558.

22 Mayne, P. E. (2019). Vitamin D in synaptic plasticity, cognitive function and neuropsychiatric illness. *Trends in Neurosciences* 42(4), 293–306.


## Chapter 31


1 C-Span (2025). Health and Human Services Secretary Kennedy Testifies on Health Care Agenda, Part 1. September 4, 2025. https://www.c-span.org/program/senate-committee/health-and-human-services-secretary-kennedy-testifies-on-health-care-agenda-part-1/664946.

2 Bach, J. F. (2002). The effect of infections on susceptibility to autoimmune and allergic diseases. *The New England Journal of Medicine* 347 (12), 911–20. doi.org/10.1056/NEJMra020100.

3 Lerner, A., Jeremias, P., & Matthias, T. (2016). The world incidence and prevalence of autoimmune diseases is increasing. *International Journal of Celiac Disease* 4(2), 151–55. doi.org/10.12691/ijcd-4-2-8.

4 Jan, Z., El Assadi, F., Velayutham, D., Mifsud, B., & Jithesh, P. V. (2025). Pharmacogenomics of TNF inhibitors. *Frontiers in Immunology* 16, 1521794. doi.org/10.3389/fimmu.2025.1521794.

5 Schwartz, D., Kanno, Y., Villarino, A. et al. (2018). JAK inhibition as a therapeutic strategy for immune and inflammatory diseases. *Nature Reviews Drug Discovery* 17, 78. doi.org/10.1038/nrd.2017.267.

6 Zhang, C., Tong, T., Miao, Dc. et al. (2021). Vitamin D inhibits TNF-α induced apoptosis of human nucleus pulposus cells through regulation of NF-kB signaling pathway. *Journal of Orthopedic Surgical Research* 16, 411. doi.org/10.1186/s13018-021-02545-9.

7 Landel, V., Millet, P., Baranger, K. et al. (2016). Vitamin D interacts with Esr1 and Igf1 to regulate molecular pathways relevant to Alzheimer's disease. *Molecular Neurodegeneration* 11(22). doi.org/10.1186/s13024-016-0087-2.

8 Liu, P. T., Stenger, S., Li, H., Wenzel, L., Tan, B. H., Krutzik, S. R., . . . & Modlin, R. L. (2011). Toll-like receptor triggering of a vitamin D-mediated human antimicrobial response. *Science 311* (5768), 1770–73.

9 Ghoreschi, K., et al (2021). Therapeutics targeting the IL-23 and IL-17 pathway in psoriasis. *The Lancet: Therapeutics* 397, 10275, 754–66.

10 Schafer, P. H., Parton, A., Capone, L., et al. (2014). Apremilast is a selective PDE4 inhibitor with regulatory effects on innate immunity. *Cellular Signalling* 26(9), 2016–29. doi.org/10.1016/j.cellsig.2014.05.014.

11 Bukvić Mokos, Z., Tomić Krsnik, L., Harak, K., Marojević Tomić, D., Tešanović Perković, D., & Vukojević, M. (2025). Vitamin D in the Prevention and Treatment of Inflammatory Skin Diseases. *International Journal of Molecular Sciences* 26(11), 5005. doi.org/10.3390/ijms26115005.

12 Liu, P. T., Stenger, S., Li, H., Wenzel, L., Tan, B. H., Krutzik, S. R., . . . & Modlin, R. L. (2011). Toll-like receptor triggering of a vitamin D-mediated human antimicrobial response. *Science 311* (5768), 1770–73.

13 Cherry, L. N., Yunker, N. S., Lambert, E. R., Vaughan, D., & Lowe, D. K. (2015). Vedolizumab: an α4β7 integrin antagonist for ulcerative colitis and Crohn's disease. *Therapeutic Advances in Chronic Disease* 6(5), 224–33. doi.org/10.1177/2040622315586970.

14 Koutruba, N., Emer, J., & Lebwohl, M. (2010). Review of ustekinumab, an interleukin-12 and interleukin-23 inhibitor used for the treatment of plaque psoriasis. *Therapeutics and Clinical Risk Management* 6, 123–41. doi.org/10.2147/TCRM.S5599.

15 Tofacitinib citrate (Xeljanz). American College of Rheumatology. https://rheumatology.org/patients/tofacitinib-citrate-xeljanz.

16 Topalova-Dimitrova, A., Dimitrov, I., Nikolov, R. (2023). Lower vitamin D levels are associated with the pathogenesis of inflammatory bowel diseases. *Medicine* 102(41):p e35505, doi.org/10.1097/MD.0000000000035505.

17 Fenercioglu, A. K. (2024). The Anti-Inflammatory Roles of Vitamin D for Improving Human Health. *Current Issues in Molecular Biology* 46(12), 13514–25. doi.org/10.3390/cimb46120807.

18 Selewski, D. T., Shah, G., Segal, B. M., et al. (2010). Natalizumab (Tysabri). *American Journal of Neuroradiology* 31 (9) 1588–90. doi.org/10.3174/ajnr.A2226.

19 Lamb, Y. N. (2022). Ocrelizumab: A Review in Multiple Sclerosis. *Drugs* 82, 323–34. doi.org/10.1007/s40265-022-01672-9.

20 Mokry, L. E., Ross, S., & Ahmad, O. (2015). Vitamin D and multiple sclerosis: A comprehensive review. *Therapeutic Advances in Neurological Disorders* 8(4), 161–72. doi.org/10.1177/1756285615586127.

21 Daniele, Stefano G. et al. (2024). Structural Basis for p19 Targeting by Anti–IL-23 Biologics: Correlations with Short- and Long-Term Efficacy in Psoriasis. *Journal of Infectious Diseases: Innovations* 4(2), 100261.

22 National Institutes of Health. (2023). *Adalimumab.* MedlinePlus. Retrieved from https://medlineplus.gov/druginfo/meds/a603032.html.

23 Pfizer. (2023). *Xeljanz (tofacitinib) prescribing information.* https://www.xeljanz.com.

24 Holick, M. F. (2007). Vitamin D deficiency. *The New England Journal of Medicine* 357(3), 266–81. https:/doi.org/10.1056/NEJMra070553.

25 Sîrbe, C., Rednic, S., Grama, A., & Pop, T. L. (2022). An Update on the Effects of Vitamin D on the Immune System and Autoimmune Diseases. *International Journal of Molecular Sciences* 23(17), 9784. doi.org/10.3390/ijms23179784.

26 Wintheiser, G. A., & Silberstein P. (2025) Physiology, Tyrosine Kinase Receptors. [Updated 2022 Sep 26]. In: StatPearls [Internet]. Treasure Island (FL): StatPearls Publishing. Available from: https://www.ncbi.nlm.nih.gov/books/NBK538532/.

27 Lacouture, M., & Sibaud, V. (2018) Toxic Side Effects of Targeted Therapies and Immunotherapies Affecting the Skin, Oral Mucosa, Hair, and Nails. *American Journal of Clinical Dermatology* 19, 31–39. doi.org/10.1007/s40257-018-0384-3.

28 National Comprehensive Cancer Network. (2023). *NCCN clinical practice guidelines in oncology: Cancer-related fatigue.* https://www.nccn.org/guidelines.

29 Paech, F., Bouitbir, J., & Krähenbühl, S. (2017). Hepatocellular Toxicity Associated with Tyrosine Kinase Inhibitors: Mitochondrial Damage and Inhibition of Glycolysis. *Frontiers in Pharmacology* 8(367). doi.org/10.3389/fphar.2017.00367.

30 Force, T., Krause, D. S., & Van Etten, R. A. (2007). Molecular mechanisms of cardiotoxicity of tyrosine kinase inhibition. *Nature Reviews. Cancer* 7(5), 332–44. doi.org/10.1038/nrc2106.

31 Shyam Sunder, S., Sharma, U.C. & Pokharel, S. (2023). Adverse effects of tyrosine kinase inhibitors in cancer therapy: pathophysiology, mechanisms and clinical management. *Sig Transduct Target Ther* 8(262). doi.org/10.1038/s41392-023-01469-6.

32 Blauvelt, A., & Chiricozzi, A. (2018). The Immunologic Role of IL-17 in Psoriasis and Psoriatic Arthritis Pathogenesis. *Clinical Reviews in Allergy & Immunology* 55(3), 379–90. doi.org/10.1007/s12016-018-8702-3.

33 Papp, K. A., Leonardi, C., Menter, A., Reich, K., Kimball, A. B., & Lebwohl, M. (2015). Brodalumab, an anti-IL-17RA monoclonal antibody, in psoriasis. *The New England Journal of Medicine* 373(15), 1391–1402. doi.org/10.1056/NEJMoa1503824.

34 Feagan, B. G., Sandborn, W. J., Danese, S., et al. (2020). Ozanimod induction therapy for patients with moderate to severe Crohn's disease: a single-arm, phase 2, prospective observer-blinded endpoint study. *The Lancet: Gastroenterology & Hepatology* 5(9), 819–28. doi.org/10.1016/S2468-1253(20)30188-6.

35 Papp, K. A., Leonardi, C., Menter, A., Reich, K., Kimball, A. B., & Lebwohl, M. (2015). Brodalumab, an anti-IL-17RA monoclonal antibody, in psoriasis. *The New England Journal of Medicine* 373(15), 1391–1402. doi.org/10.1056/NEJMoa1503824.

36 Moslehi, J. (2016). Cardiovascular Toxic Effects of Targeted Cancer Therapies. *New England Journal of Medicine* 375(15),1457–67. doi.org/10.1056/NEJMra1100265.

37 Tufail, M., Jiang, CH. & Li, N. (2025). Immune evasion in cancer: mechanisms and cutting-edge therapeutic approaches. *Sig Transduct Target Ther.* 10, 227. doi.org/10.1038/s41392-025-02280-1.

38 Papp, K. A., Leonardi, C., Menter, A., Reich, K., Kimball, A. B., & Lebwohl, M. (2015). Brodalumab, an anti-IL-17RA monoclonal antibody, in psoriasis. *The New England Journal of Medicine* 373(15), 1391–1402.

39 Sîrbe, C., Rednic, S., Grama, A., & Pop, T. L. (2022). An Update on the Effects of Vitamin D on the Immune System and Autoimmune Diseases. *International Journal of Molecular Sciences* 23(17), 9784. doi.org/10.3390/ijms23179784.

40 Zhang, Y., Xu, Y., Zhong, W., et al. (2025). Vitamin D and Immune Checkpoint Inhibitors in Lung Cancer: A Synergistic Approach to Enhancing Treatment Efficacy. *International Journal of Molecular Sciences* 26(10), 4511. doi.org/10.3390/ijms26104511.

41 Grover, S., Dougan, M., Tyan, K., et al. (2020). Vitamin D intake is associated with decreased risk of immune checkpoint inhibitor-induced colitis. *Cancer* 126(16), 3758–67. doi.org/10.1002/cncr.32966.

42 Prietl, B., Treiber, G., Pieber, T. R., & Amrein, K. (2013). Vitamin D and immune function. *Nutrients* 5(7), 2502–21. https:/doi.org/10.3390/nu5072502.

43 Carlberg, C & Campbell, M. J. (2012). Vitamin D receptor signaling mechanisms: Integrated actions of a well-defined transcription factor. *Steroids* 78(2), 127–36. doi: 10.1016/j.steroids.2012.10.019.

44 Kamen, D. L., & Tangpricha, V. Vitamin D and molecular actions on the immune system: modulation of innate and autoimmunity. *J Mol Med* 88, 441–50 (2010). doi.org/10.1007/s00109-010-0590-9.

45 Gombart A. F. (2009). The vitamin D-antimicrobial peptide pathway and its role in protection against infection. *Future Microbiology* 4(9), 1151–65. doi.org/10.2217/fmb.09.87.

46 Adebajo, A. O. (1997). Low Frequency of Autoimmune Disease in Tropical Africa. *The Lancet* 349 (9048), 361–62. doi.org/10.1016/S0140-6736(05)62867-X.


## Chapter 32


1 Uwitonze, A. M., & Razzaque, M. S. (2018). Role of magnesium in vitamin D activation and function. *The Journal of the American Osteopathic Association* 118 (3), 181–89. doi.org/10.7556/jaoa.2018.037.

2 National Institutes of Health, Office of Dietary Supplements. (2023b). Magnesium: Fact Sheet for Health Professionals. Retrieved from https://ods.od.nih.gov/factsheets/Magnesium-HealthProfessional/.

3 Gupta, A., & Gupta, J. (2017). Zinc and its relation with vitamin D: A narrative review. *Journal of Basic and Clinical Pharmacy* 8 (3), 105–9. doi.org/10.4103/jbcp.jbcp_31_17.

4 National Institutes of Health, Office of Dietary Supplements. (2023c). Zinc: Fact Sheet for Health Professionals . Retrieved from https://ods.od.nih.gov/factsheets/Zinc-HealthProfessional//

5 Institute of Medicine. (2011). *Dietary Reference Intakes for Calcium and Vitamin D.* The National Academies Press. doi.org/10.17226/13050.

6 National Institutes of Health, Office of Dietary Supplements. (2023a). Calcium: Fact Sheet for Health Professionals. Retrieved from https://ods.od.nih.gov/factsheets/Calcium-HealthProfessional/.

7 van Ballegooien, A. J., Pilz, S., Tomaschitz, A., Rios, D. L., Bakker, S. J. L., & Kiefte-de Jong, J. C. (2017). The synergistic interplay between vitamins D and K for bone and cardiovascular health: A narrative review. *International Journal of Endocrinology*, 2017, 7454376. doi.org/10.1155/2017/7454376.

8 Mladěnka, P., Macáková, K., Kujovská Krčmová, L., et al. (2022). Vitamin K—sources, physiological role, kinetics, deficiency, detection, therapeutic use, and toxicity. *Nutrition Reviews* 80(4), 677–98. doi.org/10.1093/nutrit/nuab061.

9 National Institutes of Health, Office of Dietary Supplements. (2023d). Vitamin K: Fact Sheet for Health Professionals . Retrieved from https://ods.od.nih.gov/factsheets/VitaminK-HealthProfessional/.

10 Ross, A. C. (2012). Vitamin A and vitamin D: Two retinoids for the price of one. *Journal of the American Academy of Dermatology* 66 (6), 1018–20. doi.org/10.1016/j.jaad.2012.02.012.

11 National Institutes of Health, Office of Dietary Supplements. (2023e). Vitamin A: Fact Sheet for Health Professionals . Retrieved from https://ods.od.nih.gov/factsheets/VitaminA-HealthProfessional/.

12 Colboc, H., Bazin, D., Reguer, S., et al. (2022). Chemical characterization of inks in skin reactions to tattoo. *Journal of Synchrotron Radiation* 29, 1436–45. doi.org/10.1107/S1600577522008165.

13 Jalil, B. (2012). The chemistry of tattoos. *Journal of Chemical Education* 89 (10), 1279–1282. doi.org/10.1021/ed2007798.

14 Holick, M. F. (2007). Vitamin D deficiency. *New England Journal of Medicine* 357 (3), 266–81. doi.org/10.1056/NEJMra070553.

15 McCarty, R. D., Trabert, B., Kriebel, D., et al. (2024). Tattoos and Risk of Hematologic Cancer: A Population-Based Case-Control Study in Utah. *Cancer Medicine* 13(20), e70260. doi.org/10.1002/cam4.70260.

16 Nielsen, C., et al. (2024). Tattoos as a risk factor for malignant lymphoma: a population-based case–control study. *eClinicalMedicine* 72, 102649.

17 Bouillon, R., Marcocci, F., Carmeliet, G., Bikle, D., White, J. H., Dawson-Hughes, B., . . . & Zanchi, G. (2017). Skeletal and extraskeletal actions of vitamin D: Current evidence and open questions. *Endocrine Reviews* 38 (2), 79–111. doi.org/10.1210/er.2016-1033.

18 Plum, L. A., & DeLuca, H. F. (2010). Vitamin D, disease and therapeutic opportunities. *Nature Reviews. Drug Discovery* 9(12), 941–55. https:/doi.org/10.1038/nrd3318.

19 Zhang, Y., Xu, Y., Zhong, W., Zhao, J., Liu, X., Gao, X., Chen, M., & Wang, M. (2025). Vitamin D and Immune Checkpoint Inhibitors in Lung Cancer: A Synergistic Approach to Enhancing Treatment Efficacy. *International Journal of Molecular Sciences* 26(10), 4511. doi.org/10.3390/ijms26104511.

20 Grover, S., Dougan, M., Tyan, K., et al. (2020). Vitamin D intake is associated with decreased risk of immune checkpoint inhibitor-induced colitis. *Cancer* 126 (16), 3758–67. doi.org/10.1002/cncr.32966.

21 Grant, W. B., & Boucher, B. J. (2017). Requirements for vitamin D: A critical appraisal of the Institute of Medicine and other Endocrine Society guidelines. *Reviews in Endocrine and Metabolic Disorders* 18 (2), 177–87. doi.org/10.1007/s11154-017-9411-9.

22 LeBoff, M. S., Chou, S. H., Murata, E. M., Donlon, C. M., Cook, N. R., Mora, S., Lee, I. M., Kotler, G., Bubes, V., Buring, J. E., & Manson, J. E. (2020). Effects of Supplemental Vitamin D on Bone Health Outcomes in Women and Men in the VITamin D and OmegA-3 TriaL (VITAL). *Journal of Bone and Mineral Research* 35(5), 883–93. doi.org/10.1002/jbmr.3958.

23 Food and Drug Administration. (1994). *Guideline for Industry: Dose-Response Information to Support Drug Registration*. Accessed September 25, 2025. https://www.fda.gov/media/71279/download.

24 Heaney, R. P., Recker, R. R., Grote, J. et al. (2011). Vitamin D3 Is More Potent Than Vitamin D2 in Humans, *The Journal of Clinical Endocrinology & Metabolism* 96 (3), E447–E452. doi.org/10.1210/jc.2010-2230.

25 Cekic, M., & Stein, D. G. (2010). Traumatic brain injury and aging: Is a combination of progesterone and vitamin D hormone a simple solution to a complex problem? *Neurotherapeutics* 7(1), 81–90. doi.org/10.1016/j.nurt.2009.10.017.

26 Barbarawi, M., Kheiri, B., Zayed, Y., et al. (2019). Vitamin D Supplementation and Cardiovascular Disease Risks in More Than 83,000 Individuals in 21 Randomized Clinical Trials: A Meta-analysis. *JAMA Cardiology* 4(8), 765–76. doi.org/10.1001/jamacardio.2019.1870.

27 Mathur, M. B., & VanderWeele, T. J. (2022). Methods to Address Confounding and Other Biases in Meta-Analyses: Review and Recommendations. *Annual Review of Public Health* 43, 19–35. https:/doi.org/10.1146/annurev-publhealth-051920-114020.

28 Veugelers, P. J., & Ekwaru, J. P. (2014). A statistical error in the estimation of the recommended dietary allowance for vitamin D. *Nutrients* 6 (10), 4472–75. doi.org/10.3390/nu6104472.

29 Demay, M., et al. (2024). Vitamin D for the Prevention of Disease: An Endocrine Society Clinical Practice Guideline. *The Journal of Clinical Endocrinology & Metabolism* 109(8), 1907–47, doi.org/10.1210/clinem/dgae290.

30 McChesney, C., et al. (2022). Do not routinely test for vitamin D. *British Medical Journal* 378:e070270. doi.org/10.1136/bmj-2022-070270.

31 Singer, A. G. & McChesney, C. (2023). Reduce unnecessary routine vitamin D testing. *Canadian Family Physician*, 69 (9) 620–22. doi.org/10.46747/cfp.6909620.

32 Vitamin D testing not recommended for most people. *Harvard Health Publishing.* November 26, 2024. https://www.health.harvard.edu/blog/vitamin-d-testing-recommended-people-201411267547.

33 Luo, W., Karpf, A. R., Deeb, K. K., Muindi, J. R., Morrison, C. D., Johnson, C. S., & Trump, D. L. (2010). Epigenetic regulation of vitamin D 24-hydroxylase/CYP24A1 in human prostate cancer. *Cancer Research* 70(14), 5953–62. doi.org/10.1158/0008-5472.CAN-10-0617.

34 Chen, J., Li, Y., Wang, L., Liu, Q., & Qiu, B. (2025). Neuroprotective synergy of vitamin D and exercise: a narrative review of preclinical and clinical evidence on aging-related neuroplasticity and cognitive health. *Frontiers in Nutrition*. 12. doi.org/10.3389/fnut.2025.1642363

35 Cyanotech.com. (n.d.). Benefits of Astaxanthin for Skin Health. Retrieved from https://www.cyanotech.com/pdfs/bioastin/BioAstin.Skin.Health.pdf September 12, 2025.

36 Davinelli, S., Nielsen, M. E., & Scapagnini, G. (2018). Astaxanthin in Skin Health, Repair, and Disease: A Comprehensive Review. *Nutrients* 10(4), 522. doi.org/10.3390/nu10040522.

37 Flieger, J., Raszewska-Famielec, M., Radzikowska-Büchner, E., & Flieger, W. (2024). Skin Protection by Carotenoid Pigments. *International Journal of Molecular Sciences* 25(3), 1431. doi.org/10.3390/ijms25031431.

38 Cândido, M., et al. (2022). Dietary Supplements and the Skin: Focus on Photoprotection and Antioxidant Activity—A Review. *Nutrients* 14(6), 1248. doi.org/10.3390/nu14061248.

39 Komatsu, T., Sasaki, S., Manabe, Y., Hirata, T., & Sugawara, T. (2017) Preventive effect of dietary astaxanthin on UVA-induced skin photoaging in hairless mice. *PLoS ONE* 12(2), e0171178. doi.org/10.1371/journal.pone.0171178.

40 Singh, K. N., Patil, S., & Barkate, H. (2020). Protective effects of astaxanthin on skin: Recent scientific evidence, possible mechanisms, and potential indications. *Journal of Cosmetic Dermatology* 19(1), 22–27. doi.org/10.1111/jocd.13019.

41 Singh, K. N., Patil, S., & Barkate, H. (2020). Protective effects of astaxanthin on skin: Recent scientific evidence, possible mechanisms, and potential indications. *Journal of Cosmetic Dermatology* 19(1), 22–27. doi.org/10.1111/jocd.13019.

42 Zhou, X., Cao, Q., Orfila, C., Zhao, J., & Zhang, L. (2021). Systematic Review and Meta-Analysis on the Effects of Astaxanthin on Human Skin Ageing. *Nutrients* 13(9), 2917. doi.org/10.3390/nu13092917.

43 Lademann, J., Vergou, T., Darvin, M. E., et al. (2016). Influence of Topical, Systemic and Combined Application of Antioxidants on the Barrier Properties of the Human Skin. *Skin Pharmacology and Physiology* 29(1), 41–46. doi.org/10.1159/000441953.

44 Shanaida, M., Mykhailenko, O., Lysiuk, R., et al. (2025). Carotenoids for Antiaging: Nutraceutical, Pharmaceutical, and Cosmeceutical Applications. *Pharmaceuticals* 18(3), 403. doi.org/10.3390/ph18030403.

45 Chang, M. X., & Xiong, F. (2020). Astaxanthin and its Effects in Inflammatory Responses and Inflammation-Associated Diseases: Recent Advances and Future Directions. *Molecules* 25(22), 5342. doi.org/10.3390/molecules25225342.

46 Segars, K., McCarver, V., & Miller, R. A. (2021). Dermatologic Applications of *Polypodium leucotomos*: A Literature Review. *The Journal of Clinical and Aesthetic Dermatology* 14(2), 50–60. PMC8211346.

47 Surjana, D., Halliday, G. & Damian, D. L., (2013). Nicotinamide enhances repair of ultraviolet radiation-induced DNA damage in human keratinocytes and *ex vivo* skin, *Carcinogenesis* 34(5), 1144–49, doi.org/10.1093/carcin/bgt017.

48 Shafe, M. O., Gumede, N. M., Nyakudya, T. T., & Chivandi, E. (2024). Lycopene: A Potent Antioxidant with Multiple Health Benefits. *Journal of Nutrition and Metabolism*, 2024, 6252426. doi.org/10.1155/2024/6252426.

49 Singh, B. K., Koley, T. K., Maurya, A. et al. (2018). Phytochemical and antioxidative potential of orange, red, yellow, rainbow and black coloured tropical carrots (*Daucus carota* subsp. *sativus* Schubl. & Martens). *Physiology & Molecular Biology of Plants* 24, 899–907. doi.org/10.1007/s12298-018-0574-8.

50 Gęgotek, A., & Skrzydlewska, E. (2022). Antioxidative and Anti-Inflammatory Activity of Ascorbic Acid. *Antioxidants* 11(10), 1993. doi.org/10.3390/antiox11101993.

51 Singh, B. N., Shankar, S., & Srivastava, R. K. (2011). Green tea catechin, epigallocatechin-3-gallate (EGCG): mechanisms, perspectives and clinical applications. *Biochemical Pharmacology* 82(12), 1807–1821. doi.org/10.1016/j.bcp.2011.07.093.

52 Karsten, K. B., Ferguson, G. W., Chen, T. C., & Holick, M. F. (2009). Panther chameleons, Furcifer pardalis, behaviorally regulate optimal exposure to UV depending on dietary vitamin D3 status. *Physiological and Biochemical Zoology: PBZ* 82(3), 218–25. doi.org/10.1086/597525.

53 Al Ghamdi, K., Kumar, A. & Moussa, N. (2013). The role of vitamin D in melanogenesis with an emphasis on vitiligo. *Indian Journal of Dermatology, Venereology and Leprology* 79(6), 750–58. doi.org/10.4103/0378-6323.120720.

54 Slominski, A. & Postlethwaite, A. E., (2015). Skin Under the Sun: When Melanin Pigment Meets Vitamin D. *Endocrinology* 156(1), 1–4, doi.org/10.1210/en.2014-1918.

55 Al-Smadi, K., Ali, M., Alavi, S. E., et al. (2023). Using a Topical Formulation of Vitamin D for the Treatment of Vitiligo: A Systematic Review. *Cells* 12(19), 2387. doi.org/10.3390/cells12192387.

56 Supple, W. F. (2026). *Cancer Is a Parasite: Kill it with the Safe, Over-the-Counter Antiparasitic Fenbendazole*. Skyhorse Publishing.

57 Benias, P. C., Wells, R. G., Sackey-Aboagye, B. et al. (2018). Structure and Distribution of an Unrecognized Interstitium in Human Tissues. *Scientific Reports* 8, 4947. doi.org/10.1038/s41598-018-23062-6.

58 Rettner, R. (2018). Meet Your Interstitium, a Newfound Organ. *Scientific American*, March 27, 2018. https://www.scientificamerican.com/article/meet-your-interstitium-a-newfound-organ/.

59 Slominski, A., Kim, T. K., Zmijewski, M. A., et al. (2013). Novel vitamin D photoproducts and their precursors in the skin. *Dermato-Endocrinology* 5(1), 7–19. doi.org/10.4161/derm.23938.

60 Slominski, R. M., Raman, C., Jetten, A. M. et al. (2025). Neuro–immuno–endocrinology of the skin: how environment regulates body homeostasis. *Nature Reviews Endocrinology* 21, 495–509. doi.org/10.1038/s41574-025-01107-x.

61 Holick, M. F. (2007). Vitamin D deficiency. *New England Journal of Medicine* 357 (3), 266–81. doi.org/10.1056/NEJMra070553.

62 Wortsman, J., Matsuoka, L. Y., Chen, T. C., Lu, Z., & Holick, M. F. (1998). Decreased production of vitamin D3 in skin of aged humans. *Journal of Clinical Endocrinology & Metabolism* 83 (9), 3038–42. doi.org/10.1210/jcem.83.9.5085.

63 DeLuca H. F. (2008). Evolution of our understanding of vitamin D. *Nutrition Reviews*, 66(10 Suppl 2), S73–S87. doi.org/10.1111/j.1753-4887.2008.00105.x.

64 Maroon, J. C., Mathyssek, C. M., Bost, J. W., et al. (2015), Vitamin D Profile in National Football League Players. *The American Journal of Sports Medicine* 43(5), 1241–45. doi.org/10.1177/0363546514567297.

65 Crupi, A. (2025). Proposed Pharma Ad Ban May Be a Bitter Pill to Swallow for Sports TV. *Sportico: The Business of Sports*, https://www.sportico.com/business/media/2025/proposed-pharmaceutical-ad-ban-sports-tv-1234832190.

66 Semeraro, E. (2025). Data: Pharma's Premium TV Ad Placement Strategy. *The Measure*. March 11, 2025. https://www.themeasure.net/data-pharmas-premium-tv-ad-placement-strategy/

67 Taylor, N. P. (2025). As Super Bowl nears, TV data show GLP-1 game day ads enjoyed a big year. Jan 24, 2025 https://www.fiercepharma.com/marketing/super-bowl-nears-tv-data-show-glp-1-game-day-ads-enjoyed-big-year.

68 Macy, J. T., Kercher, K., Steinfeldt, J. A., & Kawata, K. (2021). Fewer US Adolescents Playing Football and Public Health: A Review of Measures to Improve Safety and an Analysis of Gaps in the Literature. *Public Health Reports* 136(5), 562–74. doi.org/10.1177/0033354920976553.

69 Umer, M., Ali Shah, S. M., Moeckel, C., et al. (2025). Global Trends in Vitamin D Research From 1985 to 2024. *PRiMER*. 9(33). https:/doi.org/10.22454/PRiMER.2025.538113.

70 Fernandes, T. H., & Bell, V. (2024). The imprecision of micronutrient requirement values: the example of vitamin D. *Journal of Food Science* 89(1), 51–63. doi:10.1111/1750-3841.16889.

71 Máčová, L., Bičíková, M. (2021). Vitamin D: current challenges between the laboratory and clinical practice. *Nutrients* 13(6), 1758. doi:10.3390/nu13061758.

72 Sukik, A., Alalwani, J., & Ganji, V. (2023). Vitamin D, gut microbiota, and cardiometabolic diseases—a possible three-way axis. *International Journal of Molecular Sciences* 24(2), 940. doi:10.3390/ijms24020940.

73 Zhang, Y., Xu, Y., Zhong, W., Zhao, J., Liu, X., Gao, X., Chen, M., & Wang, M. (2025). Vitamin D and Immune Checkpoint Inhibitors in Lung Cancer: A Synergistic Approach to Enhancing Treatment Efficacy. *International Journal of Molecular Sciences* 26(10), 4511. doi.org/10.3390/ijms26104511.

74 C-Span (2025). Health and Human Services Secretary Kennedy Testifies on Health Care Agenda, Part 1. September 4, 2025. https://www.c-span.org/program/senate-committee/health-and-human-services-secretary-kennedy-testifies-on-health-care-agenda-part-1/664946.

75 Grant, W. B. (2018). Vitamin D acceptance delayed by big pharma following the disinformation playbook. *Orthomolecular News Service*, October 1, 2018. https://orthomolecular.org/resources/omns/v14n22.shtml.

76 Rooney, M. R., Harnack, L., Michos, E. D., et al. (2017). Trends in use of high-dose vitamin D supplements exceeding 1000 or 4000 International Units daily, 1999–2014. *JAMA*. 317, 2448–50. https://jamanetwork.com/journals/jama/fullarticle/2632494.

77 Grant W. B. (2011). An estimate of the global reduction in mortality rates through doubling vitamin D levels. *European Journal of Clinical Nutrition* 65(9), 1016–26. doi.org/10.1038/ejcn.2011.68.

# INDEX

## T

## U



## V



## W



## X



## Y



## Z